Social Work
in Health Settings:
Practice in Context

About the Author

Toba Schwaber Kerson, DSW, PhD, is Professor in the Graduate School of Social Work and Social Research at Bryn Mawr College. Educated at Chatham College, Columbia University and the University of Pennsylvania, she is the author of *Medical Social Work: The Pre-Professional Paradox* and *Understanding Chronic Illness: The Medical and Psychological Dimensions of Nine Diseases*.

Social Work
in Health Settings:
Practice in Context

Toba Schwaber Kerson
and Associates

Zelda Foster

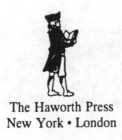

The Haworth Press
New York • London

Social Work in Health Settings: Practice in Context is #4 in the Haworth Series in Social Work Practice.

The Haworth Press, Inc., 10 Alice Street, Binghamton, NY 13904-1580
EUROSPAN/Haworth, 3 Henrietta Street, London, WC2E 8LU England

Library of Congress Cataloging-in-Publication Data

Social work in health settings : practice in context / edited by Toba Schwaber Kerson and associates.
    p.   cm. — (Haworth series on social work, ISSN 0898-0705 ; #4)
    Rev. ed. of: Social work in health settings / Toba Schwaber Kerson. c1982.
    Includes bibliographies and index.
    ISBN 0-86656-811-5. — 0-86656-851-4 (pbk.)
    1. Medical social work — United States. 2. Public health — United States. I. Kerson, Toba Schwaber. II. Kerson, Toba Schwaber. Social work in health settings. III. Series: Haworth series on social work practice ; v. 4.
HV687.5.U5S6445   1989
362.1′0425′0973 — dc19   89-1684
                                              CIP

Acknowledgements

I thank the colleagues who encouraged me to write a new edition of this book, particularly Edward A. McKinney, Kermit Nash and Jacqueline Atkins, first edition chapter authors for rewriting or allowing me to rewrite and enrich previous work, and new contributors for using the framework so effectively. Lorraine Wright and Peg McConnell contributed admirably to production and Denise DuChainey provided excellent research assistance. I look forward to her practice chapter in the third edition. As the years go by, I increasingly value the support of Larry who loves a lot and Jennie who sparkles plenty.

CONTENTS

About the Contributors

Toba Schwaber Kerson DSW, PhD, is Professor in the Graduate School of Social Work and Social Research at Bryn Mawr College. She received an MS from the Columbia University School of Social Work and doctorates in social work and sociology from the University of Pennsylvania. She is Progress Notes Editor of *Health and Social Work*, on the editorial board of *Women & Aging* and the author of *Medical Social Work: The Pre-Professional Paradox* and *Understanding Chronic Illness: The Medical and Psychosocial Dimensions of Nine Diseases*.

Susan A. Balis, MSS, ACSW, is Social Worker, Strecker Program, Institute of Pennsylvania Hospital, Philadelphia, Pennsylvania.

Margo Bare, MSW, ACSW, is Instructor, Department of Social Work, Cabrini College, Radnor, Pennsylvania.

Betsy Blades, MSW, LCSW, is Doctoral Candidate, Graduate School of Social Work and Social Research, Bryn Mawr College and Social Worker, Bon Secours Hospital, Baltimore, Maryland.

Carey Donovan, MSS, is School Social Worker, Mt. Desert, Maine.

Elisabeth Doolan, MSS, is a private practitioner in Philadelphia, Pennsylvania.

Denise DuChainey, MSS, was formerly Social Worker, Department of Obstetrics and Gynecology, Pennsylvania Hospital, Philadelphia, Pennsylvania.

Nina Millett Fish, RN, MSW, was formerly Hospice Coordinator, St. John's Mercy Medical Center, St. Louis, Missouri.

Carol Appolone Ford, ACSW, is Consultant, Comprehensive Epilepsy Program, Bowman Grey School of Medicine, Winston-Salem, North Carolina.

Zelda Foster, MS, LCSW, is Chief, Social Work Service, Veterans Administration Medical Center, Brooklyn, New York.

Susan B. Freeman, MS, LCSW, is Social Worker, Home, Health and Counseling Agency, East Bay Area, California.

Martha C. Fujimoto, MSW, is Social Worker, Rehabilitation Institute of Chicago, Chicago, Illinois.

George S. Getzel, DSW, is a volunteer at Gay Men's Health Crisis and Professor at Hunter College School of Social Work, New York, New York.

Lyne Iris Harmon, MSW, is Executive Director, Child Psychiatry Center, Northwest Corporation, Philadelphia, Pennsylvania.

Phyllis Braudy Harris, PhD, ACSW, is Postdoctoral Research Fellow, Elderly Care Research Center, Department of Sociology, Case Western Reserve University, Cleveland, Ohio.

Judith F. Hirschwald, MSW, is Director of Social Services, Magee Memorial Rehabilitation Center, Philadelphia, Pennsylvania.

Nancy V. Lotz, MSS, is Clinical Social Work Supervisor, Community Home Health Services, Philadelphia, Pennsylvania.

Susan Osteen Mercer, DSW, is Professor at the Graduate School of Social Work, University of Arkansas at Little Rock and serves on the Governor's Long Term Care Advisory Board.

Renee Weisman Michelsen, MSS, is Social Worker, Center for Geriatric Care, Morristown Memorial Hospital, Morristown, New Jersey.

Helen Peachey, RN, MSS, was formerly Director of Patient Services at Planned Parenthood of Southeastern Pennsylvania and is presently Social Worker, Community Health Affiliates, Ardmore, Pennsylvania.

Betsy Robinson, MSW, is Geriatric Clinical Social Worker at Riley's Oakhill Manor South, Little Rock, Arkansas.

Wendy Wollwage Schmid, MSW, is Coordinator of Outpatient Social Work Services, Children's Hospital of Philadelphia.

Carol Silbergeld, LCSW, is Director of Clinical Social Work at the Reiss-Davis Child Study Center and maintains a part-time private practice in Los Angeles, California.

Susan Steigner, MSW, is Social Worker at Catholic Social Services, Baltimore, Maryland.

Janet L. Taksa, MSW, is Social Work Supervisor, Thomas Jefferson University Hospital, Philadelphia, Pennsylvania.

Mona Wasow, MSW, is Professor, School of Social Work, University of Wisconsin.

Joan D. Zelinka, MSW, is Social Worker III, Department of Social Work, Francis Scott Key Medical Center, Baltimore, Maryland.

Social Work
in Health Settings:
Practice in Context

Foreword

THE FRAMEWORK

Social Work in Health Settings: Practice in Context uses a decision making model to explore a wide range of social work services in health care settings. Although the cases and settings in this book are all health related, the framework is generic and, therefore, suitable for teaching direct practice in any setting. The framework proposes, first, that social workers understand the context in which their work with clients occurs in order to be able to interpret and influence important dimensions of context. Second, the framework encourages social workers to understand the decisions which structure the helping relationship so that they can evaluate and, when necessary, alter the decisions to meet the needs of each client.

Context is a set of circumstances or facts that surround and constrain a particular event or situation. Three elements of context which influence and often limit the nature and conditions of the helping relationships are policy, technology and organization. Policy refers particularly to laws; technology, to means of diagnosis and treatment; an organization, to systems involved in the delivery of health services.

Within context, the practice decisions which structure the helping relationship are the definition of the client, goals, contrast, meeting place, use of time, treatment modality, stance of the social worker, use of concrete and other resources outside of the relationship, reassessment and transfer or termination. After termination, the social worker conducts a differential evaluation reviewing each practice decision in order to decide whether to follow the structure for the next similar client or to alter some elements in order to further the work.

1

THE FRAMEWORK APPLIED

Here, the framework is applied to twenty-two settings drawn from mental health, acute medicine, public health and long-term care. In each chapter, the practitioner has chosen a particular case to demonstrate the framework's utility. Thus, *Social Work in Health Settings* can be used as a casebook for understanding particular techniques and interventions, a means of introducing students to a range of clients, an overview of many social work settings and services in the health arena, and, perhaps, most importantly, a way to help students to consider practice and policy issues and interventions as a whole. In this framework, as in reality, practice and policy are inextricably intertwined.

CONTEXT

Policy

Unlike many other countries, the United States has no clearly demarcated and defined health policy. Primarily, health is considered the responsibility of individual states. Specific federal health policies are directed towards specific populations for which the United States government has decided it must assume some responsibility, such as present and past members of the armed services, and the elderly. Some examples are "Mutual Help Group for Emphysema Patients: Veterans Administration Medical Center" the articles relating to renal dialysis, a specific medical intervention for which the Congress decided to take funding responsibility, and chapters such as "Acute Psychiatric Unit: Two Hospitalizations in One Year," which are influenced by the relatively new Medicare policy of hospital reimbursement based on case rather than cost.

Health policy relates also to shifts in value orientation in the history of the United States. In the 1935-1944 era, when the United States was recovering from the Great Depression and participating in World War II, many categorical programs such as Maternal and Child Health ("Maternal and Child Health: Teen Mother and Well Baby Clinic") were developed through the Social Security Act of 1935. The era from 1945 to 1960 saw an investment in and expansion of health resources, facilities, manpower and research. The era of 1960-1970 focused on equity of access in part through the passage of Medicare, Medicaid and Community Mental Health Center legislation. Examples include "Community Mental Health Center: Long Term Family Therapy" and "Nursing Home: Intervention with Alzheimer's Disease." The 1970s saw the concern with the national allocation of resources, the concomitant building of an infrastructure for planning and regulation, and the concern for cost containment. The examples include "Placement of a Developmentally Disabled Man: Delegate Agency of a Regional Developmental Disability Center" and "Rehabilitation of a Quadriplegic Adolescent: Regional Spinal Cord Injury Center." Deinstitutionalization is valued (see "Psychiatric Halfway House: To Achieve Independent Living").

Competition and regulation are the themes of the 1980s, with the federal government regulating costs on the one hand and enhancing "free market" competition on the other hand. Deinstitutionalization continues with an increased number of services having cost containment as a prime objective. Hospice ("Hospice: Terminal Illness and the Quality of Life") and home services for the frail elderly ("Hospital Based Case Management for the Frail Elderly") are to cost less than their institutional alternatives. Cheaper cost will probably insure the future of such services.

Often, policies determine restraints or entitlements. For example, specific pieces of legislation entitle those with developmental disabilities to many educational and training programs while other pieces of legislation restrict driving for those with uncontrolled epilepsy. Policies regarding specific issues evolve over time, reflecting the values of a particular era of a society. At present, for example, fines and restrictions have become heavier for those arrested for driving under the influence of alcohol. Policies related to family planning seem to remain in flux (see "Family Planning Agency: An Unsuccessful Contraceptor"). For example, the use of abortion remains prominent and controversial in the political arena.

Finally, policy often determines which professionals will be part of a specific service. The inclusion or exclusion of social work in areas such as renal dialysis, hospice, home care, community mental health and health maintenance organizations is critical for the future of the profession. To be excluded removes social work from policy making as well as from service delivery. neither the profession or its clientele can afford exclusion.

Technology

Technology is the sum of the ways in which social groups provide themselves with the material objects of their civilization. It is the branch of knowledge that deals with applied science. Examples of technology include life support systems, diagnostic machinery or computer systems for monitoring foster children or the chronically mentally ill. Technology seems most applicable to health settings, but it is, in fact, important in all social service delivery. Articles which focus on high technology combinations of machinery and medication are "Psychological Recovery from Burn Injury: Regional Burn Center" "Renal Dialysis: Beyond Survival by Machine," "Confronting a Life Threatening Disease: Renal Dialysis and Transplant Program" and "Rehabilitation of a Quadriplegic Adolescent: Regional Spinal Cord Center." Medication is also a critical element in chapters such as "Acute Psychiatric Unit: Two Hospitalizations in One Year," "Epilepsy in Childhood: Pediatric Neurology Clinic" and "Pediatric Oncology: Open Communication in the Family of a Child with Leukemia."

"He's Schizophrenic and the System is Against Us: Reflections of a Troubled Parent" allows one to examine a situation in which political and technological solutions conflict. A young man who is very ill cannot be hospitalized or medicated without his consent. To do so inhibits his freedom, and the state protects this freedom. Without medication, the young man cannot manage the activities of daily living; so his life is wretched, primitive and painful but free.

Technological solutions are not only valued but expected in the United States. Thus, while spending for public health and nutrition programs has decreased, spending for "high tech" medicine such as organ transplantation and diagnostic imaging has increased. Also, as a society, we are loath to deny or end treatment, to say that someone's life quality is so poor, he should be allowed to die. The absence of a technological solution is also important for social work because our services are often valued more in those situations (see

"Gay Men's Health Crisis: Responding Effectively to the Crisis of a Gay Man with AIDS" and "Nursing Home: Intervention with Alzheimer's Disease") where there is no effective medical treatment.

The meaning of technological intervention varies according to the individual. One thinks of the example of the young man with schizophrenia who would not allow medication. At times, in renal dialysis, patients and family members name their machine, thus anthropomorphizing it. Sometimes patients refuse to return to facilities because the apparatus reminds them of their pain or vulnerability. Often, people are concerned that they will be kept alive beyond the time when they can control their futures. Thus, technology presents increased opportunities and dilemmas.

Organization

An organization is a body of persons organized for some end or work, the personnel or apparatus of an agency, business or institution. Size, hierarchy or its lack, rules and expectations regarding behavior of workers and clients or customers, ethos and values shape the entity and create parameters for work. Contrasting a very large organization with a very small one helps one understand the importance of the size of the organization. The Veterans Administration, for example, sets very different work parameters from the psychiatric half way house. In the former, an elaborate and rigid hierarchy is probably necessary for managing a huge, complex, multifaceted program. In the latter, small size and a simpler program allow professionals flexibility. Creative and excellent practice is obviously possible in both organizations but size and complexity set different parameters. Of all of the organizational arrangements described, one which presents the practitioner with the greatest freedom is private practice because the organization and the relationship between social worker and client are the same. The rules for the individual relationship are the rules of organization.

Ethos, the underlying character or spirit of an organization, is also important. This sustaining sentiment carries the assumptions and informs the beliefs, customs, and practices of a group. To be unaware of ethos is like swimming against the tide: One may be using the proper techniques, but using too much energy and getting nowhere. An example of such a situation is "Emergency Room: Help for a Family with an Abused Child," in which the ethos of the organization is changing while the service is trying to continue as before. The author points out that the organizational support for her service has changed. In fact, the ethos of the institution had changed so dramatically that it eventually became impossible to administer such a service. One wonders what will happen in a situation where the ethos of the service delivery agency and social worker differ from that of the funding agency. For example, if funding agencies for in-home services assume a certain low level of cost, and in-home service agencies assume that clients should be kept out of institutions at all costs, and cost exceeds allocation, will service cease?

The strong mission of organizations such as the Gay Men's Health Crisis and Planned Parenthood sets certain expectations for work. More than in other kinds of organizations, agency, social workers, and clients share purpose. In organizations such as acute care hospitals, while everyone might agree that the ultimate purpose is health, work objectives may vary and even be conflicting for different constituencies.

PRACTICE DECISIONS

Within the constraints of context, social worker and client make decisions which structure their relationship. Practice decisions include the definition of the client, goals, contract, meeting place, use of time, treatment modality, stance of the social worker, use of outside resources, reassessment, and transfer or termination. At times, some of these decisions are determined through policy or organization. For example, the number of days for which a person can be hospitalized in the acute psychiatric ward described in the book is determined by insurance coverage. To a great extent, the number of days for which an elderly person can be hospitalized for an acute condition is set through Medicare's system of Diagnosis Related Groups. The Gay Men's Health Crisis has the policy of helping clients for the rest of their lives. Generally, however, practice decisions are left to the social worker and client.

Definition of the Client

One first step in practice is to determine whom the client will be. Sometimes, as in the chapter on private practice, that decision is immediately clear. The person in pain who comes for the service remains the client. In the burn center chapter, since the patient is at first too ill for social work intervention and his wife needs help, the wife is the client. As the patient recovers physically, his need for social work intervention becomes greater, and he becomes the primary client. In the chapter concerning epilepsy in childhood, the patient is the child, but the primary client is his mother. She must understand her noncompliance with the medical regimen and address her own problems before her son's illness can be controlled. The child is also the client because he, too, must learn to understand his illness. In the acute psychiatric unit chapter, the patient, her parents and her children are all clients.

In some cases such as those described in the emergency room, pediatric oncology and nursing home/Alzheimer's Disease chapters, the patient is not available for direct work. Instead, relatives become the focus of intervention. At other times, the patient is too ill, and the social worker must reevaluate the person's capacity to relate as he or she recovers.

Goals

Generally, goals are related to the health or mental health problem for which the patient sought treatment. Maintaining independence, avoiding social isolation and continuing to carry one's responsibilities are general goals towards which much work is directed. As in the case in pediatric neurology, the goal can be helping the family adhere to the medical regimen. In cases such as those described in the regional spinal cord injury and developmental disabilities centers, people learn to manage profound disabilities which can affect every part of their lives. For the group with nursing home residents, the general goal was to understand and accept the aging process. In the chapters on geriatric care and home health, a goal was to maintain clients in their homes. For the family planning social worker, the goal was to have the client plan child bearing.

Goals can also be highly specific as in family planning or general as in the private practice chapter. They can be about life's beginning as in the chapters on maternal and child health and the emergency room, or about life's endings as in the chapters on hospice and AIDS. When there are many goals as there are in the chapter on community mental health, the social worker helps the clients to determine priorities and to order the work to avoid overwhelming the clients and making the work more difficult. Primarily, goals are about the shared definition of a problem, shared expectations regarding the resolution of problems, and the means for reaching resolution. In that way, goals relate directly to contract, the next decision area which explicates expectations.

Contract

A contract is an agreement between two or more parties for the doing or not doing of something specified. A contract can be an agreement between parties such as social worker and client, client and agency, social worker and agency, agency and mandating body, or agency and funding source. To some extent, all work with clients involves many contracts on various levels of relationship including clients, relatives, social workers, agencies, larger funding and oversight bodies and law making entities. An explicit contract lessens the risk of misunderstanding. Clients and social workers each often wish that the other would be or do something different or more. Contract avoids the disappointment and retreat that can result from failed but unspoken expectations. When used well, contract is flexible and changing. It should enhance rather than confine work.

In the psychiatric half way house chapter, the client who enters Shalom House also enters into an elaborate set of agreements involving many aspects of behavior. In the private practice chapter, the client contracts only to attend the session and to pay for the service. In the chapter on the mutual help group for emphysema patients, the contract is to help each other to manage their illness. Thus, contract depends on the broad purpose of the service. The degree to which it is explicated seems to depend on the social worker and the agency's expectations of the clients.

Contract is the linchpin of this framework. If it is well drawn, it will specify goals, definition of the client, modality, use of time, meeting place, use of outside resources and perhaps even the conditions of termination. Therefore, all parties can refer to it for reassessment of the success of their work.

Meeting Place

Meeting place refers to the physical space in which the relationship occurs. The most obvious distinction is between the institution and the client's home. Issues regarding privacy, space, turf, control and comfort are important here. In institutional work, the conditions of a private conversation between social worker and client must often be created in the most public of spaces. In the emergency room, for example, or in intensive care, often the patient begins to think that even his body is public property. Often, as in the discharge planning chapter, the social worker's office is too far from the patient's bedroom to make office interviews possible. If other personnel undervalue the special quality of the social work relationship, what space the social worker can construct may be fraught with interruption. Although social workers soon learn to take the problems of space and privacy for granted, the creative and innovative social worker produces a feeling of intimacy and importance for the client, whatever the physical circumstances.

The issue of control is especially powerful in the description of the spinal cord injured young man who has so little control over his body. The social worker decided that they should meet on the client's turf in the institution as much as that was possible. In another interesting solution to meeting place, the "being old" group met in the board room of the home, a place denoting high status, with a conference table and chairs in which serious business takes place.

Use of Time

The structuring of time, i.e., the spacing and duration of meetings and the length of the relationship, to a certain extent determines the nature of the work. Certainly as in the consultative function in the chapters concerning home health and suspected child abuse in the emergency room, important work may be accomplished with brief interaction. However, the depth of relationship achieved in the community mental health center, private practice or renal dialysis chapters was due, in part, to longer duration.

Little has been written in social work about the length of the individual interaction. Certainly, any experienced clinician can point to a time when she helped someone in fifteen minutes and another time when she and the client spun their wheels for an hour and fifteen minutes. There must be meaning for relationship in the concepts of "too much" or "too little" time. This is an area for further investigation.

Treatment Modality

The selection of particular methods of help involves choices regarding orientation, modality, intervention and technique. When questioned, social workers in health care generally describe themselves as eclectic and practical. They say their methods are determined by the needs of the clients.

Treatment modality is sometimes determined by the agency or funding source. For example, in the chapter describing the developmental disabilities center in California, the state designed, instituted, mandated and monitored the case management system. In the psychiatric half way house, all methods of intervention were clearly presented to social worker and client as one aspect of the contract. In the chapter on the acute psychiatric unit, one begins to understand the problems which ensue when the modality which the social worker chooses is not synchronized with that of the rest of the treatment team. Here, the work of the social worker was undermined by other, sometimes more powerful professions using different modalities.

Again, the most effective choices depend on fine interpretation of the demands of context, the needs of the client and the continued flexibility of the social worker. Interventions are adapted to the needs of the client. Thus, the emphysema patients in the veterans hospital needed peer support, so the social worker instituted a mutual support group. The nursing home resident with Alzheimer's Disease required redefined involvement from her relatives, therefore the social worker educated and supported the relatives in order to enable them to help the patient.

Stance of the Social Worker

The stance of the social worker implies that the social worker has sufficient awareness and discipline about her "use of self" to choose how to relate and behave in any particular client situation. Of course, this is not always the case even with highly experienced, well-trained and self-aware clinicians. The cases about family planning, maternal and child health and the acute psychiatric unit are especially interesting for discussion of the stance of the social worker. In the family planning chapter, the anger and disappointment of staff in relation to the client's ambivalent and other-directed behavior prevented them from offering a richer service. In the teen mother and well baby clinic, the positive identification of the social worker with the client kept her involved with the client when the rest of the staff might have offered less service. In retrospect, the overidentification of the first social worker in the acute psychiatric unit interfered with her ability to help the client. She was not sufficiently firm, and her expectations were too high.

Outside Resources

Outside resources are services located outside of the relationship, and often outside of the agency, which further the work of the relationship. The use of outside resources is perhaps most clear in situations involving case management such as developmental disability and geriatric outreach. One also sees the importance of these kinds of services in the chapters on the spinal cord injury center and the Gay Mens Health Crisis. A different use of outside resources is found in the chapter on pediatric oncology, where the family comes together and gathers strength from the process of buying a wig for the child who has lost her hair as a result of cancer treatment.

Reassessment

Reassessment allows participants to judge their work before it has concluded. The chapter on alcoholism treatment demonstrates that this process can bring clients back to treatment. The chapter about reestablishing a coordinated home care program describes this process as an opportunity for the staff team and the client group to articulate and understand what has transpired. The social worker in the chapter on patients with emphysema describes reassessment as the beginning of the termination process.

Transfer and Termination

Case transfer and termination mark an end of social worker and client's access to each other. If they work together again, the difference in time and perhaps circumstances will change the nature of the relationship. In settings such as renal dialysis and hospice, only death means termination. In other situations, as in the chapters on discharge planning, family therapy in community mental health and the "being old" group, termination occurs when the goals of the relationship have been reached.

Case Conclusion

Case conclusion refers to outcome and current functioning of the client. Reading case conclusions first is a slightly different way of conducting the discussion of a case. First being informed of a client's current functioning and then learning about the work involved in helping the client to reach that level of functioning exposes one to a larger understanding of the work of referring agencies.

Differential Discussion

Differential discussion helps the social worker to evaluate the work with the present client and to generalize to a category of similar clients. One may use a chart such as the following.

Client_____ Similar Client Group_____

	Retain	Alter	Specific Alterations
Context			
Policies			
Technology			
Organization			
Practice Decisions			
Definition			
Goals			
Contract			
Meeting Place			
Use of Time			
Treatment Modality			
Stance			
Outside Resources			
Reassessment			
Termination			

In the differential discussion of the "being old" group, the social worker decided that the next time she led such a group, she would change the meeting time and reach out more to clients who had dropped out but would otherwise follow the same structure. The social worker who wrote about epilepsy in childhood noted she would have defined the client differently by involving the father as well as the mother and child, and she may have been more confrontational with the mother. The utility of this exercise increases with experience.

THEMES EMERGING FROM FRAMEWORK, SETTINGS AND CASES

Use of this framework raises many additional themes. For example, in terms of context, mission oriented agencies such as Planned

Parenthood and geriatric outreach services help social workers to feel part of the purpose. Other organizations which have mixed purposes find the social worker sometimes siding with the client or protecting the client from the rest of the staff. Also, the many technological innovations which allow clients to live longer but which do not necessarily guarantee fine life quality raise many ethical and moral dilemmas for social workers. Perhaps, because social workers are concerned with the social roles of patients and clients after discharge, they are more caught in these dilemmas than are other professionals. Another theme related to technology is how little medical or psychiatric diagnosis informs social work practice. It is much more helpful for social workers to understand a client's functional ability and the course of his disease or disability than it is to be able to name it.

Another theme related more to practice decisions is how difficult it is to acknowledge and write about failure. The old adage, "We learn from our mistakes," somehow does not find its way into scholarly meetings and publications. I commend the clinicians who were sufficiently brave to make available their failures. A most important theme which emerges is the power of relationship to support, to expand options, to make a difference in the life of the client. In many of the situations described, the social work relationship sustained the clients in the most trying and difficult circumstances.

In retrospect, each case/setting chapter reaffirms the utility of the framework. The context of social work in health care has three primary dimensions; policy, technology and organization. Together, these elements provide parameters for the practice decisions which social workers and clients make to determine the structure of their work together. In sum, a large measure of the art of social work is the ability to structure the relationship between social worker and client in ways which maximally support the work. To do that, the social worker must be able to understand, influence and alter many dimensions of practice in context.

Part 1

Practice in Context Framework

Introduction

Social Work in Health Settings presents a framework called "practice in context" which has been developed as a tool for teaching and evaluation. This approach is called a framework because it is composed of elements the author has framed together. The primary subject of the framework is the relationship between social worker and client. As a concept, "relationship" bears considerable, intense and diverse meaning. It is an association or involvement; a connection by blood or marriage or an emotional or other connection between people. Synonyms for relationship are dependence, alliance, kinship, affinity or consanguinity; yet, each of these words suggests a different meaning, a different bond and duration. People can be related who have never met, and never will — for example, people who merely have a common membership in a religious or fellowship group or other organization.

The concept of "relationship" has many dimensions. Borrowing from and building with the dimensions described by several theorists will lead us to the definition of the social worker-client relationship used for this framework. The sociologist Erving Goffman and the anthropologist Gregory Bateson have theorized about structural dimensions of relationship such as interactional focus, connection to milieu, and rules. Bateson uses the word "interaction" and Goffman, the word "encounter" to be as precise as possible about their subjects. For our framework, "interaction" and "encounter" are seen as aspects of the broader concept of "relationship."

Goffman suggests that when studying interaction, the proper fo-

---

In this chapter, "she" is used as the third person pronoun because the majority of social workers are women. The chapters which follow are generally written in first person although some chapters have multiple authors. This format was used to enhance the notion that the practitioner is speaking about her work. With the exception of the chapters on the acute psychiatric unit and nursing home/Alzheimer's disease, additional authors were responsible for research and writing only.

cus is not on the individual and his psychology, but rather the syntactical relations among the acts of different persons mutually present to one another (Goffman, 1982, p. 2). To understand interaction, one must understand not the separate individuals but what occurs between them. Goffman further alludes to the "special mutuality of immediate interaction. That is, when two persons are together, at least some of their world will be made up out of the fact (and consideration for the fact) that an adaptive line of action must always be pursued in this intelligently helpful or hindering world. Individuals sympathetically take the attitude of others present, regardless of the end to which they put the information thus acquired" (Goffman, 1966, p. 16). Thus, in interaction, there is always a shared sense of situation, and of an ability to in some way be in the other individual's place, no matter what each participant's purpose in the interaction.

Goffman places relationship in context when he develops the notion of a "membrane" which "wraps" the interaction and, to some extent, separates it from its surroundings. "Any social encounter," he writes, "any focused gathering is to be understood, in the first instance, in terms of the functioning of the "membrane" that encloses it cutting it off from a field of properties that could be given weight" (Goffman, 1961, p. 79). Still, while the relationship can be viewed and defined in its own right, it remains intimately related to the world outside of it. Thus, Goffman says, "an encounter provides a world for its participants but the character and stability of the world is intimately related to its selective relationship to the wider one" (Goffman, 1961, p. 80).

Rules and their use are also part of Goffman and Bateson's analyses of relationship. According to Bateson, interaction is the "process whereby people establish common rules for the creation and understanding of messages" (Bateson, n.d.). Goffman adds to this definition by noting that in encounters, rules are *considered* and *managed* rather than necessarily followed: Rules may shape interaction, but they also may be influenced by the participants. He writes, "Since the domain of situational proprieties is wholly made up of what individuals can experience of each other while mutually present, and since channels of experience can be interfered with in so many ways, we deal not so much with a network of rules that must be followed as with rules that must be taken into consideration, whether as something to follow or carefully to circumvent" (Goffman, 1966, p. 42).

Helen Harris Perlman adds a psychological dimension to the more structural views of relationship posed by Goffman and Bateson. She defines relationship as "a person's feeling or emotional bonding with another" (Perlman, 1979, p. 23). Elaborating on the psychological dimension, Perlman says the relationship between social worker and client is "a catalyst, an enabling dynamism in the support, nurture, and freeing of people's energies and motivations toward problem solving and the use of help" (Perlman, 1979, p. 2). The relationship affirms and motivates the client. To these dimensions, Meyer adds *purpose*. The social worker-client relationship, she says, is not an end in itself but a tool for moving the problem situation forward (Meyer, 1976). It is formed for the purpose of meeting goals.

Thus, for this framework, the relationship between social worker and client is defined with the help of both sociological and psychological ideas. The sociological contributions have to do with structure; the focus is on interaction rather than on individual participants, on the use of rules, on the relationship's connection to (or separation from) its surroundings or context. The psychological contributions are the purposive, feeling, catalytic and enabling dimensions. Here, the relationship of social worker and client means one or more purposive encounters intended to be catalytic and enabling in which the structure of the relationship and the rules for interaction are set by dimensions of context as well as by decisions made by the participants.

PRACTICE IN CONTEXT FRAMEWORK

According to this framework, then, the two basic elements which structure the relationship between social worker and client are (1) the context in which the relationship occurs, and (2) the "practice decisions" which social worker and client make about the nature and form of the relationship. These dimensions, "context" and "practice decisions," act as a matrix for the relationship. By determining many of the rules by which the work of social worker and client proceed, "context" and "practice decisions" define the possibilities for relationship. Although elements such as personality, nature and degree of illness, psychosocial assessment and cultural background contribute to the social worker/client relationship, they are characteristics of the individuals involved and not the interaction.

This approach, or framework, is not a generic practice theory because it is not a system of ideas meant to explain certain phenomena or relations. Nor is it a model, because it does not show proportions or arrangements of all of its component parts. Here are described elements of context and practice which structure the relationship between social worker and client. The framework has three overarching purposes: (1) to help the social worker to clarify the work, (2) to understand alterable and unalterable dimensions of practice and context, and (3) to be able to evaluate work in light of these dimensions. An artist decides which medium is most suitable for a subject. In the same way, with client participation, the social worker understands and tries to influence context and constructs the relationship in ways which will help meet client goals. Thus, *Social Work in Health Settings* is about the craft of social work; the skill with which the social worker manages dimensions of practice.

CONTEXT

To a great extent, dimensions of context determine many of the rules for the helping relationship. To assume that possibilities are completely determined within the relationship is unrealistic, and may contribute to disappointment and a sense of failure on the part of the participants, evaluators of service and funding sources. Context means the set of circumstances or facts that surround a particular event or situation. Gregory Bateson defines context as a "collective term for all those events which tell the organism among what set of alternatives he must make his next choice" (Bateson, 1975, p. 289). He adds, " . . . however widely *context* be defined, there may always be wider contexts a knowledge of which would reverse or modify our understanding of particular items" (Bateson, n.d., p. 16). Therefore, context is a limitless concept and focusing on certain dimensions means ignoring others. To some extent, social sci-

entists and social workers disagree about the most salient elements
for the context of health care. For example, Strauss et al. describe
four features in the larger context of where work takes place: contemporary prevalence of chronic illness, images of acute care, medical technology and its impact on hospitals, and the hospital as a set
of work sites (Strauss et al., 1985). In her discussion of the context
of social work practice in health care, Germain includes the health
care system, the health care organization, illness and the sick role,
and the professional frame of reference (Germain, 1984). The
present framework addresses three dimensions of context thought to
have the most direct and describable consequences for the relationship between social worker and client: policy, technology, and organization. These three elements are considered most important because of the ways in which each contributes to the structure of the
social worker/client relationship. Policies often provide rules for
service — which clients may receive which service under which conditions. Organizations, also, are rule makers defining the nature of
service often at the behest of policy makers. Finally, in the cases of
many diseases and traumatic situations, dependence on technological intervention has contributed to the conditions of relationship.
Such interventions contribute to the content of the relationship and
also often constrain it. The salience of each dimension and the ways
in which dimensions are related depends on the particular setting. In
effect, these contextual factors contribute to the rules of the game,
and as they change, the constraints and possibilities for action are
altered as well.

Policy

A policy is a definite course of action which a government, an
organization or a group has decided to take in order to act in a
certain situation. Schottland defines social policy as "a statement or
social goal or strategy, or a settled course of action dealing with the
relations of people with each other, the mutual relations of people
with their government, the relations of governments with each
other, including legal enactments, judicial decisions, administrative
decisions, and mores" (Gil, 1982, p. 6).

Social work must be able to interpret and influence policy in

order to advocate for clients and the profession ("Commission
. . . ," 1986). Decisions on which populations to serve, on allocation of resources, planning and programming are too often made
before social work practitioners become involved, and it is far easier to affect the structure of a program before it is instituted than
after. These activities are also most beneficial to clients when clients and social workers advocate together. In addition, involvement
in policy formulation helps the social work profession to broaden
and strengthen its influence ("Social Work . . . ", 1985). When
policy has a negative effect on clients or the profession, a united
and concerted lobbying effort can stem the tide (Carlton, 1985).

Historically, the presence of social work has been strongest in
areas such as maternal and child health, and services to veterans
where social workers have been involved in developing policy on
national, state and local levels (Kerson, 1985; Kerson, 1980). In
one contemporary example, the Mental Health Project at the School
of Social Welfare, State University of New York at Stony Brook
and the Sayville Community Support System Program, professionals said, "Our challenge is to invite people to join us in their own/
our struggle, a task that requires us to understand the stakes/bene-
fits/costs involved for the person acting out mental patienthood as a
survival, as a way of life" (Rose and Block, 1985). Thus, patients
are empowered through advocacy. In another example, the Tennessee Conference on Social Welfare describes the strategies and
actions it used to obtain governmental approval for increases in the
Aid to Families with Dependent Children standard of need and level
of payment (Granger and Moynihan, 1987).

A contemporary example of a policy which has directly affected
the relationship of social worker and client is the federal creation of
Diagnosis Related Groups or DRGs (for a discussion of DRGs, see
the chapter on discharge planning) in which Medicare and participating insurers pay hospitals according to case diagnosis rather than
cost (Fein, 1986). Formerly, the hospital charged the insurer what it
had cost to care for the patient. Now, the insurer pays the hospital
based on the patient's diagnosis. According to DRGS, if the diagnosis indicates four days of hospitalization, the hospital will be paid
for four days of hospitalization only, even if the patient stays in the
hospital longer. For example, when the patient is hospitalized be-

yond the number of days indicated in the schema, the hospital must absorb the extra cost. Consequently, there is great pressure on the hospital to discharge the patient, and great pressure on the social worker to make prompt and appropriate arrangements for the patient to return to the community. Thus, a social worker who previously may have had weeks to develop a relationship with and an adequate discharge plan for a patient, now may have a matter of days to accomplish the same task.

"Practice and politics mix," as Bailis said, ". . . solid health policy makes for strong social work practice in health care and those . . . concerned with practice issues must focus on the objective of improving policy. Politics is the vehicle for getting there" ("Health Experts . . . ," 1984). Thus, interpreting and advocating are prime social work tasks. Policy is a key element in the context of social work in health care.

Technology

Technology is applied science: the ways in which a social group satisfies its material needs. In the broadest sense, technology means the concrete, practical solutions people invent or discover. In the present framework, technology refers to medical/scientific inventions which are used for diagnosis or treatment: medication, surgical techniques, life-sustaining machinery or ways of viewing or measuring bodily functions.

For contemporary health care, the development and cost of technology relate directly to policy formulation. Technology and the organizations which house and/or distribute it account for a good deal of the astronomical costs of medical care today (Aaron and Schwartz, 1984). The United States' love for, rapid acceptance and diffusion of "high tech" solutions means that hospitals, health professionals, patients and families want the best available to them no matter what the cost (Russell, 1979). From the end of World War II, until very recently, the federal government spent massive sums of money to develop medical technology, train health professionals and build facilities. From the 1960s until the mid 1970s, the purpose of much federal health policy such as Medicare, Medicaid and the Community Mental Health Centers Act was to insure access to health care and expensive technology. Since the beginning of the 1980s, most federal health policies have been generally directed toward controlling health care costs with specific attention to expensive technological interventions.

For social workers, sometimes the very lack of medical means to intervene in an illness creates opportunities for psychosocial intervention. Historically, social workers had important roles in the care of people with venereal diseases and tuberculosis in part because medical interventions were inadequate to treat the illnesses. Before the discovery of penicillin permitted treatment of syphilis at an early stage with a single injection, treatment required many outpatient visits over eighteen months. The social worker's role was to be sure that patients returned for prolonged outpatient treatment and to educate them and others in the same network who might have been infected. Now, the task might be purely epidemiological or educational (Kerson, 1980).

Contemporary situations provide like opportunities. With diseases like AIDS and Alzheimer's for which there is not yet adequate medical treatment, social workers help garner the social support needed to live with the illness. With other conditions, such as End Stage Renal Disease and severe burns, technology provides life support, and the social worker helps the patient and family to live with both the illness and the technology.

The development of life sustaining technology has also raised perplexing ethical and legal problems in health care (President's Commission, 1983; Callahan, 1986; Reamer, 1985; Elliott, 1984). Sometimes, the extension of life can mean greatly diminished life quality. In other situations, medical solutions may be dehumanizing and/or produce negative side effects. Each of these circumstances provides opportunities for social work intervention. Thus, the presence or absence of technological solutions shapes the parameters of the relationship between social worker and client.

Organization

An organization is a body of people structured for some end or work, the administrative personnel or apparatus of an agency, business or institution (French, Bell and Zawacki, 1983). Organization, too, structures practice. The role of a social worker in a prison for the criminally insane is necessarily different than it is in a community mental health center. Prison walls, guards and garb must affect the relationship with the client.

Formal dimensions of organization are size, division of labor, degree of bureaucratization, degree of centralization of control, and role structure. Changes in structure and design carried out in the names of efficiency and cost-effectiveness can restrict services and creativity (Lynn, 1980; Mahler and Nicholson, 1987). For example, when told to spend less money, one county agency fired all of its first line supervisors, saying their tasks could be carried out by two or three administrators. The following year, problems with staff morale and poor, undirected practice caused almost a 100% turnover in line staff.

Informal dimensions include "mores," the unwritten rules about behavior which people know implicitly but rarely discuss, such as ways in which to relate to members of other professions or whether it is acceptable to have a meal at a client's home. Also important are the networks which people develop outside the formal organizational structure in order to accomplish tasks. Often, the establishment of such a network means being able to enlist those with expertise or power regarding matters which are critical to clients. Such power does not necessarily reside with high office. Sometimes it can be held by a chief of service, other times by a clerk. Although it is generally easier to make exceptions or bend the rules in a smaller organization, those who work for large, highly bureaucratized organizations also learn to develop informal networks. Intimate knowledge of an organization increases the possibility of making it more responsive to clients' needs (Germain, 1984; Gortner, Mahler and Nicholson, 1987).

PRACTICE IN CONTEXT

Within "context" is located the relationship between social worker and client. The framework suggests that specific elements in the context (policy, technology and organization) structure the relationship between social worker and client. Similarly, the framework suggests that specific elements within the relationship, which are to a degree determined by the participants in that relationship, provide structure and regulate interaction (Goffman, 1981). In the framework, the elements are called "practice decisions" because they are often determined by decisions made by social worker and client which determine the pattern for their relationship. "Practice decisions" means that the participants themselves have the power to create the vehicle which will enable them to accomplish their goals. The term stresses the notions of activity, judgement and responsibility implicit in such choices.

In some situations, practice decisions may be constrained by elements of context. For example, in order to receive funding, an organization may have to adhere to policies set by a funding source regarding use of time or even goals. The organization would therefore constrain its social workers in those ways. Also, practice decisions are not always discrete, and can recur as the relationship evolves. Alterable, they act as a flexible structure which can guide the relationship and help the participants to judge the quality of their work.

The ten practice decisions in this framework are: (1) definition of the client, (2) goals, (3) use of contract, (4) meeting place, (5) use of time, (6) treatment modality, (7) stance of the social worker, (8) use of outside resources, (9) reassessment, and (10) transfer or termination.

Definition of the Client

Defining the client involves the choice of a client unit: deciding with whom one works in a situation. The client can be any unit such as an individual, a family, couple, parent and child, group, committee, housing project or clinic. While a case is open, the definition of the client can change as needs change. Sometimes, one may intervene with the most troubled people in the situation, and in other instances, the social worker may work on the client's behalf because that person is not available for work (Chetnik, 1980). For example, the person who is most dependent or most troubled may be too young, demented or ill to be directly involved. At times, broadening the definition of the client from an individual to a larger unit enhances the social support of the ill person and strengthens the whole (Pilisuk and Parks, 1986).

Goals

Goals refer to solutions which the social worker and client work to attain. In the literature, these points of attainment are referred to by various terms such as treatment objectives or outcomes (Hollis and Woods, 1981; Hepworth and Larsen, 1986; Germain, 1984; Carlton, 1984). Primarily, goals reflect the needs and desires of the client (Goldstein, 1983; Leader, 1981). Of all, the practice decisions, goals are owned primarily by the client. The client is helped by the social worker to articulate goals and the social worker, with the client's help, uses the rest of the practice decisions to structure the relationship in ways which will support the work. If they are the goals of the social worker, family members or other staff, but not those of the client, they are less likely to be attained.

The relationship between social work goals and diagnosis is important in that diagnosis is often made by another profession, usually medicine, with which social work collaborates. In some ways, when diagnosis is imposed, it becomes part of context, an organizational issue which informs social work practice. Often, a diagnostic term such as schizophrenia, arthritis or epilepsy is a label which provides very little information about functional capacity. If the social worker employs this kind of information to limit the use which she thinks a client can make of the relationship or even to discard certain clients into a category which receives no service, she is allowing diagnosis to restrict her work.

Goals may be as concrete as obtaining an apartment or a prosthesis or as intangible as feeling better about oneself or feeling happier. If some of the goals in each client situation are concrete, then they are measurable, and the social worker and client are provided with a means of assessing progress. Being able to call attention to some success such as "arriving at work on time nearly every day" or "screaming at the children less than five times a week" is helpful in encouraging a client to continue to work in the relationship.

Additionally, goals should be separated from wishes or dreams of client and social worker. Goals are realistic and attainable aims rather than fantasies for which one would hope in the best of all possible worlds. However, while setting realistic expectations for work, the social worker must also "lend a vision," that is, help the client to envision a more satisfying life (Schwartz, 1971).

Contract

Contrast means agreement between social worker and client about the means used to obtain goals as well as the description of the goals themselves (Rothary, 1980; Mallucio and Marlow, 1974; Seabury, 1976). It is the keystone, cynosure and linch pin of the social worker-client relationship and of this framework. Comprised of mutually agreed upon obligations and expectations, a contract is a way of establishing norms for the relationship (Goffman, 1972). Norms also exist for the relationship between client and agency (Stewart, 1984; Weissman et al., 1983). Increasingly, there are contracts between funding source, agency and client. For example, many drug abuse treatment centers require that clients sign agency formulated contracts stipulating the conditions of treatment.

Whether verbal or written contracts are more effective remains a matter for debate and most probably depends on the nature of the agency, work and clients (Klier, 1984). Certainly, written form clarifies the agreement, and having all participants sign adds formality and, perhaps, importance to the matters at hand. Some would argue that this very formality stultifies the interaction, interfering with creativity, transference or other aspects of the relationship. Because contract requires that each party articulate goals and norms, it includes each of the elements of relationship structure. Participants in a helping relationship always have some expectations of each other. Use of the dimensions of contract allows the expectations of all parties to be made explicit and helps prevent misunderstanding.

Meeting Place

Meeting place refers to the physical space in which the relationship happens. Most work occurs in the institution/agency or in the client's home. Increasingly, meeting place is determined by the organization rather than by the needs of the clients. In these cost-cutting days, the major portion of some services such as home care, foster care and hospice is dispensed in the home while other services such as dialysis, discharge planning and community mental health are offered almost entirely within the institution.

Meeting place can influence assessment by limiting or increasing the amount of information made available about the client. Social scene provides some information about identity (Goffman, 1972). When meetings take place outside of the client's habitat, the social worker relies on the person's appearance and the details she provides about her life. The sight of an institutionally gowned person lying in bed in a hospital room provides no clues to individual identity. Personality, memories, experiences and style are all obscured. Often in such situations, the social worker assumes information which she does not have.

When the client is seen at home, the social worker learns something about the client's means, organizational abilities, values, neighborhood and, perhaps, her relationships with family members and neighbors (Cohen and Egen, 1981; Bloom, 1983). No other means compares to home visits for assessing the life of a client or, sometimes, for empowering her (Whittington, 1985; Bregman, 1980; Moynihan, 1974). One sees the impact of problems, illnesses and disabilities on daily living. Through home visits, social workers can help collaborating professionals and aides to understand a client's life and problems. Unfortunately, many organizations think that home visits are too expensive and do not allow them.

Two important aspects of meeting place are space and privacy. In many institutional or agency settings, space and privacy are at a premium. Where none exist, social workers create private space for themselves and their clients using undivided attention, eye contact, voice and body language. When other professionals ignore the need for privacy, social workers have to educate them in order to protect their clients and foster the work.

The telephone, too is another "place" in which to help people who cannot come to the organization and whom the social worker cannot visit. It has proven effective as a means of support and treatment for isolated clients (Shepard, 1987; Ranan and Blodgett, 1985; Stein, 1986). Again, decisions about meeting place are determined to a degree by the rules of the setting and the needs of the clients.

Use of Time

Decisions about time concern the duration and spacing of each meeting and of the relationship. Since use of time is a means of structuring the relationship, sharing this information with clients empowers them (Lemon and Goldstein, 1978). In the broadest sense, orientation in time and space "is felt as a protection rather than a strait jacket, and its loss can provoke extreme anxiety" (Mead and Bateson, 1942). The importance of time is no less diminished in single encounter work in a hospital emergency room than it is in group work or long term psychotherapy (Alissi, 1985).

In many instances, the use of time is determined by the organization or funding source. For example, policy may determine the duration of a session, how many sessions a client may be seen or the number of days for which a patient is hospitalized. Time is also an important dimension of contract. No matter who determines duration, using time to structure the relationship and having the client participate in the structure aids the work (Smalley and Bloom, 1977; Perlman, 1979).

Treatment Modality

Treatment modality refers to the selection of particular methods of care which are most appropriate for specific clients in particular situations (Hanrahan and Reid, 1984; Meyer, 1983; Carlton, 1984; Hartman, 1983; Lemon, 1983; Rushton and Davies, 1984). In every situation, the social worker makes decisions about the ways in which the client can best be helped. These decisions involve choices about orientation, modality, technique and intervention.

To some degree, choice of treatment modalities relates to definition of client and client unit. Thus, designating an individual as client might indicate that one would do individual work, while designating the family as the client would indicate family work. However, the more general decision to work with a certain client unit opens the possibility of a plethora of decisions regarding particular theoretical orientations such as a psychodynamic, cognitive or behavioral approach (Rosenblatt and Waldfogel, 1983; Hollis and Woods, 1981; Carlton, 1984; Hepworth and Larsen, 1986; Germain, 1984; Turner, 1986; White, 1981; Wletner, 1982; Shazer, 1986; Birdman 1981). Such orientations often reflect beliefs and world views of the social worker which may relate little to particular client problems. For example, because it is common in our society to believe that elderly people are not amenable to psychodynamic work, these approaches are unusual in work with the elderly; yet, some programs for the elderly report excellent psychodynamic work (Lewis, 1987; Milinsky, 1987; Kaminsky, 1985). This practice decision cautions social workers to choose treatment modalities which reflect needs and goals of clients rather than their own world view or beliefs.

In turn, choice of a particular theoretical orientation and treatment modality brings one to decisions regarding specific techniques or interventions such as the use of ritual, life story or sculpting (Fox, 1983; Laird, 1984; Jefferson, 1978). Techniques such as these are tools to bring a theoretical model into action. Monitoring their use offers the social worker another way to assess ongoing work because strategies such as these tend to have specified outcomes (Russell et al., 1984). At times, interventions which are used are different from ones that had been anticipated because client's needs may be redefined as the work progresses (Rosen and Mutschler, 1982). Articulating practice interventions enhances the social worker's control of her medium.

Treatment method is sometimes determined by dimensions of context such as organization or funding policy. For example, one facility may extol a particular form of family therapy to treat an illness such as bulimia and another may use a specific form of individual therapy to treat the same illness. These choices seem to arise from differing beliefs about etiology and/or cure.

At times, the nature of the illness or disability affects the choice of modality. For example, an illness or disability which leaves an individual physically dependent such as advanced rheumatoid arthritis or emphysema may require that the social worker work with family members as well as the ill person. In the case of advanced

Alzheimer's disease or with a seriously ill infant, the social worker may work only with family members. Use of time, another practice decision, sometimes may be a dimension of treatment modality. Since the 1960s, short-term, brief and crisis-oriented work has been conventional, but within each of these orientations, there are a myriad of practice decisions regarding modality and specific technique (Turner, 1986; Rosenblatt and Waldfogel, 1983; Kanter, 1983; Shazer, 1982).

One modality often thought to be different from the rest is case management (Weil, Karls and Associates, 1985; Rubin, 1983). Developed for client groups such as the frail elderly, chronically mentally ill and foster children, this modality is one response to the complexity of service delivery systems (Weissman, Epstein and Savage, 1983). It can be used to organize the services of an entire agency, a national program of immense proportions or a single caseload; but, properly defined, case management should never exclude clinical work. In fact, "case management is both a concept and a process. As a concept, it is a system of relationships between direct service providers, agency administrators and clients. As a process, case management is an orderly, planned provision of services intended to facilitate a client's functioning at as normal a level as possible and as economically as possible" (Weil, Karls and Associates, 1985).

Practitioners generally suggest that their approach is both pragmatic and eclectic; that is, they do what they must depending on the circumstances, needs and capabilities of their clients, and they tend to draw from many modalities and techniques. Sometimes, it is difficult to distinguish between the style of the social worker and the choice of treatment modality. Social workers who are more comfortable in a listening and supporting mode may report their orientation as Rogerian or psychoanalytic. Those who are highly structured and/or directive may say they use crisis intervention or a task oriented approach. In some ways, this is like self type-casting. One plays the ingénue or bad guy because it is comfortable. Again, the allusion to an art form is meant to underscore the notion that conscious decisions about modality are more likely based on the client need than in the style of the social worker.

Stance of the Social Worker

Stance of the social worker is closest to the old fashioned term "conscious use of self," an understanding of one's self, motivations, place in and impact on relationships (Lammert, 1986; Baldwin and Satir, 1987; Robinson, 1978). It implies that the social worker has sufficient self-awareness, experience and discipline to be able to choose how to behave in a particular client situation. Unlike some other practice decisions shared with the client, the social worker is totally responsible for this choice. Experience and self-awareness provide the social worker greater mastery of "stance" so that, within realistic limits, the social worker can be what the client and situation need her to be. Just as an actor learns to assume a role, the social worker adapts and refines her stance according to the needs of the client situation.

Some elements of stance are the worker's degree of activity or passivity, amount of advice-giving, use of authority, self-disclosure and touch (Lackie, 1983; Goldberg, 1986; Ewalt and Katz, 1976; Gourse and Cheschier, 1981; Borenzweig, 1984; Reynolds, 1983; Leader, 1983). Other elements such as transference and counter-transference, prejudices and false assumptions which may support action different from the needs of the client situation are part of the stance of the social worker as well (Saari, 1986; Brown, 1984; Googins, 1984; Atwood, 1982; Hardman, 1975).

Outside Resources

Outside resources are the services used by client and social worker which are outside of the relationship, often external to the agency and which further the work of the relationship (Germain, 1983; Hollis and Woods, 1981). These services can range from the protective work of a state or county child welfare agency to assistance with obtaining an apartment, walker or prosthesis. Determination of the client's ability to broker her own services is an issue in the use of outside resources. Sometimes, the client and/or family can grow stronger by managing outside resources themselves. In some instances, the social worker can enhance the relationship by arranging services, and at other times, the social worker must procure outside resources because the client/family is unable to manage (Bates, 1983).

Reassessment

Reassessment presents an opportunity for social worker and client to evaluate their work during the course of the relationship. Here, like artists, they are asked to step back from their work and examine it. Reassessment is the process of reexamining the dimensions of the framework as well as other issues which participants have deemed important. It can be made part of the pattern of each meeting or set aside to be brought into the work at certain intervals. Technique can be as simple as discussing how the work is going or as sophisticated as using standardized measures of success (Corcoran, 1987; Reid and Hanrahan, 1982; Blom and Fischer, 1982; Levitt and Reid, 1981; Ivanoff, 1987; Thomlinson, 1984). Also, reassessment can be a way to reactivate a stalled relationship or to slow one which seems to be speeding along almost out of control. Schwartz's questions, "are we working?" and "what are we working on?" are helpful here (Schwartz and Zalba, 1971). Finally, reassessment provides the social worker an opportunity to assess and obtain feedback about her performance (Gummer, 1984).

Transfer and Termination

Transfer and termination mark the end of relationship between client and social worker, the fact that they will not be meeting in this way any longer (Levinson, 1977; Sanville, 1982; Hepworth and Larsen, 1986; Hollis and Woods, 1982). Goffman noted that greetings and farewells are ritual displays that mark a change in degree of access (Goffman, 1972). Here, social worker and client will not have the same kind of access to each other as they would have had if the work continued. Ideally, termination is a decision which social worker and client have made together because goals have been accomplished and their work is finished. Often, when clients terminate before the social worker is ready, it is because the client has perceived work more positively than the social worker (Toseland, 1987). Even when the client wants to terminate before the social worker thinks work is finished, it is important to end the relationship positively so that the client may return to the agency (or to another one) if she needs further help.

Sometimes, termination signals the end of the relationship between client and agency. At other times, the social worker is leaving the organization, and the client will continue with another social worker (Super, 1982). Vacations, too, evoke issues about termination (Webb, 1983). Often a difficult period, termination has great potential for growth through use of the relationship.

Case Conclusion

Conclusion, here, refers primarily to outcome and current functioning of the client. Client and social worker summarize their work together so that each can leave the relationship with knowledge of accomplishments. In addition, they finish in a positive manner which will allow the client to seek help again if necessary.

Differential Discussion

Here, all of the previous framework decisions are reviewed in order for the social worker to analyze her work. Differential discussion allows the social worker to be a "Monday night quarterback," to look back on the case to decide which elements would remain the same the next time she worked with a client with similar capacity, personality and problems. Differential discussion encourages the social worker to generalize from a specific client to a category of like cases with whom she can use similar structure and techniques. For example, in retrospect, the social worker may decide she was too confrontational with a client; the coldness of the meeting place might have been a detriment; or the client may have been asked to coordinate more resources than she was able to manage. Emphasis on the social worker's ability to (1) generalize from a particular case and (2) alter elements in the relationship between social worker and client makes differential discussion the most useful dimension of the framework. This step moves the social worker out of the present relationship and on to the next.

PRACTICE IN CONTEXT

A review of the overarching conception of practice in context brings the framework full circle. The first article is a summary which reviews the framework providing examples from the setting chapters. Here, themes drawn from setting articles are developed for a broad discussion of social work in health settings. Constraints on the setting, the influence that these constraints have had on the relationship and the series of decisions which determine the structure of the relationship enable social workers to map their work and, as a result, enhance action.

This review also helps to identify areas of advocacy and social action for the social worker.

Using the framework described above, *Social Work in Health Settings* acts as a casebook, a collection of real cases in settings described by and reflecting the style of each experienced social work practitioner. Altogether, twenty-two health and mental health settings demonstrate "the cadence and pattern" of social work in health (Mead, 1973). Each setting article follows the "practice in context" framework as its outline.

The settings are presented in four broad based sections based on related settings; acute medical, long term care, mental health and public health. Reflecting the funding arrangements of the times, this second edition contains a new section called long term care, and the public health section is shorter than its predecessor. Also, because acute medical problems are now often managed in settings other than the traditional hospital organization, the section that was referred to formerly as hospital-based practice is called acute medical care. These sections are not discrete. As a matter of fact, many of the settings overlap into two or more sections. For example, renal dialysis is a treatment for End Stage Renal Disease which has acute episodes but requires long term care. Settings include an emergency room, community mental health center, burn unit, private practice, renal dialysis center, AIDS self-help organization, nursing home, channeling project, epilepsy clinic, developmental disability center, veterans hospital, alcoholism treatment facility, spinal cord injury center, teen mother-well baby clinic, psychiatric halfway house, hospice, acute medicine, home health, acute psychiatry, pediatric oncology and family planning.

A fifth section with two special articles provide an insider's view of social work in health settings. The papers are written by social workers who have personal and professional interests in a particular setting. The author of the first is a social worker whose husband was maintained on renal dialysis for almost twenty years and who has been the social worker in a dialysis unit. The second is written by a social worker with many years of experience as a practitioner and educator whose son has chronic schizophrenia.

Ideally, the format for this book would be a three-ringed notebook in which case/setting articles and dimensions of context and practice could be arranged and rearranged for teaching purposes. One can use these case/settings to discuss issues around settings and populations such as short term and long term care, institutional and home care, physical and mental health, services for children, adults and the elderly, or trauma and disease. In addition, one can examine a particular practice decision such as use of contract or stance of the social worker across twenty-two practice settings. Overall, *Social Work in Health Settings* has one primary purpose: To help the social worker to clarify and explicate practice in context in order to best ply her craft.

REFERENCES

Aaron, H.J. and Schwartz, W.V. *The painful prescription: Rationing health care.* Washington, D.C.: The Brookings Institution, 1984.

Abramson, M. and Black, R.B. "Extending the boundaries of life: Implications for practice." *Health and Social Work*, 10(3), 1985, pp. 165-173.

Aiken, L.H. and Mediance, D. *Applications of social science to clinical medicine and health policy.* New Brunswick, N.J., 1986.

Alissi, A.S. and Caspar, M. "Time as a factor in group work." *Social Work in Groups*, 8(2), 1985, pp. 3-16.

Allphin, C. "Envy in the transference and countertransference." *Clinical Social Work Journal*, 10(3), 1982, pp. 151-164.

Ashford, J. et al. "Advocacy by social workers in the Public Defender's Office." *Social Work*, 32(3), 1987, pp. 199-203.

Atwood, N. "Professional prejudice and the psychotic client." *Social Work*, 10(2), 1982, pp. 172-177.

Baldwin, M. and Satir, V., eds. *The use of self in therapy*. New York: The Haworth Press, 1987.

Bates, M. "Using the environment to help the male skid row alcoholic." *Social Casework*, 64, 1983, pp. 276-282.

Bateson, G. "The natural history of an interview," unpublished manuscript.

_____. *Steps to an ecology of mind*. New York: Ballantine, 1975.

Birdman, S., ed. *Forms of brief therapy*. New York: Guilford Press, 1981.

Birdwhistell, R.L. *Kinesics and context: Essays on body motion communication*. Philadelphia: University of Pennsylvania Press, 1970.

Bloom, M. "Usefulness of the home visit for diagnosis and treatment." *Social Casework*, 54, 1973, pp. 67-75.

_____ and Fischer, J. *Evaluating practice: Guidelines for the accountable professional*. Englewood Cliffs, N.J.: Prentice-Hall, 1982.

Borenzweig, H. "Touching in clinical social work." *Social Casework*, 64, April 1983, pp. 238-242.

Bregman, A. "Living with progressive childhood illness: Parental management of neuromuscular disease." *Social Work in Health Care*, 5(4), Summer 1980, pp. 387-407.

Briggs, D. "The trainee and the borderline client: Countertransference pitfalls." *Clinical Social Work Journal*, 7, 1979, pp. 1-20.

Brown, F. "Erotic and pseudoerotic elements in the treatment of male patients by female therapists." *Clinical Social Work Journal*, 12(3), 1984, pp. 244-257.

Callahan, D. "How technology is reframing the abortion debate." *Hastings Center Report*, 16(1), 1986, pp. 33-42.

Carlton, T.O. *Clinical social work in health settings*. New York: Springer, 1984.

_____. "Highlights of a decade." *Health and Social Work*, 10(4), 1985, pp. 308-312.

_____. "Understanding and choice of treatment procedures." In *Clinical social work in health settings*. New York: Springer, 1984, pp. 422-445.

Chetnik, M. "The treatment of a preschooler via the mother." In *Psychotherapy and training in clinical social work*, J. Mishne (ed.). New York: Gardner Press, 1980, pp. 135-149.

Christoffel, T. *Health and the law: A handbook for health professionals*. New York: The Free Press, 1982.

Cohen, S. and Egen, B. "The social work home visit in a health care setting." *Social Work in Health Care*, 6(4), 1981, pp. 55-67.

"Commission allies with lobby seeking healthy budget policy." *NASW News*, April 1986, p. 6.

Conrad, P. and Kern, R., eds. *The sociology of health and illness*. New York: St. Martin's Press, 1986.

Corcoran, K. *Measures for clinical practice: A sourcebook*. New York: The Free Press, 1987.

Coulton, C. "Person-environment fit as the focus in health care." *Social Work*, 26(1), 1981, pp. 26-35.

Dear, R. B. and Patti, R.J. "Legislative advocacy: Seven effective tactics." *Social Work*, 26, 1981, pp. 289-296.

Ehrenreich, J. *The altruistic imagination: A history of social work and social policy in the United States.* New York: Cornell University Press, 1985.

Elliot, M.W. *Ethical issues in Social Work: An annotated bibliography.* New York: Council on Social Work Education, 1984.

Ewalt, P. and Katz, J. "An examination of advice-giving as a therapeutic intervention." *Smith College Studies in Social Work*, 47, November 1976, pp. 3-19.

Fein, R. *Medical care: Medical costs.* Cambridge, Mass.: Harvard University Press, 1986.

Fortune, A.E. "Grief only? Client and social worker reactions to termination." *Clinical Social Work Journal*, 15(2), 1987, pp. 159-171.

Fox, R. "The past is always present: Creative methods for capturing the life story." *Clinical Social Work Journal*, 11, 1983, pp. 368-378.

French, W.H., Bell, C.H. and Zawacki, R.A. *Organization development: Theory, practice and research.* Plano, Texas: Business Publications, Inc., 1983.

Germain, C. "The ecological approach to people-environment transactions." *Social Casework*, 62(1), 1981, pp. 67-76.

_____. "Using social and physical environments." In *Handbook of clinical social work*, A. Rosenblatt and D. Waldfogel (eds.). San Francisco: Jossey-Bass, 1983, pp. 26-57.

Gil, D. *Unravelling social policy: Theory, analysis and political action towards social equality*, 2nd ed. Cambridge: Schenkman, 1982.

Goldberg, F. "Personal observations of a therapist with a life threatening illness." *International Journal of Group Psychotherapy*, 34(2), 1984, pp. 289-296.

Gortner, H.F., Mahler, J., and Nicholson, J.B. *Organization theory: A public perspective.* Chicago: The Dorsey Press, 1987.

Goffman, E. *Asylums: Essays on the social situation of mental patients and other inmates.* New York: Doubleday, 1961.

_____. *Behavior in public places.* New York: The Free Press, 1966.

_____. *Encounters: Two studies in the sociology of interaction.* New York: Macmillan, 1961.

_____. *Interaction ritual: Essays in face to face behavior.* New York: Pantheon, 1981.

_____. *Presentation of self in everyday life.* New York: Doubleday, 1959.

_____. *Relations in public.* New York: Harper & Row, 1972.

Goldstein, H. "Starting where the client is." *Social Casework*, 64, 1983, pp. 267-275.

Googins, B. "Avoidance of the alcoholic client." *Social Work*, 29(2), 1984, pp. 161-166.

Gourse, J.E. and Cheschier, M.W. "Authority issues in treating resistant families." *Social Casework*, 62(2), 1981, pp. 60-68.

Granger, B.P. and Moynihan, L. "Successful engagement in social legislation." *Administration in Social Work*, 11(1), 1987, pp. 37-45.

Gummer, B. "How'm I doing?: Current perspectives on performance appraisals and the evaluation of work." *Administration in Social Work*, 8(2), Summer 1984, pp. 91-101.

Hanrahan, P. and Reid, W. "Choosing effective treatment interventions." *Social Service Review*, 58, 1984, pp. 244-258.

Hardman, D.S. "Not with my daughter you don't." *Social Work*, 20(4), 1975, pp. 278-285.

Hartman, A., Section Ed. "Theories for producing change." In *Handbook of clinical social work*, A. Rosenblatt and D. Waldfogel (eds.). San Francisco: Jossey-Bass, 1983, pp. 97-279.

Haynes, K.S. and Mickelson, J.S. *Affecting change: Social workers in the political arena*. New York: Longman, 1986.

"Health experts take policy to task." *NASW News*, 1(10), July 1984.

Hepworth, D.H. and Larsen, J.A. "The final phase: Termination and evaluation." In *Direct social work practice: Theory and skills*. Homewood, Ill.: Dorsey Press, 1986, pp. 319-342.

_____. "Negotiating goals and formulating a contract." In *Direct social work practice: Theories and skills*. Chicago: Dorsey Press, 1986, pp. 300-335.

Hiatt, H.H. *America's health in the balance: Choice or chance*. New York: Harper & Row, 1987.

Hollingshead, J.R. *A political economy of medicine: Great Britain and the United States*. Baltimore: The Johns Hopkins University Press, 1986.

Hollis, F. and Woods, K.M. *Casework: A psychosocial therapy*. New York: Random House, 1981.

_____. "Reflective discussion of the person-situation configuration." In *Casework: A psychosocial therapy*, pp. 146-160.

_____. "Understanding and choice of treatment objectives." *Casework: A psychosocial therapy*, 405-421.

Ivanoff, A. et al. "The empirical clinical practice debate." *Social Casework*, 68(5), 1987, pp. 290-298.

Jansson, B. and Simmons, J. "The survival of social work units in host organizations." *Social Work*, 31, Sept./Oct. 1986, pp. 339-343.

Jeffersen, C. "Some notes on the use of family sculpture in therapy." *Family Process*, 17, 1978, pp. 69-75.

Johnson, P. and Rubin, A. "Case management in mental health: A social work domain." *Social Work*, 28, 1983, pp. 49-55.

Kaminsky, M. The Arts and Social Work: Writing and Reminiscing in Old Age, *Gerontological Social Work in the Community* (ed. Dobrof, R.). New York: The Haworth Press, 1985, pp. 225-246.

Kanter, J.S. "Reevaluations of task-centered social work practice." *Clinical Social Work Journal*, 11(3), 1983, pp. 228-244.

Kerson, T.S. *Medical social work: The pre-professional paradox*. New York: Irvington Publishers, 1980.

_____. "Responsiveness to need: Social work's impact on health care." *Health and Social Work*, 10(4), Fall 1985, pp. 300-307.

_____. "The social work relationship: A form of gift exchange." *Social Work*, 23, July 1978, pp. 326-327.

_____. *Understanding chronic illness: The medical and psychosocial dimensions of nine diseases*. New York: The Free Press, 1985.

Klier, J., Fein, E. and Genero, C. "Are written or verbal contracts more effective in family therapy?" *Social Work*, 29, 1984, pp. 298-299.

Lackie, B. "The families of origin of social workers." *Clinical Social Work Journal*, 11, 1983, pp. 309-322.

Laird, J. "Sorcerers, shamans and social workers: The use of ritual in social work practice." *Social Work*, 29(2), 1984, pp. 123-129.

Lamb, H. "Therapist-case managers: More than brokers of services." *Hospital and Community Psychiatry*, 31, 1980, pp. 762-764.

Lammert, M. "Experience as knowing: Utilizing therapist self-awareness." *Social Casework*, 67, 1986, pp. 369-376.

Leader, A. "The relationship of presenting problems to family conflict." *Social Casework*, 62(8), Oct. 1981, pp. 451-457.

_____. "Therapeutic control in family therapy." *Clinical Social Work Journal*, 11(4), 1983, pp. 351-361.

Lemon, E.C., Section Ed. "Education and methods for clinical practice." In *Handbook of clinical social work*, A. Rosenblatt and D. Waldfogel (eds.). San Francisco: Jossey-Bass, 1983, pp. 281-548.

Lemon, E. and Goldstein, S. "Use of time limits in planned brief treatment." *Social Casework*, 59(19), 1978, pp. 588-596.

Lenrow, P.B. "The work of helping strangers." In *Things that matter*, H. Rubenstein and M. Bloch (eds.). New York: Macmillan, 1982, pp. 42-57.

Levinson, H. "Termination of psychotherapy: Some salient issues." *Social Casework*, 58(10), 1977, pp. 480-489.

Levitt, J.L. and Reid, W. "Rapid-assessment instruments for practice." *Social Work Research and Abstracts*, 17(1), 1981, pp. 13-19.

Levy, C.S. "Labelling: The social worker's responsibility." *Social Casework*, 62(6), 1981, pp. 332-342.

Lewis, M. "Sex Bias Dangerous to Women's Mental Health," *Perspective on Aging* 16(2), March/April, 1987, pp. 9-11.

Lynn, L. *The state and human services: Organizational change in a political context*. Cambridge, Mass.: M.I.T. Press, 1980.

Mahaffey, M. and Hanks, J.W., eds. *Practical politics: Social work and political responsibility*. Silver Spring, Md.: National Association of Social Workers, 1982.

Mailick, M. "The impact of severe illness on the individual and family: An overview." *Social Work in Health Care*, 5(2), Winter 1979, pp. 117-128.

Mallucio, A. and Marlow, W. "The case for contract." *Social Work*, 19(1), 1974, pp. 28-35.

Mead, M. *An anthropologist at work*. New York: Equinox Books, 1973.

Mead, M. and Bateson, G. *Balinese character*. New York: New York Academy of Sciences, 1942.

Meyer, C. "Selecting important practice methods." In *Handbook of clinical social work*, A. Rosenblatt and D. Waldfogel (eds.). San Francisco: Jossey-Bass, 1983, pp. 731-749.

Meyer, C.H. *Social work practice*. New York: The Free Press, 1976.

Milinsky, T.S. "Stagnation and Depression in the Elderly Group Client," *Social Casework*, 68, March 1987, pp. 173-179.

Miller, R. and Rehr, H. *Social work issues in health care*. Englewood Cliffs: Prentice Hall, 1983.

Milne, C. and Dowd, E. "Effect of interpretation style and counselor social influence." *Journal of Counseling Psychology*, 30, 1983, pp. 603-606.

Mintzberg, H. "Organizational design: Fashion or fit." *Harvard Business Review*, Jan./Feb. 1981, pp. 103-116.

Moynihan, S.K. "Home visits for family treatment." *Social Casework*, 55(12), 1974, pp. 612-617.

Palombo, J. "Spontaneous self-disclosures in psychotherapy." *Clinical Social Work Journal*, 15(2), 1987, pp. 107-120.

Patti, R. "In search of purpose for social welfare administration." *Administration in Social Work*, 9(3), Fall 1985, pp. 1-15.

Perlman, H.H. "The helping relationship: Its purpose and nature." In *Things that matter*, H. Rubenstein and M. Bloch (eds.). New York: Macmillan, 1982, pp. 7-27.

_____. Relationship: The heart of helping people. Chicago: University of Chicago, 1979.

Pilisuk, M. and Parks, S.H. *The healing web*. Hanover, New Hampshire: University Press of New England, 1986.

Pinderhughes, E. "Empowerment for our clients and ourselves." *Social Casework*, 64, 1983, pp. 331-338.

President's Commission. *Summing up: Final Report on studies of the Ethical and Legal Problems in Medicine and Biomedical and Behavioral Research*. Washington, D.C.: U.S. Government Printing Office, 1983.

Ranan, W. and Blodgett, A. "Using telephone therapy for unreachable clients." *Social Casework*, 64(1), 1983, pp. 39-44.

Reamer, F.G. "The emergence of Bioethics in Social Work." *Health and Social Work*, 10(4), 1985, pp. 271-281.

Reid, W. and Hanrahan, P. "Recent evaluation of social work: Grounds for optimism." *Social Work*, 27, 1982, pp. 328-340.

Reynolds, C. and Fischer, C. "Personal versus professional evaluations of self-disclosing and self-involving counselors." *Journal of Counseling Psychology*, 30, 1983, pp. 451-454.

Robinson, V.P. *The development of a professional self: Teaching and learning in professional helping processes*. New York: AMS Press, 1978.

Reiser, S. and Anbar, M., eds. *The machine at the bedside: Strategies for using technology in patient care*. New York: Cambridge University Press, 1984.

Rose, S. and Block, B.L. *Advocacy and empowerment*. Boston: Routledge & Kegan Paul, 1985.

Rosen, A. and Mutschler, E. "Correspondence between the planned and subsequent use of interventions in treatment." *Social Work Research and Abstracts*, 18, 1982, pp. 28-34.

Rosenblatt, A. and Waldfogel, D. *Handbook of clinical social work*. San Francisco: Jossey-Bass, 1983.

Rothary, M.A. "Contracts and contracting." *Clinical Social Work Journal*, 8, Fall 1980, pp. 179-186.

Rubin, A. "Case management in mental health: A social work domain?" *Social Work*, 28(1), 1983, pp. 49-56.

Rushton, A. and Davies, P. "Social work methods in health settings." In *Social Work and Health Care*. London: Heineman Educational Books, 1984, pp. 48-63.

Russell, C., Atilano, R., Anderson, A., Jurich, A. and Bergen, L. "Intervention strategies: Predicting family therapy outcome." *Journal of Marital and Family Therapy*, 10, 1984, pp. 241-251.

Russell, L.B. Technology in hospitals: Medical advances and their diffusion. Washington, D.C.: The Brookings Institution, 1979.

Saari, C. "The created relationship: Transference, countertransference and the therapeutic culture." *Clinical Social Work Journal*, 14(1), 1986, pp. 39-51.

Sanville, J. "Partings and impartings: Towards a non-medical approach to interruptions and terminations." *Clinical Social Work Journal*, 10(2), 1982, pp. 123-130.

Schwartz, W. "On the use of groups in social work practice." In *The practice of group work*. New York: Columbia University Press, 1971.

Seabury, B. "The contract: Uses, abuses and limitations." *Social Work*, 21, 1976, pp. 16-21.

Shazer, D. et al. "Brief therapy: Focused solution development." *Family Process*, 20(3), Sept. 1982, pp. 281-289.

Shepard, P. Telephone therapy: An alternative to isolation." *Clinical Social Work Journal*, 15(1), 1987, pp. 56-65.

Simos, B. *A time to grieve*. New York: Family Service America, 1979.

Smalley, R. and Bloom, T. "Social Casework: The functional approach." In *Encyclopedia of social work*, J.B. Turner (ed.). New York: National Association of Social Workers, 1977, pp. 1280-1290.

Smith, V. "How interest groups influence legislators." *Social Work*, 24, 1979, pp. 234-239.

"Social services in the year 2000." Washington, D.C.: U.S. Documents, 1985.

"Social work in hospitals expanding." *NASW News*, Oct. 1985, p. 14.

Sosin, M. "Social work advocacy and the implementation of legal mandates." *Social Casework*, 60(3), 1979, pp. 265-273.

———— and Caulum, S. "Advocacy: A conceptualization for social work practice." *Social Work*, 28(1), 1983, pp. 12-17.

Steidl, J. "What's a clinician to do with so many approaches to family therapy?" *The Family*, 4(2), 1977, pp. 60-65.

Stein, D.M. and Lambert, M.J. "Telephone counseling and crisis intervention: A review." *American Journal of Community Psychology*, 12(1), 1986, pp. 101-126.

Stewart, J. "The treatment relationship: Real or symbolic?" *Clinical Social Work Journal*, 13, 1985, pp. 171-181.

Stewart, R. "Building an alliance between the family and the institution." *Social Work*, 29, 1984, pp. 386-390.

Strauss, A. et al. *Social organization of medical work*. Chicago: University of Chicago Press, 1985.

Super, S. "Successful transition: Therapeutic interventions with the transferred client." *Clinical Social Work Journal*, 10(2), 1982, pp. 113-121.

Thomlinson, R. "Something works: Evidence from practice effectiveness studies." *Social Work*, 29, 1984, pp. 51-56.

Toseland, R. "Treatment discontinuance: Grounds for optimism." *Social Casework*, 68(4), pp. 195-204.

Turner, F., ed. *Social work treatment: Interlocking theoretical approaches*. New York: Free Press, 1986.

Weaver, D. "Empowering treatment skills for helping black families." *Social Casework*, 63, 1982, pp. 100-105.

Webb, N. "Vacation separations: Therapeutic implications and clinical management." *Clinical Social Work Journal*, 11(2), 1983, pp. 126-138.

Weil, M., Karls, J.M. and Associates. *Case management in human service practice*. San Francisco: Jossey-Bass, 1985.

Weissman, H., Epstein, I. and Savage, A. *Agency-based social work: Neglected aspects of clinical practice*. Philadelphia: Temple University Press, 1983.

Whittington, R. "House calls in private practice." *Social Work*, 30(3), 1985, pp. 261-264.

Wing, K.E. *The law and the public's health*. Ann Arbor: Health Administration Press, 1985.

Part 2

Acute Medical Settings

Emergency Room: Help for a Family with an Abused Child

Martha Fujimoto
Toba Schwaber Kerson

DESCRIPTION OF THE SETTING

Presbyterian-University of Pennsylvania Medical Center is a 254 bed, acute care medical facility located in a moderately depressed, predominantly black neighborhood in the shadow of the University of Pennsylvania. In order to become financially viable, Presbyterian is changing its image from a community hospital to a highly specialized, regional tertiary care facility. As the hospital expands into profitable enterprises, they have "overlooked or modified their commitment to the sick who have little or no insurance coverage" (Rehr, 1985). Part of this transformation has meant curtailing many of the supports on which I depend in the emergency room, especially services for children.

The emergency room, located in the outpatient clinic building adjacent to the main hospital, handles more than 30,000 visits per year. Many of the patients are black and on low, fixed incomes. In the emergency room, my tasks include pre-admission psychosocial assessments of patients, discharge planning, and work with crisis situations such as abuse (Clement and Klingbeil, 1981).

I am one of eleven social workers in the hospital. The social work department head reports to an assistant administrator. Our department also includes an outreach program which works with families alleged to be abusing or neglectful. The program provides intensive visits in the home to engage the families in alternatives to discipline, to teach life skills, to assist in obtaining concrete services, and to provide support to parents (Wolfe and Sandler, 1981; Kelly,

1983). It is funded through the SCAN Center, a large network of services dealing with problems of abuse and neglect, under contract to the Department of Public Welfare of the City of Philadelphia (Pennsylvania, 1985). On all cases of suspected abuse or neglect, we work closely with the Department of Public Welfare Child Protective Unit, as that is the city's mandated investigatory unit (Stein and Rznepnicki, 1984).

Policy

According to the Child Protective Services Law of the State of Pennsylvania, "Any persons who in the course of their employment, occupation, or practice come into contact with children shall report or cause a report to be made when they have reason to believe or suspect, on the basis of their professional training and experience, that a child (aged seventeen and under) is being abused and/or neglected" (Nelson et al., 1980). This mandate affects many professionals such as school teachers, police, social workers, physicians and nurses. The hospital emergency room is one of the places in which suspected abuse is most often identified (CPS Law, 1975; Stein, 1984; United States, 1986).

A toll free hotline, "Childline," is accessible at all times. Additionally, those who report abuse are protected by laws regarding "acts of good faith" from legal liability. The mandate also allows hospitals to take protective custody without court order for up to twenty-four hours. Most states have similar systems.

Child abuse and neglect can be broadly defined as those accidental or nonaccidental situations in which a child sustains physical trauma, deprivation of physical and mental needs (neglect), sexual abuse, or psychological abuse, as a result of an act or omission by a parent, caretaker, or legal guardian. Examples of neglect are abandonment; repeated failure to meet a child's physical needs, such as malnutrition not due to organic disease (failure to thrive); failure to seek (or unnecessary delay in seeking) medical care for a significant problem, or noncompliance with necessary follow-up; and gross lack of adequate supervision of the child, resulting in an injury or illness. Sexual abuse includes molestation or incest committed by a family member or caretaker, or precipitated by parental neglect in supervising the child. Another significant but more ambiguous area is emotional or psychological abuse and/or neglect, where the parent(s) contribute to or do not seek help for a child's emotional disturbance, or where there is gross failure on the parents(s) part to meet the emotional needs the child requires for normal development (DHHS, 1986).

The most frequently documented area of abuse is physical trauma, with symptoms such as bruises, scars, burns and fractures. Other abuse situations present more subtly. Medical indicators may raise suspicion about the possibility of abuse and neglect, without providing conclusive evidence: They must be considered within the context of available information. Some of the common indicators are traumatic injuries to children under the age of five such as head trauma, burns, bruises and fractures; discrepancies between the history give by the parent(s) and the degree, age, or type of injury; injuries for which there are no explanations at all; injuries occurring as a result of poor supervision; malnutrition, dehydration, or delayed development without obvious organic cause; severe and untreated disease; and the use of inappropriate food, drink, or drugs. Observations of interfamily interactions should also be documented (Russell and Trainor, 1984). For example, a cause for concern would be when parents sit in the corner of the room while their infant is being examined.

Based on medical and social assessment, hospital staff plans the patient's discharge from the emergency room. If the child's medical condition requires admission, he is admitted. Child Protective Services (CPS) is notified of any suspected abuse/neglect cases, and the disposition and treatment of the child is determined by their assessment. If home and family pose an immediate risk and the child is discharged home, CPS is immediately notified. A restraining order for temporary custody can be petitioned by CPS, which means that a detention hearing is scheduled within seventy-two hours. Hospitalization is helpful particularly when the child's medical and social conditions are uncertain or are not considered critical enough to warrant a restraining order.

Organization

Fiscal decisions made by the hospital's board of trustees have affected the organization of services within the hospital, including my capacity to help families with abused children. For example, emergency room service is severely limited by a lack of adequate psychiatric staff and facilities. Although there are several attending psychiatrists in the hospital, they are not always available or interested in seeing emergency room patients. Unless these patients can be admitted to a psychiatric hospital because they are suicidal or homicidal, they are referred to the community mental health center outpatient service in their catchment area for follow-up.

Several years ago, the hospital closed an eight bed pediatric unit. Since then, it has been difficult to maintain consistent care. When children in the emergency room require admission, they are transferred to Children's Hospital located about ten blocks away. The obstetrics-gynecology inpatient service was also closed because of the low number of deliveries. Those patients in acute distress are stabilized and transferred to the nearest hospital with OB-GYN facilities, generally the Hospital of the University of Pennsylvania which is located about six blocks away. From 1976 until 1980, our emergency room was one of two rape centers in Philadelphia helping approximately 500 victims a year. With the closing of OB-GYN, this program was also terminated. As part of our child abuse protocol, whenever a child is suspected to have been abused or neglected, emergency room or pediatric clinic staff can admit the child to the hospital as a "social admission" with the consent of parents or guardians, even though there is no acute medical problem. With no pediatric or maternity (nursery) unit, the child may be admitted to any adult floor. This solution presents problems because many of the staff are unaccustomed to working with children and even less accustomed to working with abused or neglected children and families.

Case Description

Bobby Woods is a fifteen-month-old black male who was brought to the emergency room by a policeman accompanied by the child's paternal aunt, Mrs. Jones, Mrs. Jones's daughter, and Bobby's half sister. The initial complaint was that the child had been beaten. On examination, the attending physician found an unexplained temperature of 104°, multiple lacerations of different ages about the eyes, forehead, and chin, partly healed lacerations the shape of belt buckles, several healed scars on the back, and possible "failure to thrive," indicated by a weight less than the third percentile for a child his age (Alderette and deGraffenreid, 1986). Mrs. Jones said that Bobby's mother had dropped him off at her house, where she noticed the bruises and called the police to bring Bobby to the hospital. Bobby's mother left before Mrs. Jones had a chance to ask her what happened.

Bobby lives with his mother, Ms. Woods, aged twenty-six, three siblings (Jerry, aged, four, Mary, aged two, and Annette, aged four months), and Ms. Allen, a former paramour of his father. Bobby's half sister added that she had seen Bobby's mother hit Bobby and often leave the home for days. Mrs. Jones was very concerned about Bobby's condition and safety. She said that Bobby's mother had four older children (aged five through eight) who are in foster care through a court order.

The doctor completed a report of suspected abuse/neglect and advised that the child be admitted for observation and social evaluation. We had to obtain Ms. Woods' consent for admission and could not locate her. At that moment, we received a telephone call from Bobby's father, incarcerated at Camden, New Jersey prison, who had heard about Bobby from his family and gave consent for admission. Child Protective Services was notified that Bobby was being admitted.

Just prior to Bobby's admission, two policewomen from the juvenile aid division came to the emergency room who had been notified by the police officer who had brought the family to the hospital. Concerned about the siblings still at home, they visited and reported that the children were in good health and being looked after by Ms. Allen. The following day, Ms. Jones called to say that Bobby's mother had been arrested at 1:30 that morning and was in jail on charges or assault and battery and recklessly endangering the life of a minor. Ms. Allen was planning to post bail.

Later that day, Bobby's mother came to see me. Ms. Woods is an attractive, short, young woman. We discussed the events leading up to Bobby's admission and the filing of the abuse report. Ms. Woods said that she had left Bobby with his aunt so that she could visit his father in prison. After visiting him, she went shopping and came home in the early evening to find that Bobby was in the hospital. She came to the hospital after visiting hours and was given my name by the security guard. Ms. Woods denied any anger or upset about her arrest, the child abuse report or the hospital admission. I felt, however, that she was barely in control. She was anxious to see her son. On seeing Bobby, she seemed scared and anxious. Bobby began to cry and then assumed a rather flat, emotionless expression. Ms. Woods stayed for only a few minutes, and we arranged to meet the following day.

DECISIONS ABOUT PRACTICE

Definition of the Client

In many respects, Bobby is the identified client. He is the patient presented in the emergency room with the complaint, and his medical record is documented accordingly. Similarly, hospital social service records are compiled under the patient's name, and the child abuse reporting form is documented under the name of the child suspected of being abused and/or neglected. If there is more than one child involved (siblings or unrelated children), each child has a separate "case" or report filed. In child abuse or neglect, however, the unit of intervention is the family system. It may include natural parents, legal guardians, responsible caretakers such as grandparents or extended family members as well as others in the household. The reporting form asks for the name of an "alleged perpetrator" of the abuse/neglect and the person responsible for the child at the time the incident or incidents occurred (Butz, 1985).

I work to develop a relationship with the child and family as quickly as possible. Once the child is medically cared for, I turn my attention to the parents' problems, needs and concerns. Exclusive focus on the child's condition further exacerbates the parent's sense of failure and rejection.

My work with relatives is not limited to the people who have been defined as clients. Several of Bobby's relatives came to see me during his hospitalization because they were concerned with his welfare. These contacts were brief, and after I listened to their concerns about how Bobby was treated at home, I referred them to the CPS worker. This happens often when there are caring relatives, but one must be careful to keep the parents' information confidential (Mouzakitis and Varghese, 1985).

Goals

One goal is ensuring the safety of the child and seeing that he or she receives proper medical attention. The child's best interests are paramount. Some children fear a parent and do not want to return home. When others want to return to a dangerous situation, we ask that temporary, alternative living arrangements be found. If possible, we involve parents or supportive family members in this transition.

Another goal is the preservation of the family system. Often, this goal is not shared by other service providers. In fact, sometimes, the highly emotional, insensitive and ill-considered response of providers interferes with the proper provision of care, and disrupts the nonpunitive relationship which the social worker is trying to establish (Ebeling and Hill, 1983). Ms. Woods' arrest and detention is a good example. Parents and families, particularly abusing families, are acutely sensitive to these interactions, in part because they are concerned that their children will be taken from them (Hill, 1975). The majority of cases, however, do not involve police or court action.

Contract

Early identification of the crisis precipitating the child's coming to the attention of the hospital is helpful in engaging the parent in a "contract," a verbal agreement to achieve mutual goals. To be open, honest, sympathetic and compassionate with the abusing family while providing information is difficult, but imperative. With Ms. Woods, I explained the way Bobby came to our attention, what our concerns were, and the contents of our child abuse report. Then, I described the investigative process of the CPS worker and explained that discharge and treatment plans for Bobby would be worked out by the hospital team, parent and CPS worker. I told Ms. Woods that the CPS worker would contact her for a home evaluation, gave her the name of the pediatrician treating Bobby, and introduced her to the nurses on the floor. From the outset, I tried to involve her in the treatment process (Friedrich and Wheeler, 1982).

The first interview with parents is important in the development of the contract. Establishing the treatment plan provides social worker and clients with the opportunity to explore issues such as how the parents were raised and disciplined, the extent and pattern of isolation, interrelationships between parents and significant others, and parental perceptions of the child in question. Ms. Woods related that she was an only child and both of her parents were deceased. Her first four children were placed in foster care as a result of a child abuse report seven years ago. Ms. Woods expressed a desire to have her children returned to her. She felt that Bobby was a difficult child; he would not eat and would not mind her. She described his abrasions and old scars as accidental, said that Bobby fell a lot and kept bumping into things. She did not seem to have any problems with her other children, and indicated that he was "different" (Frodi, 1981).

Bobby's father was incarcerated for assault several months earlier, and she visited him often. His family has been her primary support as she has no relatives in the area. She had no friends because her children kept her occupied most of the time, and she felt she could not trust most people.

The contract we made was based on identified problems and appropriate interventions. As Bobby's eating and developmental skills began to improve during his hospitalization, I used these aspects of his care to extend the contract to finding a way to help him to continue to progress after discharge. Possibly, Ms. Woods could benefit from a special day-care center for assistance with Bobby's growth and development.

The CPS worker and I also established a contract after the hospital team determined the course of medical treatment. Generally, follow-up is managed by the CPS worker and, if the family is agreeable, the outreach program or family health worker (Kempe and Kempe, 1978). Often, the CPS worker, the parent and I begin to plan for follow-up during hospitalization. If the child is not hospitalized, the CPS worker becomes the case manager, and I take the role of consultant and have minimal contact with the family.

Meeting Place

The emergency room is chaotic and hectic. Interruptions by staff, diversions created by other patients, police sirens and the general atmosphere of crisis aggravate the already sensitive nature of the relationship between social worker and family. In this community, however, many families cannot afford private physicians, and the emergency room is often used as the "family doctor." It remains the most accessible place for attention, comfort, relief and human contact, a place where asking for help is acceptable. Across from the emergency room is a room set aside for family members in extraordinary situations such as death or sexual assault.

My office is on the same floor as the emergency room. Although I share it with the social workers and students whom I supervise, we try to avoid interruptions when we see clients. Furnished with a round table and four chairs, it can be cramped. In an interview with a single parent, there is more opportunity to rearrange the seating so there can be touching (Borenzweig, 1983). I saw Bobby's relatives and, later, Ms. Woods in my office.

When the child is hospitalized, it is common to see relatives in the child's room or on the medical floor. Although it is not conducive to a relaxed and neutral interview, this highly charged atmosphere greatly contributes to the social worker's observations of family interaction. Meeting away from the child may feel more supportive to the parents but is less based in reality.

It would be ideal to include a home visit as part of the assessment, because the hospital presents an authoritarian image, and is an intimidating place in which to explore sensitive personal issues. Home visits are not made, however, because of time constraints.

Use of Time

Generally, the relationship is short term. When the child is hospitalized, the duration of hospitalization dictates the duration of the relationship. Bobby was hospitalized for nine days, now considered a long period. Few admissions necessitate a long hospital stay. For the children who are not admitted, it is difficult to continue contact beyond the initial assessment of about two hours, particularly if the child does not require medical follow-up. Once the medical emergency has been resolved, child welfare or other agencies which have been mandated to do so follow the client.

To avoid emotionally wearing interviews, much of the literature recommends short sessions with the parents. My first contact is generally one to one and a half hours. After that time, the length of the session depends on information requirements or new developments.

Treatment Modality

The primary treatment modality is crisis intervention: actively promoting psychosocial functioning during a time of disequilibrium or "medical crisis." This modality is generally well-suited to work in the emergency room, and specifically suited to emergency room work with child abuse. It is time-limited, highly focused, direct, fast paced and works well when people feel vulnerable. The social learning model with the identification of behavioral goals, specific techniques, constant evaluation and intervention with environmental factors is also helpful (Tracy and Clark, 1974). One common response of abusing and neglecting families is that they only brought the child to be seen by a doctor and suddenly all these other things come up. It requires tremendous skill to communicate concerns beyond the medical problem, to assess not only the complaint but background and history, and to gather appropriate resources to enable the patient to cope with the stress and its effects (Bonnefil, 1980; Duggan, 1984; Goldberg, 1975).

Stance of the Social Worker

My stance is affected by the decision to hospitalize and the responsiveness of the parents in the initial interview. Hospitalization means that I will actively treat the family. Discharge means that I will basically support the family in medical follow-up and act as consultant to the CPS worker. Some parents verbalize their problems, concerns and need for help while others remain guarded, suspicious and mistrusting. Ms. Woods remained very guarded during our contacts. Although she responded to my questions, she rarely raised questions or offered comments. With parents like Ms. Woods, I do not confront, but I actively and directly elicit feelings and responses (Faller, 1981).

At one point in our work, Ms. Woods asked whether I had any children, and I said no. This is often asked of social workers. She replied that I could not understand what it was like to have children. I shared the fact that I was one of many children in my family and that I remembered what my parents experienced. I am still not sure whether this had any effect.

I have found it helpful to respond to my immediate impression of the parent in the interview. That is, if the parent appears fearful, anxious, angry, happy, etc., I address those feelings at that moment. Particularly as new situations arise during the treatment period, it has been helpful to remain clear about the event which precipitated the protective service referral. The need for this is evident in situations where a restraining order has been filed for protective custody, and the parents are informed that the child will not be returning home until a hearing is held. Generally, information about procedures and changes in treatment plans must be communicated as directly as possible, and with understanding and concern. Even if the parent becomes hostile and belligerent, calmness and clarity have proven to be more effective than confronting and reacting to the anger (DeMaria, 1986).

Outside Resources

The SCAN Center described earlier has been most helpful in long-term follow-up with abusing families. Paraprofessionals work intensively with parents in their home on the problems identified by the multidisciplinary team and the parents themselves. Decisions regarding the provision of services are ultimately made through the CPS evaluation. Team members contribute their assessments, and joint decisions are made regarding available resources. Medical follow-up is arranged by the pediatrician. This may include referral to an extended care facility for long-term care (Faller, 1987; Faller, 1982).

When the parent has difficulty navigating through the system, I assist. For example, one child was placed in a long leg cast for treatment of his broken leg. I made arrangements for transfer to an extended care facility, accompanied the mother to the interview at the new facility (she was hard-of-hearing and borderline mentally retarded), and helped her learn the system of public transportation so that she could visit her son.

Each discipline involved indicates the kinds of services required to support the child and/or family, and the parent participates significant in the planning. Outside resources may include day-care, psychotherapy, referrals for housing, financial or legal assistance, special equipment, visiting nurses, alcohol and drug counseling and homemaker service. The hospital social worker helps arrange for medical management services while the CPS worker manages child welfare services such as special programs for parents.

Reassessment

Since the relationship between the child and family and the hospital social worker is so limited in time, reassessment takes place between the CPS worker and the family health worker. If there is no family worker involved, reassessment is more difficult.

If the family is being followed by a health worker, there is more opportunity to assess progress. If the child is hospitalized for a reasonable amount of time, both goals and contract can be reevaluated. The majority of our cases of child abuse and neglect are managed by CPS, however, and it is difficult for me to determine whether goals are met. CPS caseloads are very large, the monitoring system is over-extended, many families are lost to follow-up, and reassessment commonly occurs only during the next crisis (Besherov, 1985). Even with court supervision and scheduled evaluation hearings, delays within the court schedules interfere with necessary alterations in treatment plans (Goldstein, 1986).

Transfer or Termination

In most of my emergency room cases, termination occurs when mutually agreed upon goals are met. In child abuse cases, termination seems less complete. When the child is hospitalized, I can discuss the referral with the family and introduce them to the CPS worker. In outpatient situations, I am not afforded this opportunity. Sometimes, a month passes before the parent is contacted by a child welfare worker. During this time, the family is always given the opportunity to contact me. Termination of my role with the family generally occurs when the CPS social worker has made an assessment, the treatment plan has been instituted, and there appears to be no further need for involvement because the plan is working (Nelson, 1984).

Because our hospital thus far continues to function as a community hospital, I find that I see the family or the parent in the hospital waiting area or cafeteria, and we talk informally about how they are managing. Sometimes, a parent is admitted to the hospital for a medical problem and will ask to see me, or a mother will deliver another child and I will see her then.

Case Conclusion

Bobby quickly gained the weight more normal for his age. Developmentally, he became lively and animated, and displayed better social and motor skills. His fever disappeared immediately after admission. Medicine was prescribed for anemia due to iron deficiency. As with all children who fail to thrive, it was recommended that his weight be monitored through pediatric outpatient visits. The nursing staff worked closely with the mother to involve her with her child. Progress was slow, but Ms. Woods came to visit Bobby often.

After much discussion between team members, Bobby was discharged to his mother with follow-up by a family health worker and case management by the CPS worker. The contract between Ms. Woods and the family health worker included the following: Help with management of the children, assistance in caring for Bobby, possible day care, referral for psychotherapy, and work on child rearing and alternate forms of discipline (Baxter, 1985).

The family health worker worked with Ms. Woods and her family for almost three years. Ms. Woods is seeing a therapist at a mental health center (Wolfe et al., 1987). Bobby is progressing well in a special developmental disabilities program in which Ms. Woods participates. Two other siblings are in day care. Bobby's father was released from prison and is living in the home, and Ms. Woods has had another child. Ms. Woods' other children remain in foster care, and it is unclear whether she will continue to try to regain custody. The case was closed by CPS. The family health worker has periodic contact by phone with Ms. Woods, and the family seems to be coping.

Differential Discussion

I am pleased with the outcome of our interventions (Salter, 1985). Both the CPS worker and I were inexperienced with child abuse at the time, and my inexperience interfered with my relationship with Ms. Woods. I remember the biases in my first contact with Ms. Woods. First, the overwhelming deluge of relatives, including those who brought Bobby into the emergency room, subsequent phone calls from other relatives, and visits from neighbors including a hospital employee painted a very negative picture of Ms. Woods as an irresponsible, inconsiderate parent who beat her children regularly. Second, Ms. Woods' unexpected arrival at my office after being released from jail caused me some worry about my own security. Third, our initial contact was much too long (approximately two hours), and I passively confronted her. I wanted her to admit that she had inflicted injuries on her son. Actually, I wanted her to admit to anything at that point, but her passivity and lack of apparent emotion baffled me. When we went to see Bobby, I remember her asking him inane questions such as "Aren't you glad to see Mommy?"

The events leading up to our initial interview, then, had already influenced my impression of Ms. Woods. It was difficult for me to be objective and to try to understand her feelings of mistrust and anger. My expectations were delusions. I expected the "confession" and began to feel like the interrogator. Not until later did I discover that Ms. Woods thought the hospital had alerted the police to arrest her. Additionally, the coordinator of the outreach program was present at our first meeting and left in the middle of the session. I imagine that I was so distressed I sought support in conducting the interview. I should have spoken to Ms. Woods alone.

Limiting our initial meeting might have helped lessen anxiety for both of us. I could have offered more support and asked fewer questions. In terms of collaboration, although I helped Ms. Woods relate to the nursing staff and the CPS worker, I did not help her relate to the pediatrician. Responsibility for communicating medical management was left to the nursing staff. The hospital staff's reception of Ms. Woods was mild to angry.

Ms. Woods has nine children. No one raised the issue of birth control with her. I am not sure whether that should have been the task for me, the CPS worker, the family health worker or all of us. She is a young woman who is capable of giving birth to many more children. Even with the kind of support she had for the three years of CPS involvement, I do not know how she will cope with more children (McMurtry, 1985).

PRACTICE IN CONTEXT

The hospital has changed dramatically since my involvement with Ms. Woods, including the recent sale of the emergency room to a private entity, so that it is now financially separate from the rest of the hospital. When that change first occurred, there was no social worker assigned to the emergency room. Recently, however, a social worker has been reassigned.

Because there was no longer a pediatric service in the hospital, after its reorganization the emergency room medical staff was unfamiliar with treating children and families. Children who came during evenings and weekends were seen by medical staff ill-equipped to diagnose adequately and forced to rely on phone consultations with Children's Hospital. Additionally, in order to be seen in the emergency room, children had to be accompanied by a parent who gave consent unless symptoms were life-threatening or the child was an emancipated minor.

These organizational changes created severe disruptions for the community, and for the internal operation of the child abuse program. When there were pediatric beds, we could use the automatic admission policy to admit children for social evaluation, and a bed was always available. Now, with the tremendous bed shortage and no designated pediatric beds, our opportunities for intervention are fewer. In one situation, a child was to be admitted under this policy but there was no room in the entire hospital, and the father took the child out of the emergency room having waited for five hours.

The hospital had originally committed itself to the child abuse program, but nonmedical admissions generate no revenue. In the past, we had time to assess and develop plans for the family while the child was hospitalized, but now we cannot even have the child admitted. The hospital did allow one social admission of a fifteen-month-old child recently; however, the child was placed on an adult floor where staff had no experience with pediatric care.

During my work with Ms. Woods, visiting hours on the pediatric unit were the same as for other services. The physician had to order exceptional visiting privileges. Hospital policy did not allow anyone under sixteen years of age to visit patients on the floor, so patients would come to the first floor to visit their minor relatives or friends. I could facilitate more liberal visiting hours by accompanying the parent to the floor or requesting that the family visit with my supervision. This allowed the child more accessibility to his or her family and lessened the isolation of being hospitalized. Even though the nurses on the floor were treating elderly patients, there were certain staff informally assigned to the children, and this allowed for close relationships and collaborative efforts. The nursing staff would often go out of their way to spend more time with the children or contact the volunteer office to recruit a playmate for the child.

Policies existing at the time of my relationship with Ms. Woods allowed us valuable time to begin exploring the issues and problems surrounding Bobby's admission. There was no great pressure to discharge Bobby as soon as he was medically ready. Instead, emphasis was placed on devising an appropriate plan of treatment. Hospitalization meant that I did not have to transfer Ms. Woods quickly to the less permissive and perhaps less nurturing CPS worker. It also provided me an opportunity to meet with Ms. Woods in my office and several times on the floor before visiting hours. The contract was developed jointly. Although it was a long and slow process, we were fortunate to have the family health worker become involved with Ms. Woods and her family, meeting with them almost daily to reach defined goals.

Concern for financial survival has profoundly affected the organization and policies of the hospital. Altered priorities have resulted in decreased support for social work in terms of services and consultation. On the other hand, the hospital has been responsive to the social work department's request for more social workers. Thus, the role of the social worker is continually redefined and refocused. Knowledge of the system allows me greater flexibility in my relationships with clients. Despite the limitations, there is a challenge to be creative in developing a contract to achieve common goals.

AUTHOR'S NOTE: This article was written during my employment at the hospital. In May, 1984, I left the hospital and moved to Chicago, where I am now employed at the Rehabilitation Institute of Chicago (RIC) as the outpatient social worker for the pediatric service, with responsibilities for some inpatient cases.

The Rehabilitation Institute of Chicago is a private, non-profit hospital with 176 beds, serving all ages in the areas of spinal cord and head injury, stroke, amputation, cerebral palsy, and arthritis. It is the Mid-West Regional Spinal Cord Injury center and is affiliated with the McGaw Medical Center of Northwestern University. Newborns to teenagers are treated for such conditions as cerebral palsy, neuromuscular diseases, spina bifida, head or spinal cord injury due to trauma or illness, orthopedic problems, and brain-related conditions such as near drowning or systemic infection.

It is a teaching hospital with a residency program in physical medicine. The social work staff is comprised of a director, two clinical supervisors, and eleven social workers. The multi-disciplinary team includes pediatric psychiatrist, nurses, social workers, occupational, physical, therapeutic and communicative therapies, vocational rehabilitation counselors, psychologist, and chaplain.

Within this special population, we work with, the occurrence of suspected child abuse and neglect is becoming more frequent. Often, the origin of the child's injuries or medical condition or issues of neglect in the treatment process are identified at an acute care facility prior to their transfer to the rehabilitation hospital. As the outpatient social worker, I am involved with the coordination of services between RIC, the family, and CPS, and all children followed by CPS are considered "high-risk" follow-up. The number of reports we file of suspected abuse/neglect are much fewer than those identified in acute care. When we do file or report, it is usually for neglect; more specifically, poor medical follow-up and inability of the parent to follow treatment plans, promote school attendance, and so on.

All states have reporting mechanisms for child abuse and neglect. Chicago is a much larger city than Philadelphia, and thus, the child welfare system is much more complicated to negotiate. There are similarities in that there is a 24-hour hotline in the state capital for reporting, and mandates for intervention and follow-up are similar. There is no specific program similar to the hospital-based program at Presbyterian, as the CPS contracts out to private community agencies to provide intensive home visiting and follow-up.

In considering whether we need to file a report, we pursue all avenues of assisting the parent in getting access to medical recommendations. My work often involves the school system in facilitating the child's needs for education and related therapeutic interventions. Since my employment in 1984, I have noticed an increase of CPS involvement with both hospitalized and outpatient children. Because some children have such special medical and therapeutic needs, family teaching is the most important means to ensure that the parent has the knowledge and understanding needed to take care of the child. Family teaching is provided by all the team members, whether individually or jointly. Parents are given written instructions on how to properly care for their child. Yet, there are some parents who are unable to carry through with these treatment plans and who require help from CPS. The psychiatrist calls the hotline and is usually notified within 24 hours of the findings by CPS. The parent is informed and we begin our coordination with the family, RIC, and CPS.

REFERENCES

Alderette, P. and D.F. deGraffenried. "Nonorganic failure-to-thrive syndrome and the family system." *Social Work*, 31,3 (1986), pp. 207-211.

Baxter, A. *Techniques for Dealing with Child Abuse*. Springfield, Ill: Charles C Thomas, 1985.

Belsky, J. "Child maltreatment: an ecological approach." Edited by S. Chess and A. Thomas. *Annual Progress in Child Psychiatry and Child Development*. New York: Brunner/Mazel, 1981, pp. 637-665.

Besharov, D.J. "An overdose of concern: child abuse and the over-reporting problem." *Regulation: AEI Journal on Government and Society* 9 (1985), pp. 2528.

Bonnefil, M.C. "Crisis intervention with children and families." Edited by G.F. Jacobson, *Crisis Intervention in the 1980's*. San Francisco: Jossey-Bass, 1980.

Borenzweig, H. "Touching in clinical social work" *Social Casework*, 64 (1983), pp. 238-242.

Butz, R.A. "Reporting child abuse and confidentiality in counseling." *Social Casework*, 66, 2 (1986), pp. 83-90.

"Child Protective Services Law" Act 124, State of Pennsylvania, 1985.

Clement, N. and Klingbeil, K.S. "The Emergency Room." *Health and Social Work*, 6 (Supplement) (1981), pp. 83-90.

Conde, J. and L. Bekliner. "Sexual abuse of children: implications for practice." *Social Casework*, 62,10 (1981), pp. 601-606.

De Maria, R. "Family therapy and child welfare." *Family Therapy Networker*, 75 (1986), pp. 31-32.

Duggan, H.A. *Crisis Intervention: Helping Individuals at Risk*. Lexington, Massachusetts: D.C. Heath and Company, 1984.

Ebeling, N.B. and D.A. Hill, Editors. *Child Abuse and Neglect: A Guide with*

Case Studies for Treating the Child and Family. Boston, Massachusetts. John Wright, 1983.

Faller, K.C., Editor. *Social Work with Abused and Neglected Children: A Manual of Interdisciplinary Practices*. New York: The Free Press, 1981.

Faller, K.C. *Multidisciplinary Team Functions*. Ann Arbor, Michigan: Interdisciplinary Project in Child Abuse and Neglect, 1982.

Faller, K.C. "Protective services for children." A. Minahan, Editor, *Encyclopedia of Social Work*, Silver Spring: National Association of Social Work, 1987.

Friedrich, W.N. and A.N. Einbender. "The abused child: a psychological review." *Journal of Clinical Child Psychology*, 12,3 (1983), pp. 244-256.

Friedrich, W.N. and K.K. Wheeler. "The abusing parent revisited: a decade of psychological research." *Journal of Nervous and Mental Disease* 170,10 (1982), pp. 577-587.

Frodi, A.M. "Contribution of infant characteristics to child abuse." *American Journal of Mental Deficiency* 85,4 (1981), pp. 341-349.

Goldberg, G. "Breaking the Communication Barrier: The Initial Interview with an Abusing Parent." *Child Welfare* (1975), pp. 274-282.

Goldstein, J. et al. *In the Best Interests of the Child*. New York: The Free Press, 1986.

Kelly, J.A. *Treating Child-Abusive Families*. New York: Plenum Press, 1983.

Kempe, C.H. and Helfer, R.E., Eds. *The Battered Child*. Chicago: University of Chicago Press, 1980.

Kempe, R.S. and Kempe, C.H. *Child Abuse*. Cambridge: Harvard University Press, 1978.

Kinard, E.M. "Child abuse and neglect" in A. Minahan, Editor, *Encyclopedia of Social Work*. Silver Spring, Maryland: National Association of Social Work, 1987.

Korbin, J.E., Editor. *Child Abuse and Neglect: Cross Cultural Perspectives*. Berkeley, California: University of California Press, 1981.

McMurtry, S.L. "Secondary prevention of child maltreatment: a review." *Social Work*, 30 (1985), pp. 42-48.

Mouzakitis, C.M. and T. Varghese, Editors. *Social Work Treatment with Abused and Neglected Children*. Chicago: University of Chicago Press, 1985.

Nelson, B. J. *Making an Issue of Child Abuse: Political Setting for Social Problems*. Chicago: University of Chicago Press, 1984.

Nelson, G., Dainauski, J. and Kilmer, L., "Child Abuse Reporting Laws: Action and Uncertainty." *Child Welfare* (1980), pp. 203-212.

Parton, N. *The Politics of Child Abuse*. New York: St. Martin's Press, 1986.

Pelton, L.H., Editor, *The Social Context of Child Abuse and Neglect*. New York: Human Sciences Press, 1981.

Pennsylvania Department of Public Welfare, Office of Children, Youth and Families. *Child Abuse Report*. Harrisburg, Pennsylvania, 1985.

Rehr, H. "Medical Care Organization and Social Service Connection." *Health and Social Work*. 4 (1985), pp. 245-258.

Russell, A.B. and C.M. Trainor. *Trends in Child Abuse and Neglect: A National Perspective*. Denver, Colorado: American Humane Association, 1984.

Salter, A.C., C.M. Richardson, and P.A. Martin. "Treating abusive parents." *Child Welfare*, 64,4 (1985), pp. 327-341.

Stein, T.J. and T.L. Rzepnicki. *Decision Making in Child Welfare Services*. Hingham, Massachusetts: Kluwer-Nijhoff Publishing, 1984.

Tracy, J. and E.H. Clark. "Treatment for Child Abuser." *Social Work*, 5 (1974), pp. 338-342.

United States Department of Health and Human Services. *Joining Together to Fight Child Abuse*, pamphlet, Washington, D.C.: United States Government Printing Office, 1986.

United States Department of Health and Human Services. *Child Abuse Prevention and Treatment Act: Public Law 93-247 as Amended*, pamphlet. Washington, D.C.: United States Government Printing Office, 1986.

United States House Committee on Government Operations, Intergovernmental Relations and Human Resources. 99th Congress, 2nd Session. *Child Abuse and Neglect and Child Sexual Abuse Programs* Hearing, March 1, 1986.

United States Select Committee on Children, Youth and Families. 98th Congress, 2nd Session, *Violence and Abuse in American Families*, June 14, 1985.

Wolfe, D.A. and J. Sandler. "Training abusive parents in effective child management." *Behavior Modification*, 5 (1981), pp. 320-335.

Wolfe, D.A. et al. "Intensive behavioral patient training for a child abusive mother." *Behavior Therapy*, 13 (1982), pp. 438-451.

Psychological Recovery from Burn Injury: Regional Burn Center

Betsy C. Blades

DESCRIPTION OF THE SETTING

The Baltimore Regional Burn Center is a tertiary care facility of the Maryland Emergency Medical System for the treatment of seriously burned patients. It has twenty beds organized in a ten bed intensive care unit (BICU) serving critically ill adults and children, with a contiguous ten bed intermediate care unit. The intermediate care area serves both as a stepdown unit for adults from the critical care area and as the site of care for less seriously burned adult patients. There are additional beds on the general pediatric unit for less seriously burned children and for those transferred from the intensive care unit. Approximately 250 to 300 patients are admitted to the burn center annually; their average length of stay is slightly more than 16 days. The Baltimore Regional Burn Center is one of the few facilities in the nation to be designated a burn treatment center and is the only one in the state of Maryland.

Policy

Maryland has a highly sophisticated emergency medical system. The Maryland Institute for Emergency Medical Services Systems, commonly known by its acronym MIEMSS, is established as an autonomous state agency to plan, implement and coordinate the

The author would like to thank those from the Baltimore Regional Burn Center who assisted with the updating of information for this chapter: Gail Horowitz, MSW, James Scheulen, RPA and Andrew M. Munster, MD.

system. The system includes such tertiary facilities as a shock trauma center, neonatal units, a hand center, and a spinal cord center. The burn center is designated by MIEMSS as the facility to receive patients from throughout the state with major burns. The American Burn Association has established criteria for burn care facilities, and the burn center designation is reserved for the highest level facility. A burn center is required to maintain the highest level of services, equipment, teaching program and research. The American Burn Association criteria mandates, for example, that a burn center have a nurse/patient ratio of 1:1 or 1:2.

MIEMSS has an arrangement with the state police to provide patients with air transportation to the centers on a priority basis. A central communications system connects centers and helicopters, ambulances or other hospitals. Although patients are admitted directly from the hospital's catchment area and from local hospitals, they are also transported by ground or air from the scene and from distant hospitals.

MIEMSS policy, which is consistent with American Burn Association recommended guidelines, sets the following criteria for admission to the burn center: second- and third-degree burns of 10 percent or more for persons under 10 and over 50 years of age; burns of greater than 20 percent for other age groups; burns requiring special attention, such as those involving the face, hands, feet, joints, or perineal areas; or chemical and electrical burns. This policy allows professional discretion; patients meeting the criteria for admission may be treated at local hospitals if they are not transported directly from the field to the center. Patients may also be admitted from beyond the state boundaries.

Financial policy is becoming an important part of any discussion of inpatient hospital care, and state and federal policies are extremely important in tertiary care. Prospective payment systems of reimbursement which are in current use in most states under Medicare and in many states under Medicaid are viewed as a particular threat to burn care facilities as well as to access for many persons in need of such care (Rees and Dimick, 1987; Hunt and Purdue, 1986). The cost of burn care is very high—on average the highest of all diagnostic related groups (DRGs) (Fleming et al., 1985). When the DRGs were developed, there were an insufficient number of burn cases to accurately predict resource utilization. However, the nature of burns demanded that they be placed in their own diagnostic group (DRG). Thus under the current DRG system, the reimbursement to cost ratio is very high for the person with a major burn who dies shortly after admission, but reimbursement is often lower than costs and charges for the survivor who requires high resource utilization. There is some concern among burn professionals that the current system could provide a disincentive to aggressive treatment for the individual with a low probability of survival. A particular threat to the survival of burn care facilities would occur if all third party payers adopted the current prospective reimbursement categories, as younger patients are more likely to survive a more extensive injury and injuries with more serious complications. A facility such as a burn center which does not have an average case mix but treats a disproportionate share of the severely injured would be severely affected by the projected losses that would occur with a universal system of prospective payments based on the current DRGs. There has been a great deal of activity among burn care facilities and groups that represent them, to document the potential impact of such reimbursement systems, to develop alternate strategies and to lobby for change (Rees and Dimick, 1987). There have also been some additional efforts to attempt to shorten the length of stay for survivors by changes in the technology of care. In some areas of the country, there have been some short-term efforts to circumvent this reimbursement policy by reclassifying beds from tertiary care to rehabilitation beds for which there are currently no DRGs in effect.

Maryland currently has a Medicare waiver so that hospitals are reimbursed by all payers according to the same methodology rather than by the prospective payment formula. Designated facilities in the emergency medical system in Maryland have a Medicaid waiver which removes the limits on coverage for inpatient hospital days that are applied to general hospital services. The Medicaid waiver thus serves as an incentive to provide treatment in designated facilities for those with Medicaid and for those who are uninsured. Medicaid reimbursement policies for inpatient hospitalization vary by state. Although it does not appear to be a problem in Maryland, reimbursement policies in some states without an emergency medical system with strong protocols, provide an incentive for non-designated hospitals to transfer patients with potential for low reimbursement to specialized facilities while "creaming" or keeping those with potential for higher reimbursement. Such conditions pose a threat of access to the most appropriate facilities for those with the need for specialized care and threatens the future viability of specialized centers.

An additional financial policy consideration related to Medicaid that varies among the states is participation in optional programs such as Medicaid for the medically needy and Medicaid for two parent families. Maryland participates in both of these programs. Thus, the uninsured or inadequately insured individual with low income or the person who has no income once he becomes ill can easily "spend down" to the level of eligibility by accumulating a hospital bill which relieves him of responsibility for all charges above that level. Because the cost of burn care is so high, a family with a modest income, such as one with a middle-to-low income working spouse, may also be eligible for Medicaid. A state's participation in such optional programs will have an important impact on both the patient and on the facility which provides treatment for those without insurance or with inadequate coverage. Additional factors that may vary from state to state include state programs for catastrophic illness, state sponsored insurance pools, and other programs to cover the cost of uncompensated care.

In many states, including Maryland, patients must be admitted into the emergency medical system based on their needs for treatment without prior inquiry as to ability to pay. The federal Emergency Medical Services Systems program that formerly existed to promote development of emergency systems (EMS) set this as a condition of receiving federal grants, and many states have included this in comprehensive EMS laws (Emergency Medical Systems Act, 1981). Also under the federal program was a requirement that individuals have access to facilities in neighboring states when appropriate and necessary. Such an agreement exists, for example, between the state of Maryland and the District of Columbia so that an individual may be admitted directly to the closest facility, and the facilities in these jurisdictions serve as back-up facilities if the closest facility lacks available beds. The state Medicaid program reimburses designated facilities in the District of Columbia on the same basis as those in the state. In many states such agreements do not exist, and there are problems collecting reimbursement from state programs across state lines. There are also reimbursement problems for out-of-state patients when neighboring states have differing Medicaid policies, such as limits on days of reimbursement or eligibility of two parent families (Joe et al., 1985). These situations all have the potential for limiting access to the most appropriate facility for the injured person's need. Hospitals, for example, may respond to the threat of loss of revenue by denying access to out-of-state residents. In states without comprehensive EMS laws and protocols, cooperation in a system of emergency medical services is voluntary, and hospitals may refuse access to patients according to their own rules in order to limit potential loss. The problem would be intensified in sparsely populated areas where a single tertiary care center such as a burn center may be the only appropriate facility within a multi-state area for the patient's needs.

However, for Maryland residents hospitalized at the burn center, the direct costs of burn care are minimized for the poor and uninsured through the Medicare and Medicaid waivers and by state participation in optional Medicaid programs to extend coverage to two parent families and the medically needy. Financial losses to designated facilities are minimized under the all-payer system, which also covers a portion of uncompensated care. In addition, the hospital provides "uncompensated care" to those in need through Hill Burton and other programs. However, there are still costs that may be unmet such as the cost of non-prescription supplies for outpatients, which may be substantial; the cost to families for lodging away from home, and the loss of income during the recovery period. Persons with inadequate insurance coverage, such as policies that provide only 30 days of inpatient care, may sustain substantial loss of savings and other financial resources before "spending down" to Medicaid eligibility levels. All of these situations will vary depending on the policies in different states.

Technology

Because a burn injury affects all aspects of the human system, the technology involved is very complex. A burn most obviously affects the skin, the largest organ of the body, which acts as a first line of defense against infection, controls temperature, and serves to contain fluid.

The severity of a burn is determined by its depth and the percent of the body surface involved. A full thickness, or third-degree, burn is the deepest and involves all layers of the skin. Nerves, hair follicles, and sweat glands are all destroyed. The capacity to regenerate skin is lost; skin must be grafted. A second-degree burn is a partial thickness burn where nerve endings are exposed. With no complications, the skin will regenerate within several weeks. First-degree burns are similar to sunburns, and, because they do not cause systemic damage, are not considered in calculating burn size.

An important consideration in determining the depth of a burn is the source of the injury. Typical sources are flame, electricity, chemicals, scalds and contact with a hot object. Burns may involve muscles, tendons and other underlying structures in the case of very deep injuries, such as electrical burns. Burn size, burn depth, and the age of the patient are significant factors in determining mortality, as are other general physiological conditions.

A partial thickness or second-degree burn is very painful, as nerves are partially damaged and the endings are exposed. All of us have experienced partial thickness skin loss when the skin is scraped, as with, for example, a "skinned knee" or a brush burn, or when burned by a grease splatter, an oven pan, or a hot iron. The seriousness of the burn obviously increases with the size of the surface involved.

A third-degree, or full thickness, burn, because it destroys the nerves, is not painful. There are, however, few burns that are entirely third-degree. Frequently there are patches of second-degree burns within and around third-degree areas. Donor areas from which partial thicknesses of skin have been removed for grafts are the equivalent of second-degree injuries.

When the patient is admitted, he is brought directly to the burn center, where the burn size and depth are estimated. He is placed in a tub of water, washed, and dead skin is removed. The burned areas are covered with an antibiotic cream and wrapped in gauze dressings. The patient is then x-rayed, and catheters and needles are inserted to monitor all body functions. Depending on the circumstances of the injury, the patient may require an endotracheal tube to assist his breathing, in which case he will be unable to talk.

Burned extremities are elevated in slings, and rigid splints are required to maintain proper position. A heat radiating shield is placed above the bed to help compensate for the diminished ability to control body temperature. For patients with burns on the back or buttocks or for those with potential for skin loss from pressure, an air fluidized support system may be used. This is essentially a bed on which the patient "floats" so that no pressure is exerted on the body. While the bed prevents further skin loss and permits healing, the experience is unique and can exacerbate disorientation which is particularly a problem for many elderly patients.

For the first few days, patients are placed in protective isolation, and all who enter the room are required to wear gowns, gloves, and masks. Vascular changes as a result of the injury cause the patient to swell massively; if the face is burned, the patient may be unable to open his eyes and will be largely unrecognizable to friends and family during this initial period. Patients are nevertheless usually quite lucid and are often talkative; however, few if any are able to understand the seriousness of their injuries.

Dressings and creams are changed at least twice each day during the acute phase of the injury. The patient is usually "tubbed" once daily. This procedure involve several staff members washing the patient and removing creams and dead skin. Physical and occupational therapy are instituted daily to exercise joints to aid in the prevention of contractures which result from the tightening of healing skin. All of these necessary procedures cause additional pain for the patient. Many feel that the tub water burns. Wounds are covered with cream before they are wrapped, and washing or wiping the creams off is very painful for the patient, some preferring to do this themselves. Nurses and therapists are sometimes referred to as torturers. There is also pain involved in positioning and with maintaining a position for a period of several days while grafts heal. Healing burns itch and often continue to itch for months. Some patients feel that this experience is more stressful than the pain.

Pain does vary from individual to individual. Patients who are relaxed, for example, find exercising far less painful than those who are tense, because anxiety, fear of pain and visual stimuli compound the feeling of pain. Patients do often cry, moan, swear, etc., but despite the seriousness of the injuries and discomfort of the treatment, burn centers are not filled with constant expressions of pain.

While healing, patients need massive amounts of calories to maintain normal body temperature and to promote healing. This requires that patients with large calculated calorie requirements be fed high-calorie substances continuously through nasogastric tubes. Those who can must eat as much as possible.

Patients with full-thickness injuries require skin grafting. This operation is performed with general anesthesia and involves the excision or removal of dead skin from the burned area and its replacement with a partial thickness layer of skin from an unburned area. At times, pigskin or cadaver skin is used as a temporary wound covering. The first of often multiple grafting procedures may take place within a few days to several weeks following admission. Following grafting, the patient must remain immobile without pressure to grafted or donor areas until a blood supply has formed to the grafted skin. Dressings over grafts are not changed but must be kept constantly wet with antibiotic solutions. Once the graft takes, tubbings and exercises resume until the time for the next grafting procedure. A recent change in procedure that is partially related to financial policies which create pressures to decrease the length of stay is the trend of burn care facilities to do more extensive early excision and grafting within the first few days of admission.

Throughout the time the patient has areas of unhealed burns, infection is a constant threat. This can be minimized to some extent by various medications and procedures. However, organisms that normally exist within and on the healthy human almost inevitably reach the burn wound. If the infection reaches the blood stream, the patient may become quite ill and may die.

With this available technological arsenal, even the fatally injured patient can be supported for quite some time, in some cases more than a month, during which time he is often quite alert and oriented. The course of treatment for those not fatally injured is often, at best, marked by ups and downs. Pain, periods of immobility, therapeutic exercises, physical isolation and interrupted cycles are all necessary throughout the treatment process. Psychological defenses, which are all mobilized initially, are often depleted after a month of this regimen, and this frequently leads to lowered ability to tolerate further treatment. Physicians try to minimize discomfort. Medications are often used to dull the pain, to control infection, to aid sleep and promote relaxation, to promote healing, and to minimize itching in healing areas.

Once the wounds are covered or healed, the patient is fitted with custom-made pressure garments to minimize scarring. These garments are worn over affected areas for 20 hours a day for one to one and a half years, the period during which scarring is most likely to occur. Additional splints may be necessary, as well, to prevent contractures. Plastic surgery may also be required after discharge for reconstruction of burned areas or for release of contracted scars over joints.

Social work involvement with the patient, as well as with the family, must begin immediately after admission with an assessment of the circumstances of the injury, the pre-injury functioning of the patient and family, and their initial responses to the injury.

Organization

The burn center is located in the Francis Scott Key Medical Center, a community teaching hospital which has been a part of the Johns Hopkins Medical System since 1984. The hospital was formerly owned and operated by the City of Baltimore, and many of the staff members were formerly city employees.

The general hospital attending physicians are employed by a professional association, the Chesapeake Physicians Professional Association (CPPA). This association also employs some of the center's supporting staff, such as the physician's assistant and research personnel. The director of the burn center is a general surgeon and professor on the faculty of the Johns Hopkins University School of Medicine. The physician house staff is assigned on rotation from the Johns Hopkins Hospital. A chief resident in plastic surgery is assigned for six months; an assistant resident and an intern have one month rotations. Additional residents are assigned from three area teaching hospitals. There is usually a burn fellow who is employed by the hospital for one year. There are no community attending physicians.

A head nurse is responsible for the BICU and the Intermediate Care Unit. One nursing staff serves both, and is organized on a primary nursing model. Nursing and other team members, who are hospital employees, include a burn nurse clinician who is responsible for staff education; occupational and physical therapists; a dietician, and a social worker. Other professional disciplines are available on a consultation basis as needed.

Virtually all of the patients are followed in the burn clinic after discharge. The clinic is located in the outpatient surgery department and is staffed by surgical clinic nurses. Patients are seen by the center's director, the physician's assistant, the burn fellow and inpatient house staff. The center's social worker also has responsibility for the clinic patients. Patients requiring reconstruction are usually referred to the attending plastic surgeons, who are able to see the patients in the burn center or in the burn reconstruction clinic which is held on burn clinic days.

The social work department has approximately 25 social workers who are assigned by the department's director on a nonrotating basis to medical services and units. The burn center's social worker, who requested this position, is assigned full-time and has an office adjacent to the center.

The treatment program is organized on a team model with a clear commitment that the whole patient must be treated. The expectation is that all team members will become involved with the patient within three days of admission. Weekly team rounds in which each patient is discussed in a comprehensive manner are well attended. Individual patient care conferences are held as needed. The director of the center is most accessible to patients, staff and families. Family education classes are offered by the staff, and families are encouraged to approach staff members with questions and concerns. Visits are restricted to one five hour periods per day.

The demands of caring for burn patients can be quite stressful to the staff. Burn nurses often regard their work as more demanding and requiring more comprehensive knowledge than other critical care areas. However, nursing turnover and staffing can be a problem. While there have been waiting lists of nurses wishing to work in the burn center in recent years, there is currently a desire on the part of many nurses to work in non-hospital settings which leads to nursing shortages in many regions. And when shortages occur, there are often financial incentives for nurses to move to hospitals with more generous salary structures. When there are nursing shortages in the burn center, there seems to be more of a demand to concentrate on wound care with less emphasis on total patient and family care.

A high level of professionalism is encouraged, which at times can turn a feeling of isolation into an attitude of exclusiveness or specialness. Many burn team members teach in the hospital and in the community. Students from most disciplines, including social work, receive training at the center. Professional association memberships, meeting attendance, and research are encouraged for all team members. Logo patches, t-shirts, baseball caps, and parties also serve to promote team identity.

There is a certain amount of anxiety about burns on the part of many people in the hospital, as well as the community. This creates some problems obtaining resources for patients. It is difficult, for example, to arrange inpatient interviews for some services when the interviewer does not visit, is afraid to visit, or is bothered by burns.

Patients and staff generally address each other by first names. Former patients frequently visit and correspond with the staff, sometimes for several years. An informal support group meets on clinic days, and the structure can be more formal when there is a need for support for a particular patient or group of patients. Staff members are able to utilize the continued interest of former patients by having them visit the newly burned. In the past, this was formalized into a group of former patients who visited and sponsored diversionary events; however, this practice was discontinued in favor of the individual approach.

Case Description

Paul was a thirty-two-year old male at the time of his admission to the burn center with a flame burn over 40 percent of his body surface. He was injured when his car burned and ignited his clothing. He suffered full- and partial thickness burns on his head, face, chest, arms, and neck, very deep burns on his hands, and a severe injury to his lungs from the inhalation of smoke, superheated air, and toxic fumes from the burning car upholstery. He was admitted via helicopter transport from the scene, approximately fifty miles from the center. His condition was critical; he required a lengthy period of respirator support and was unable to talk for the first ten days. Taking into account only his age and burn size, his survival estimate was 85 percent. However, the injury to his lungs was a complicating factor which significantly lowered this estimate.

Paul's face and head were burned and what remained of his beard and hair in the burned areas was shaved to facilitate treatment. On the day following his admission when I first saw him, his face was extremely swollen. Although he is a small-framed man, he appeared to be very large, almost massive. His eyes looked like slits because of the swelling of the lids and surrounding areas. His lips and lower face were so swollen that the lower lip stuck out and the inside surface was exposed. His head and face were covered with white cream, and his hands and arms, which also appeared very large, were wrapped in dressing and suspended in slings.

Initial assessment information was obtained primarily from his wife, Marsha, on the day following his admission. Paul lived with his wife, to whom he had been married for five years; they had one four-year-old daughter. He had a nine-year-old son from a previous marriage, who lived with his first wife and with whom he had limited contact. His mother lived about fifty miles from the hospital in the opposite direction from the patient. Paul's parents were divorced when he was fourteen, and he had had no subsequent contact with his father. He had two older sisters who were living outside the state; he and Marsha lived in the same community as Marsha's parents and one sister. Although they individually had friends through work and other activities, Paul and Marsha did not have close friends with whom they socialized as a couple. The entire family, including their parents, enjoyed aquatic activities. Paul had his own boat, which he kept docked near his mother's home, and this was their main source of recreation.

Paul worked as a mechanic specializing in diesel engines. He had been with the same firm for eight years, and was a supervisor. Marsha had a job as a department administrator in an office where she had started as a secretary.

Paul was described by both his wife and his mother as a quiet person who tended to keep his concerns to himself and to withdraw under stress. His wife described him as a heavy drinker. This had been a source of discord between them; she had threatened to leave him if he did not seek help. He had attended several meetings of Alcoholics Anonymous, but his wife felt he never acknowledged that he was an alcoholic. This was later confirmed by the patient. They had not been involved in any other counseling or therapy.

Before he was burned, Paul had wanted to buy a house in a rural waterfront area near where his mother lived. He thought a space of their own and the opportunity to pursue their water-related interests would solve their marital problems. They had recently contracted to purchase such a house and, at the time of his injury, were awaiting final financial arrangements for possession.

Marsha saw herself as the stronger of the two and the decision maker of the family. She felt she had a close relationship with her family and a positive relationship with Paul's mother. His mother was very protective of the patient and denied that there were any pre-existing problems.

The circumstances of the injury were somewhat obscure. Paul had been drinking with friends while they worked on a car they were restoring. The friends had left him to close up the garage after they had finished their work for the evening. He was next seen several hours later running from the scene with his clothes in flames. Although he maintained later that the car exploded when he turned on the ignition switch, he had no recall of the events surrounding the explosion, and he could not account for the lapse in time. There was some speculation by the staff, based on the severity of his respiratory injury, that he had been sitting in the car while the upholstery smoldered, perhaps from a cigarette.

Several significant facts were learned from the initial assessment. The patient's injuries were potentially lethal, and, at best, would result in physical limitations to his hands. An obscure account such as the one he gave often indicates that the person was drinking heavily. I interpreted Paul's use of alcohol as, at least in part, an attempt to cope with stress. His difficulty verbalizing his concerns and his search for magical solutions (in which his wife collaborated to some extent) were significant in light of the task he faced of reconciling himself to his losses. In addition, Marsha was quite angry with him; she blamed him not only for injuring himself but also for disrupting their lives and plans. Positive factors were his supportive family system, his history of employment stability and success, and his apparent desire to maintain his marriage.

DECISIONS ABOUT PRACTICE

Definition of the Client

A traumatic event such as a severe burn injury constitutes a crisis for the entire patient-family system; each part of the system is affected in different ways, and each must be addressed. It is the patient's physical, psychological, and social recovery toward which team efforts are primarily directed, not only because of his physical injury but also because his available emotional resources become the most depleted. However, the patient can not be separated from his family, and intervention at any point takes place along a continuum of client definitions, ranging from patient only at one end to family only at the other. The degree of social work involvement along this continuum changes throughout the course of time, depending upon the urgency of the need and the accessibility of family members and patient.

Paul's psychosocial recovery was my primary concern from the time of his admission. However, he was unable to talk because of the need for respirator support. Because of the burns, his face was quite swollen initially, he was unable to open his eyes, and he could not make himself clearly understood by moving his lips. His hands were in splints and elevated in slings, so he could not write, and he had a limited ability to gesture. During this time, therefore, he was not directly accessible to me.

Marsha was overwhelmed by a sense of helplessness. She was able to visit and was aware that he could hear her, but she could not understand his attempts to communicate, and she could not anticipate his concerns. He became agitated when she visited. She was accessible to me and expressing a need. By helping her, I could also provide for some of Paul's needs. If Marsha could reduce her anxiety and regain a sense of control, she could be supportive to him, and, in turn, help reduce his anxiety. When Marsha gained control over her anxiety, it became obvious that she was angry with Paul. She had been trying to force him to make family financial decisions when he was barely able to communicate with her. By my accepting her feelings as legitimate and encouraging her to express herself, she was able to recognize that she wanted to punish him, when his suffering was already great, and she was able to stop trying to increase his burden. Also, by helping Marsha focus her anger early, she was less likely to express it in a more detrimental way later toward Paul, his family, or the center's staff.

Later, Marsha did become much more comfortable visiting Paul, and also resumed her responsibilities at home and work. Paul, on the other hand, felt very frustrated and helpless. He required high levels of pain medication, ate poorly, and was withdrawn. I decided that Paul's stress might be eased with an opportunity to verbalize his concerns, a task which had been difficult for him in the past. He now became the primary focus, and Marsha's progress of adaptation was merely monitored.

These decisions represented different points of intervention along the patient-family continuum. There are many times when the most accessible point of intervention or the need in the client-family system is more difficult to define. In another case, I became involved with a grief-stricken and guilt-ridden husband whose critically injured wife had requested that he not be permitted to visit. They had separated on the day of her injury. Because of her condition, she was not accessible to me at that point, and he was requesting help. He could not see her, and although he was experiencing the loss of separation, he could not comprehend the effect of her severe injuries. By becoming involved with him, the opportunity to develop a relationship of trust with her at a later point was destroyed.

Goals

The team has general goals for every patient. Whether these become the goals for the patient-social worker relationship depends on how well the patient is able to negotiate the tasks involved without intervention and on the decisions made by the patient and the worker.

The most general goal for the treatment program is to help the patient and family achieve the best possible level of functioning. Functioning is defined in terms of physical, social and psychological goals, primary among them the ability to pursue one's usual work and be independent. This general goal includes an important recognition that the physical survival of the patient is not the exclusive focus of treatment. While life-saving and life-maintaining efforts are priorities, intervention in psychological, social and physical functioning must begin even before survival is assured.

To achieve these goals, the patient and family must undergo a process of adjustment (Steiner and Clark, 1987; Goodstein, 1985). They must first recognize that something terrible has happened to the patient. The next step is to try to explain the injury and to place it in a rational framework. Patients ask questions such as: What did I do to deserve this? Why am I being punished? Why have I been chosen? They must understand that they did nothing to *deserve* their injuries and that there is no rational explanation of this sort for why they have been injured. Patients must accept that the injury is unrelated to punishment, malign fate or divine wrath before they can fully participate in their own rehabilitation. Then they can consider how their lives have been changed and how they will adjust their lives for the future. These steps are not discrete and may be reached at different rates. The adjustment process is marked by periods of great anxiety, depression, regression, and associated behaviors. The social worker's goal is to help the patient negotiate this process.

Burn patients define their goals predominantly in physical terms. Patients and families generally feel that once the patient leaves the hospital, all their past, present, and future problems will be solved. Intervention often begins without clearly defined mutual goals, but the patient is helped to comprehend his situation more realistically and to participate in defining goals for psychosocial adjustment.

Paul initially thought only of surviving the pain, discomfort and frustration of physical recovery. He often could see no further into the future than the time for his next pain medication. When he first thought about leaving the hospital, he thought about operating his boat. As he began to think about actual hospital discharge, however, he began to think more realistically about what post-injury life would be like for him. At this point, we were able to begin to define mutual goals for our work.

Contract

Contracts with patients are usually broad in the beginning, unless there is a particular, immediate need. They are almost always oral and must be flexible to accommodate the treatment process and the physical and emotional fluctuations that frequently arise between interviews.

Patients and families have rarely had another experience to compare to a burn or other major trauma. Their knowledge of social work is also often limited. For my initial assessment, I ask clients for information about themselves, particularly about how the patient and family respond to stress. When family members know their information is important to the patient's care, they begin to become involved in the treatment plan. I explain that the patient's recovery process will be difficult for everyone, but I can assist them by answering questions, explaining the process, and providing support. I often see family members daily for the first few days.

My introduction to the patient is often limited to asking him about the circumstances of the injury. Reviewing the experience helps the patient incorporate the reality of what has happened. The first loss the patient experiences is his preinjury sense of invulnerability. After verbalizing his thoughts about the experience and the loss, the patient is surprised by the relief he feels through talking. This recognition of the importance of talk helps me explain my role.

As the patient progresses physically, social and psychological goals become better defined. Patients are usually attuned to the present, however, so planning far into the future is not a realistic expectation. If we do establish a contract, it is to remind us of the tasks on which we agreed to work.

Paul could not recall the circumstances of his injury or the first ten days of his hospitalization. His increasing awareness that he had "lost" ten days of his life was very alarming to him, and this awareness needed to be incorporated into his recovery process and our discussion. He was also concerned that his limited hand function would make it hard for him to be a father to his daughter. He presented a long list of things he could not do with her. I agreed that it might be difficult for him to do these things but suggested that there were other things he could do with her, things we could figure out together. I could help him think of options he had never considered. We agreed to focus on what he really needed to be able to do and on what he could do. For his part of the contract, Paul agreed to work between our sessions on tasks which used his hands, such as holding a glass.

Clearly, one does not need hands to be a good father, but Paul was focusing on his pre-injury situation and present experience exclusively in those terms. He could learn to think in other ways. In establishing a contract to focus on his hands—on tasks, needs and realistic abilities—Paul was willing to commit himself to this relearning and thinking process. His desire to be a good father helped me motivate him to cooperate in his physical therapy and to begin to deal realistically with his rehabilitation.

Meeting Place

Both the injury and the treatment process frequently dictate where the meetings can take place. For example, a patient interview could take place in the patient's room when he is in bed in the morning. However, this may be a time when he is anticipating tubbing and dressing changes. In the afternoon, the patient may be seated in a lounge chair in the hallway, feeling less anxious and therefore better able to participate in the process.

Privacy is more often a concern for me than for the patient. There are few private moments in the patient's treatment process, and the patient frequently loses his sense of need for privacy through exhaustion, regression, or adaptation. Families are less likely to have lost this need, and office meetings are frequently arranged for them. During the first few days following the patient's admission, however, families are often reluctant to leave the visitors' waiting area. Early meetings may take place there, if there is an opportunity and need for privacy.

Use of Time

The length of hospitalization is an important issue for burn patients. When patients ask how long this will last, they are also expressing their concerns about their ability to endure the physical process. At this point, they do not anticipate emotional difficulties beyond enduring the pain and discomfort of physical recovery, or any other problems beyond hospitalization. We tell patients that they will be changed by this experience and that their physical, emotional and social functioning can improve for at least a year and often for much longer (Blades et al., 1979; Blades et al., 1982). The date of discharge is the one time that should be clearly inflexible, once that date has been determined. No matter how much they talk about going home, patients and families experience a very high anxiety level at this time and frequently attempt delaying tactics. Altering this date for any reason other than a medical one reinforces the feeling that he is not ready. It is necessary for the social worker, the patient, the family, and other staff members to work with physicians in making this determination, so that there is adequate time to carry out necessary tasks without having to postpone the date.

Treatment Modality

I most often use the problem-solving approach. Although the patient must complete a lengthy process of adjusting to his losses, he accomplishes this process by solving a series of problems which he experiences individually and in his "present." This approach meets the patient's need for short-term goals and solutions. Solving problems helps reduce anxiety and provides the patient with a sense of control.

This modality can also be expanded from a brief crisis intervention model to a longer problem-solving model. I used a long-range version of the problem-solving approach when Paul expressed his concern about fulfilling his role as a father to his daughter. He was recovering and was better able to tolerate working toward a longer-range goal. That approach allowed him to think about what he wanted to do as a father. He was already losing contact with his son, as his own father had lost contact with him; Paul did not want to repeat this with his daughter.

When considering the choice of modalities, the social worker needs to recognize the enormous effects of the burn. The patient relates everything to the burn itself, and it takes a long time before he and his family are able to recognize that pre-injury problems will recur. So much has changed for the patient that they feel everything has changed. Paul imagined that his marital conflicts had ended and that he would never want to drink again. Modalities such as family therapy are not often useful until much later in the recovery process.

Stance of the Worker

When I began working with Paul, I encouraged him to talk about his experience. I gave him minimal direction, listening instead. I knew he needed to incorporate what had happened to him. Verbalization assists this process, helps to relieve some of the patient's anxiety and reduces the frequency of dreams or nightmares of the injury event which are often indistinguishable from reality. I took a rather passive stand with Paul because that was all he needed to carry out the task.

I was more active with the family, but I also encouraged them to express their feelings. They required reassurance that their feelings were legitimate. I also had to interject notes of reality, which are important to counter feelings of overoptimism and guilt about feeling pain. I helped the family regain their sense of control by passively listening to their descriptions of how they learned about Paul's injury, by being attentive to the individual experiences they were describing. I was also active in teaching them about the burn center and the ways in which Paul could be helped. They had many questions about treatment and the physical process. Although medical and nursing staff members had previously explained the situation and answered questions, the family's anxiety had blocked their incorporation of some of this information, which would have helped them to feel somewhat more in control of this experience. My understanding of the treatment and recovery process enabled me to answer questions that simplified or clarified what they had heard.

My initial stance, therefore, may be active, passive, or a combination of both. Techniques of teaching, clarification, listening and support are frequently all that are needed to help the patient and his family negotiate the early stages of the treatment process.

I could be more directive and confrontational with Paul when he was having difficulty negotiating a step. For example, as Paul recovered, he became obsessively concerned about the loss of hair from his head. Without minimizing the importance of this change for Paul, I knew that the loss of hair was in the configuration of natural baldness and was clearly not his major loss. Paul talked about it incessantly, however, as it was related to his worry that his daughter would not recognize him. At the same time, he regarded his hands with detached interest. He looked at them and tried to use them, but he did not talk about his losses in terms of either appearance or function. The reality of the situation was that his hands did not work very well and were not likely to work well in the near future. He could wear a hat in public, but people would stare at his hands. By confronting Paul with his avoidance, I enabled him to move to the next step of his adjustment process.

Outside Resources

Decisions about concrete services are based on whether or not patient and family involvement is necessary and whether their involvement would increase their sense of competency. A worker can help the family become involved in the recovery process by assisting them with various tasks. Marsha, a capable person striving to regain control, needed some assistance to make a list of tasks she could implement. She was then able to arrange for Paul's sick and insurance benefits, obtaining the necessary information from doctors without any further assistance.

Paul did not require any appliances for exercising or function. He did have a hand splint to maintain position and to apply pressure to his palm. Patients rarely require any special equipment at home as they usually leave the hospital with maximal function which they must work to maintain. Thus, wheelchairs and other assistive devices would potentially contribute to loss of function as scarring and contractures develop. If outpatient therapy is required, it is primarily to maintain function that may be lost as healing (scarring and contracting) continues. Arrangements were made for Paul to receive physical therapy at a hospital near his home. They negotiated a schedule and Marsha arranged the necessary transportation. Marsha's needs and abilities were determining factors in my not offering assistance in making these arrangements.

Reassessment

Reassessment may be either formal and comprehensive or informal and problem-related. Decisions about reassessment relate to when it should and should not take place. Paul experienced periods of depression and regression that are typical in the recovery process (Steiner and Clark, 1987). Attempts to help the patient recognize progress through reassessment at times like these may result in the patient viewing the worker's attempts at reassessment as false reassurance. In timing reassessment with the patient, I take into account his pre-injury style of coping, the duration of regression and depression periods, and his awareness of the recovery process.

A formal reassessment took place at regular intervals following Paul's discharge. Originally instituted as part of a research protocol, the assessment involved discussing the patient's preinjury functioning with him and assessing change in relation to that level. A comprehensive assessment, it included work, independence, physical functioning, family and social relationships, psychological functioning and subjective concerns. The patient and social worker individually and together identified problems and growth areas.

The benefit of this type of comprehensive reassessment approach can be seen in Paul's case. He was focusing on his diminished hand function as an indicator of his lack of progress. He had not considered the fact that he was not drinking and that his relationship with his family had improved. When he did, he was able to view his progress in a new light, and it helped to increase his sense of efficacy. We identified his inability to work as a problem but not one accessible to intervention at that point.

Transfer or Termination

When Paul left the hospital, he and Marsha were seen regularly each time he returned to the clinic or for further surgery. After the typical high anxiety they experienced at the time of his discharge, he found the home environment to be quite supportive. He avoided some of the problems that patients often face when returning home to friends and acquaintances because they moved to their new home and were far from former associations. If a need had been identified for family counseling or therapy for Paul and Marsha, they would have been referred to an agency near their home because of the distance and decreasing frequency of their hospital visits.

As Paul became more independent, Marsha stopped accompanying him, so there was no formal ending with her. Paul and I reviewed his progress for the last time one year after discharge. He had exceeded or achieved his pre-injury levels of functioning in most areas. He was still not employed; however, he regarded this as a future goal and not a problem that was causing him distress. He was able to acknowledge that apart from the possibility that he might not ever be able to do the type of work he had been doing, he had found the work stressful and had not really enjoyed it. In his decision to consider a more satisfying type of work in the future, he had made a positive step. We agreed that he could and would contact me if he required assistance in this or other areas in the future.

Case Conclusion

Several years have elapsed since Paul's burn injury. The injuries to his hands were severe. He required several reconstructive surgical procedures to achieve the maximum degree of function. At this point, Paul's only physical limitations involve his right hand where all of the digits are partially absent. Although he has developed a "grip" with his palm, he is limited in the size of objects he can pick up with that hand. The left hand is now dominant, but functions requiring bilateral fine movements are limited.

When Paul left the hospital, his hair had grown back on the sides, but he was bald over the crown. His nose was red, which is the color of actively healing skin. He wore a hat and long-sleeved shirt to avoid exposure to the sun and a custom-made glove on his left hand to apply pressure to minimize scarring. His right hand was very dark red and somewhat swollen. The skin on his arm was also red. I do not know what Paul looked like before his injury. He describes his hair prior to the injury as thinning at the forehead. He is now bald on top of his head and deep over the crown. He has some scarring on his nose that would not be immediately obvious or remarkable except that the contour of his nose is somewhat changed (the end is larger and slightly lumpy). He has some flat scars on his chest and left arm. The grafted areas of his arm have a meshed appearance. His right hand is as described, with thumb and fingers completely or partially absent. His skin is tanned now, and he has a full beard.

Paul talks more with Marsha now and recognizes when things ought to be discussed. These discussions are still not easy for him, however, and he often must rehearse before he begins. Paul at first felt sexually awkward, but as he became more comfortable with himself and more accepting of his limitations, he and Marsha were able to resume a satisfactory sexual relationship.

Paul did not return to his former job. Upon his discharge, he quickly assumed responsibility for the care of his daughter while Marsha worked. He received Social Security Disability Insurance payments for two and a half years. Although he did not solicit contact with his son, coincidentally his former wife returned him to live with him. He welcomed this opportunity to be a father to his son as well as to his daughter.

Paul also found a new drive for mastery. He quickly learned to drive his car and to operate his boat. He developed a new interest in woodworking, which he was able to sustain, even though it took him several hours to do an hour's work. Eventually he was able to develop a new career, built on his interest in boating. He did not require any special training program, but, rather, he was able to figure out how to do the work by persistent trial and error, and he devised the adaptive equipment he needed to do the work himself. Paul's adjustment to his losses is considered good, both in terms of the measures he has taken for himself and in terms of his ability to reassess his situation. He has not resumed drinking, and he and Marsha both describe their relationship in positive terms.

Differential Discussion

The impact of the burn injury is such that most of the patient's energy is directed toward coping with the present. Paul and Marsha had difficulties prior to the injury, but their marriage had not collapsed. As in many such cases, they felt their pre-injury difficulties would not recur. For this reason, problems such as Paul's drinking, chronic communication difficulties, and problems assuming responsibility were not focused on directly. If a patient's pre-injury functioning is chronically chaotic and results in intensification of preexisting problems (Bowden, 1973), I intervene only in major crises that interfere with his ability to participate in the treatment program. In these cases, I help the patient do some problem-solving, but I know he will probably still have major areas of dysfunction when he leaves the hospital.

When an individual has difficulty negotiating the steps of adjustment, the process may halt at any point. Because Paul was expected to have physical limitations that would require his dependence on others to be able to eat and to carry out other basic functions initially, regression was a likely complication. When Paul did regress, it might have been possible to introduce behavior modification or other directive techniques (Simons et al., 1978); however, I chose to stay with my original problem-solving approach. Paul's early involvement in the problem-solving process increased his sense of competence during a very stressful period; his involvement possibly helped him to avoid persistent regression.

A major role for social workers is early and ongoing psychosocial assessment of the patient and family (Cook, 1982; Talabere and Graves, 1976). Through a comprehensive assessment, preinjury problems which are often associated with hospital adjustment and long term adjustment may be identified (Andreason et al., 1972; Bowden, 1979). Such assessments can be used to guide planning of multiple interventions by the entire team, both to identify immediate needs and as a basis for early post-hospital planning. By meeting with Marsha and Paul's family on the day after his admission, their immediate needs for education were assessed and arrangements were made to meet those needs with the assistance of several team members. Marsha's need to be in more control of her anxiety and to focus her anger were identified and addressed. Communicating with the staff that Marsha was angry, enabled the staff to be observant for indications that she may be using this in a detrimental way which could then be communicated to the social worker for intervention. There was no evidence of this reported after the first few days. A great deal was learned about Paul and his usual methods of coping that staff members were able to use to guide their communication with him even before he could tell us about himself. For example, knowing that Paul enjoyed water sports and found boating relaxing, enabled the staff to evoke relaxing memories for him when he became agitated.

Paul was in many respects an unusual patient in that his injuries were more disabling than most. In general, the long term loss of function is less of a problem for the burned patient than disfigurement (Bernstein, 1976). However, the long term emotional outcome for most patients is good, and the most important factor associated with good long term outcome is perceived social support (Davidson et al., 1981; Knudson-Cooper, 1981). The long term effects of both burn size and visible disfigurement appear to be mediated by social support. In Paul's case, the initial assessment indicated that his family had a strong potential for providing social support although his non-family support system did not appear strong. The task was to bolster this support system by meeting their immediate needs and to monitor their on-going response to avoid over-protectiveness or other behavior that would interfere with his engaging in his treatment in his own behalf. Because the family unit remained supportive, minimal intervention was required with them after the initial period although other families require more extensive intervention (Abramson, 1975; Brodland and Andreason, 1974); Reddish and Blumenfield, 1986). In Paul's case, the only direct psychosocial intervention focus was provided by the social worker, although this would vary with the patient and the setting depending on policy and available resources (Morris and McFadd, 1978; Miller et al., 1976). Paul was not evaluated by an alcoholism counselor or other professional. This decision was based on a knowledge of available resources and on the belief that he was not amenable to intervention during hospitalization. Although he did not resume his drinking after hospitalization, patients often do return to former behaviors in the post-hospital period, and it may well be possible and desirable for intervention to be planned during hospitalization.

Although I favor a flexible approach, a more strict and structured approach to goals, contract, meeting times, and other practice considerations may provide a greater sense of security for the patient. That I feel a more flexible approach is less stressful to the patient may reflect my own need, which is also a factor in decision making.

PRACTICE IN CONTEXT

The burn center's context is most obviously shaped by its technology. Although patients now leave the hospital after shorter lengths of stay and with less disfigurement than a few years ago, the treatment remains long, painful, and emotionally draining for the patient and his family. The center's multidisciplinary team focus not only saves lives and promotes healing but also works to achieve a high quality of life for survivors. The social worker's involvement from the beginning helps to anticipate and prevent problems that may develop in the patient's adaptation process.

Because Maryland requires all designated facilities to maintain the highest level of technology and expertise, the center was able to diagnose and treat the severe injury to Paul's lungs, an injury that would have been rarely seen or treated in a rural community hospital. Although his initial prognosis was not good, it was improved by his speedy admission to the center where expertise and experience in treating similar injuries was available. Paul is in some ways an exceptional patient in that his injuries were particularly handicapping. However, the treatment team at the center included therapists and other staff who were familiar in working with these unusual injuries. At the time of discharge, he had maximal function; his present function is excellent, considered in the light of potential disability. Tertiary care facilities do have the disadvantage of removing the patient from friends and family, and it is also difficult to ease the transition to outpatiency and to identify resources when the person is from another part of the state. However, the advantages outweigh the disadvantages.

Financial policies will continue to be a threat to access in many areas of the country. Although some of the policies that affect burn care are national in scope, most vary with the state and will affect both the insured and the uninsured directly and indirectly. Likewise, policies that affect the organization and delivery of emergency medical services in each state will affect access. Changes in financial policies, in general, are contributing to changes in technology and other measures to reduce the length of stay of patients. While Paul was hospitalized for 42 days, a shorter length of stay would likely have altered some of the decisions about practice.

In this case the organization of the center was supportive of the social worker's role. While support from the director of the center was probably most important in beginning to establish a role in this setting, ongoing support and cooperation from the entire staff are most important in further development of the role for both direct and indirect intervention. There have been subtle changes that are associated with nursing staffing and patient loads for example. Additional changes may relate to the physical organization of the setting. For example, the expansion of office space reduced the family waiting area so that informal group meetings with families are no longer possible, the opportunity for informal meetings with individual families has been reduced, and the opportunities for families to be supportive to each other has been reduced.

The problem-solving approach proved effective in reducing Paul's anxiety and providing him with a feeling of competence. By beginning my work with him early in his hospitalization, I was able to help him establish a pattern of problem solving early in his recovery and adaptation process. Later, he was able to define problems and establish long-range goals independently. My awareness of the burn center's technology and resources and my knowledge of the process of adaptation to losses associated with burn injuries helped me define problems and goals that could be realistically met.

REFERENCES

Abramson, Marcia. "Group Treatment of Families of Burn Injured Patients." *Social Casework*, 1975; 50(4), 235-241.

Andreasen, Nancy J., Noyes, Russell, and Hartford, Charles E. "Factors Influencing Adjustment of Burn Patients During Hospitalization." *Psychosomatic Medicine*, 1972; 34(6), 517-525.

Bernstein, Norman R. *Emotional Care of the Facially Burned and Disfigured*. Boston: Little Brown, 1976.

Blades, Betsy, C., Jones, C.A., and Munster, A.M. "Quality of Life After Major Burns." *Journal of Trauma*, 1979; 19(8), 556-558.

Blades, Betsy C., Mellis, N., and Munster, A.M. "A Burn Specific Health Scale." *Journal of Trauma*, 1982; 22(10), 872-875.

Bowden, M.L. "Family Reactions to a Severe Burn." *American Journal of Nursing*, 1973; 73(2), 317-319.

Bowden, M.L. *Psychosocial Aspects of a Severe Burn: A Review of the Literature*. Ann Arbor: National Institute of Burn Medicine, 1979.

Brodland, Gene A. and Andreasen, N.J.C. "Adjustment Problems of the Family of the Burn Patient." *Social Casework*, 1974; 55(1), 13-18.

Cook, Tom. "Psychosocial Assessments of Families on a Pediatric Burn Center." *Journal of Burn Care and Rehabilitation*, 1982; 3(2), 105-108.

Davidson, T.N., Bowden, M.L., Tholen, D., James, M.H., and Feller, I. "Social Support and Post Burn Adjustment." *Archives of Physical Medicine and Rehabilitation*, 1981; 62: 274-278.

Dimick, Alan R., Potts, L.H., Charles, E., Wayne, J., and Reed, I.M. "The Cost of Burn Care and Implications for the Future in Quality of Care." *Journal of Trauma*, 1985; 26(3), 260-265.

Emergency Medical Services Systems Act of 1973, Pub. L. No. 93-154, 87 Stat. 594 (1973) (repealed 1981).

Fleming, Steven, Kobrinske, E.J., and Lang, M.J. "A Multidimensional Analysis of the Impact of High Cost Hospitalization." *Inquiry*, 1985; 12(2), 178-187.

Goldstein, Richard K. "Burns: An Overview of Clinical Consequences Affecting Patient, Staff, and Family." *Comprehensive Psychiatry*, 1985; 26(1); 43-57.

Hunt, J.L. and Purdue, G.F. "Cost Containment/Cost Reduction: The Economic Impact of Burn DRGs." *Journal of Burn Care and Rehabilitation*, 1986; 7(5), 417-421.

Joe, Thomas C.W., Melzer, Judith, and Yu, Peter. "Arbitrary Access to Care: The Case for Reforming Medicaid." *Health Affairs*, 1985; 4(1), 59-74.

Knudson-Cooper, Mary. "Adjustment to Visible Stigma: The Case of the Severely Burned." *Social Science in Medicine*, 1981; 15B: 31-34.

Miller, William C., Gardener, Nancy and Mlott, Sylvester. "Psychosocial Support in the Treatment of Severely Burned Patients." *Journal of Trauma*, 1976; 16(9), 722-725.

Morris, James and McFadd, Adrienne. "The Mental Health Team on a Burn Unit: A Multidisciplinary Approach." *Journal of Trauma*, 1978; 18(9), 658-663.

Reddish, Patricia and Blumenfield, Michael. "A Typology of Spousal Response to the Crisis of Severe Burn." *Journal of Burn Care and Rehabilitation*, 1986; 7(4), 328-330.

Rees, Joseph M. and Dimick, Alan R. "Will Burn Centers Survive Another Round of Budget Cuts?" *Journal of Burn Care and Rehabilitation*, 1987; 8(3), 240-241.

Rees, Joseph M. and Dimick, Alan R. "Will Burn Centers Survive PPS?" *Journal of Burn Care and Rehabilitation*, 1987; 8(2), 155-156.

Simons, R.D., McFadd, A., Frank, H.A. et al. "Behavioral Contracting in a

Burn Care Facility: A Strategy for Patient Participation." *Journal of Trauma*, 1978; 18(4), 150-156.

Steiner, Hans and Clark, William R. "Psychiatric Complications of Burned Adults: A Classification." *Journal of Trauma*, 1987; 17(2), 134-143.

Talabere, L. and Graves, P. "A Tool for Assessing Families of Burned Children." *American Journal of Nursing*, 1976; 76(2), 225-227.

Confronting a Life-Threatening Disease: Renal Dialysis and Transplant Programs

Margo Regan Bare

DESCRIPTION OF THE SETTING

The Hospital of the University of Pennsylvania (HUP) is a six-hundred bed teaching Hospital affiliated with the University. The Renal Dialysis Unit at HUP was created in 1952 for the treatment of patients with acute renal failure. In 1963, a three-bed unit for chronic dialysis and research was set up. There is now an eight-bed hospital-based hemodialysis unit for inpatients and patients whose medical problems preclude being dialyzed in the outpatient dialysis unit. In 1977, HUP initiated a home training program for peritoneal dialysis. Initially, a three-bed unit was located in the Inpatient Unit, patients were trained for continuous ambulatory peritoneal dialysis (CAPD) and intermittent peritoneal dialysis. Because of the increasing number of patients diagnosed with ESRD a freestanding hemodialysis unit affiliated with HUP was opened in 1979 and all medically stable patients who were dialyzed in the Inpatient Program were transferred to the Outpatient Unit. Then, in 1984, the CAPD Program was moved to the Outpatient Unit and because of space limitations was reduced to two beds for training.

One of the major functions of the Inpatient Dialysis Unit is to provide dialysis treatment to both pre- and post-renal transplant patients. The first renal transplant at HUP was performed in 1966, and that year a total of four transplants were done. Since that time the Program has grown substantially and the number of transplants done in 1986 was one hundred and twenty two. Approximately forty-five percent of the recipients had living related donors (LRD), with the remaining fifty-five percent receiving kidneys from cadaveric donors.

All patients being considered for maintenance hemodialysis, home peritoneal dialysis or transplant are referred to the social worker for a full psychosocial evaluation to assess the appropriateness of a given treatment alternative. Factors which are important in determining appropriateness include the emotional stability of patients and their families, their ability to cope with the stress which accompanies a given treatment modality, and available support systems. As the renal social worker at HUP, I also participated in a number of multidisciplinary meetings in both the dialysis unit and the transplant unit, which facilitate communication between different members of the treatment team.

Policy

Before 1972, a person in need of chronic dialysis who lacked substantial personal resources or insurance coverage was compelled to forgo the treatment, with physical deterioration and death the inevitable result. Because of limited funding and equipment, dialysis was simply not available to all who required it. Decisions regarding which particular patients would receive dialysis were made by admissions/uremia committees, which were multidisciplinary groups composed of medical, legal, religious and lay representatives who assessed a candidate's value to society and determined whether dialysis would help the individual remain a productive member of society (Fox and Swazey, 1974). The decisions of these so-called "death committees" had an adverse effect upon certain racial and income groups and upon patients suffering from such systemic diseases as diabetes and lupus, who were likely to continue to suffer serious medical complications despite dialysis.

In 1972, however, the need for such life-and-death decision making was largely eliminated by the enactment of Public Law 92-603, Section 2991 (known as HR 1), which amended the Social Security Act to provide Medicare coverage for persons with End-Stage Renal Disease (ESRD) (Adams, 1978). The legislation provided funding for in-center hemodialysis after the first three months, coverage for transplant surgery, kidney donor costs and one year's postoperative coverage. In the ensuing years, technological advances made home peritoneal dialysis a viable, lower-cost treatment alternative for many renal patients. In 1978, Congress amended HR 1, extending Medicare coverage to include peritoneal dialysis (with no waiting period if the patient dialyzes at home) and three years of posttransplant coverage. Many of the gaps in the Medicare program's insurance coverage have also been filled by the Pennsylvania State Renal Program, which is based on income eligibility and provides funds for renal-related medications and the initial three-month period of hemodialysis not covered by Medicare.

These legislative changes reflected a shift in social policy which led legislators to conclude that no person suffering from renal disease should be denied treatment because of prohibitive costs or limited resources. This broadened public funding is a major factor in making it possible for HUP's dialysis and transplant units to exist and to offer a wide-ranging panoply of treatments and services to renal patients.

It is interesting to note that HR 1 represents a rare singling out by Congress of a particular disease for such funding assistance. For no other disease have patients been so targeted by Congress for such extensive insurance coverage of their treatments. Even more uniquely, in 1976 the Federal Regulations titled "Implementation of Coverage of Suppliers of End Stage Renal Diseases" mandated the availability of social work services to patient with ESRD (Fortner-Frazier, 1981). It is entirely possible that this requirement that social services be available in renal units makes the social worker a more viable and accepted member of the treatment team then might otherwise by the case.

Technology

There are four general treatment alternatives available for the patient suffering from End-Stage Renal Disease: hemodialysis; peritoneal dialysis; transplantation; and lastly, no treatment, which will eventually result in death.

Any form of dialysis provides only a substitute for impaired or lost kidney function; it does not restore kidney function. Dialysis is designed to compensate for two of the functions the damaged kidney is failing to carry out. One function is the removal of waste substances produced by normal body activities. The other function is the removal of fluid (salt and water) from the body. Dialysis cannot perform either of these functions as well as a healthy kidney. It is therefore necessary to supplement dialysis with additional measures, such as medication and dietary restrictions (Fortner-Frazier, 1981).

During hemodialysis, which may be performed in the hospital, at a dialysis center, or at home, blood flows through tubing attached to the patient's access route into a machine which filters out accumulated waste products. Before beginning hemodialysis, the patient must undergo a surgical procedure to create an access route, to make his or her circulatory system accessible to the machine tubing. The cleansed blood is then returned to the patient through another line of tubing. This continuous circulatory cleansing process lasts between three and five hours and is done three times a week, fifty-two weeks a year.

The other form of dialysis is peritoneal dialysis, which prior to 1968 was done only in acute cases. In 1968, the advent of the Tenchkoff Catheter, a permanent plastic catheter which can be placed in the patient's abdomen, made peritoneal dialysis a treatment alterative for chronic renal failure which may be performed in the hospital or at home. In this treatment, tubing is attached to the permanent catheter and the diffusion of excess wastes occurs through the peritoneum, the sac surrounding the intestines. This waste filtration does not require removal of any blood from the body (Brey and Jarvis, 1983).

There are three forms of peritoneal dialysis available: intermittent peritoneal dialysis (which is done on an inpatient basis); continuous ambulatory peritoneal dialysis (CAPD), developed in 1976; and continuous cyclic peritoneal dialysis (CCPD). Only IPD and CAPD are done at HUP, although other institutions train patients in CCPD.

In IPD, concentrate is introduced through the tubing into the abdomen, where it bathes the peritoneal membrane. Patients are admitted to the hospital for this form of dialysis; the procedure takes approximately forty-eight hours and is usually done one time a week. IPD is intended as a temporary form of dialysis until the individual is either transplanted or starts a chronic hemodialysis or CAPD training program.

The other form of peritoneal dialysis, CAPD, does not involve any machinery, and the patient is essentially dialyzing twenty-four hours a day, seven days a week. The patient has a permanent catheter with tubing attached to a two-liter bag of concentrate which empties into the abdomen through the tubing and remains there for approximately four hours, drawing off wastes from the body. The patient then replaces the bag with a fresh bag of concentrate, performing four such exchanges a day. It requires approximately three to seven days to train an individual to handle CAPD independently. Once trained in CAPD, an individual only returns to the hospital once a month for clinic visits, where he or she is seen by the entire dialysis team, including the nurse, the social worker, the dietician, the physician, and the administrator.

The third treatment alternative is kidney transplantation, which involves surgically placing a new kidney in the patient's pelvic area. Whenever possible, it is preferable to procure the new kidney from a living, related donor, in which the kidney survival rate at one year is ninety-five percent as opposed to a cadaver donor, in which case, the kidney survival rate is seventy-five percent (interview with Diane Jorkasky, MD, 1987). The major threat in transplantation is rejection, which may be temporary or permanent and may occur at any time. Rejection occurs when the body's natural defensive mechanisms against foreign bodies attacks and attempts to destroy the transplanted kidney. In some cases rejection can be reversed with massive doses of immunosuppressants. The recently developed immunosuppressant cyclosporine has essentially revolutionized organ transplant. The success rate for both living related and cadaveric kidney transplants has increased dramatically with this drug. In cases where immunosuppressants are unsuccessful in reversing rejection, however, the transplanted kidney must be removed, and the patient is forced to return to chronic dialysis. He/she may or may not opt to attempt transplant again. When the transplant is successful, the patient is able to resume a relatively normal lifestyle. The patient receiving a transplant is hospitalized an average of nine days to three weeks and must take immunosuppressant drugs for the life of the transplanted kidney.

Both dialysis and transplant have serious, though different, physiological and psychological ramifications for the patient. Dialysis is merely a maintenance treatment and not a cure for renal failure.

Unless the patient undergoes successful transplant surgery, dialysis will be necessary for the remainder of the patient's life. Transplantation, on the other hand, is the nearest available thing to a cure for renal failure.

The dialysis patient faces a wide range of chronic and periodic medical problems, including, but not limited to, weakness, fatigue due in part to anemia, bone disease, clotting of access routes, and sexual dysfunction arising from both physiological and psychological reasons. The patient on dialysis is also placed on a restrictive diet that limits fluid intake as well as many foods high in potassium and sodium. Additionally, patients must take medications to supplement certain functions the diseased kidney no longer performs (Frazier, 1981).

Transplant patients also encounter medical problems, although they are not generally as severe as those confronting dialysis patients. Most of these problems result from the continuous use of immunosuppressants. Side effects may include fat deposits in the cheeks, abdomen and back of the neck; increased susceptibility to opportunistic infections, steroid-induced diabetes mellitus; acne; elevated blood pressure, increased appetite; excessive hair growths or loss of hair; gastric irritation; and altered mental states such as lability, irritability, and nervousness (Fortner-Frazier, 1981). Cyclosporine can be nephrotoxic (toxic to the kidney) and consequently the levels of the drug must be closely monitored.

With either transplant or dialysis, the threat of death is omnipresent. Among the dialysis patients there is a mortality rate of approximately ten percent each year, and a transplant patient has a one to five percent mortality rate depending on whether they have a living related donor transplant or a cadaver transplant. Those receiving transplants from living related donors have a lower mortality rate (interview with Diane Jorkasky, MD, 1987).

Organization

I was one of thirty-one social workers who covered all services in the hospital. My assignment was limited to the dialysis unit and the transplant program.

Case Description

Robert Jones, a handsome, muscular, twenty-four-year old black man, presented himself as self-assured and in control, but was actually quite anxious and depressed. He began dialysis in 1978 and was being dialyzed three times a week at the Inpatient Unit at HUP. Partly because of his manipulative behavior, Mr. Jones made a less than satisfactory initial adjustment to hemodialysis. Before the onset of his illness, he had maintained a high level of activity and had never been seriously ill or hospitalized. The onset of his renal disease was quite sudden and was accompanied by multiple complications. When his condition finally stabilized, he was unable to cope with the limitations imposed by chronic hemodialysis, and he responded by being demanding with the staff.

Mr. Jones was aware that renal transplant was a treatment alternative for him. During the initial stages of his illness, his entire family was tissue-typed to determine whether any member would be a good donor candidate. However, because of medical and personal problems, none of them volunteered to donate, so Mr. Jones was placed on the list of those waiting for a cadaver donor.

Mr. Jones had undergone multiple surgeries as a result of his renal disease. He did not cope well with the stress of hospitalization and often became quite nervous, exhibited regressive behavior, and acted out his emotions. Additionally, he had never been able to deal with any sort of pain, most notably that caused by the needles used for hemodialysis. The staff had attempted several methods to alleviate his pain but achieved only moderate success. Mr. Jones admitted to taking none of his medications, asserting that he did not perceive any appreciable difference in his condition when he took the medications and therefore did not see the need to take any. He also felt that taking medications reminded him of his illness, which, when not on dialysis, he denied.

Mr. Jones lived alone in an apartment in Philadelphia, having been separated since 1977, and he has an eight-year-old son. Although a high school graduate, at the time of our initial interview he was unemployed. He had a series of odd jobs, but although he professed a desire to work, he rarely followed through with referrals which might have led to employment.

Mr. Jones is the eldest of four children. His parents are divorced and both are remarried. His siblings, a brother and two sisters, all in their late twenties, live independently, and he sees them occasionally. Mr. Jones did not describe a particularly happy childhood. He was essentially raised by his paternal grandmother; consequently, his closest relationship was with her, and she tended to dote on him. Despite their closeness, however, Mr. Jones resented the continual advice she gave him. He was not particularly close to his mother, toward whom he harbored a great deal of anger for her neglect of him when he was young. Mr. Jones had, however, recently become close to his father.

Mr. Jones was a very active person before the onset of his illness, and in fact was quite an accomplished athlete, holding a black belt in karate. Since most of his interests and energies were channeled into physical activity, it was difficult for him to settle into a more sedentary lifestyle. Mr. Jones is an intelligent, sensitive individual who was unable to cope with the multiple stresses of chronic illness, including loss of his independence, and, most importantly, changes in his body image. He could be quite charming, and his appearance had always been very important to him. Consequently, his multiple surgical scars altered his body image and diminished his self-concept.

Mr. Jones was, then, markedly depressed and in intense emotional pain. He denied this, however, and his psychic pain manifested itself in physical pain. This accounted for his repeated requests for pain medication and his analgesic abuse. At that point, pain medication was the only way Mr. Jones could cope with the severe depression resulting from the onset of his illness.

DECISIONS ABOUT PRACTICE

Definition of the Client

In every case the primary focus, in terms of client population, is the patient himself. As a renal social worker, it is the patient with whom I have the closest continuous contact. However, renal disease by its nature affects the patient's family, and so the family is also usually included in the definition of the client (Gorman and Anderson, 1982).

In Mr. Jones' case, as with many others, several family members have been part of the client system. Actually, the definition of the client has been fluid, depending on which members of his family are active in his case at any given point. For instance, when Mr. Jones was first diagnosed, all the members of his family expressed concern and the possibility of donation for transplant was discussed. Although several members of his family, including his mother, were indicated by tissue-typing to be suitable matches, no one volunteered to donate. At that point, his mother's involvement in Mr. Jones' case virtually ceased, as did her inclusion in the client group. Later, however, when Mr. Jones suffered a cardiac arrest and nearly died, his mother "rallied around," so to speak, and for a time became more involved with her son, thereby becoming part of the client group again.

This phenomenon of family members dropping in and out of the patient's case and thus in and out of the client group, depending on whether the patient is at a crisis point, is a common one. As a patient stabilizes and adjusts to renal disease and its treatment, some nonpatient members of the client group tend to distance themselves from the patients and get on with their own lives.

Goals

My role was to assist Mr. Jones to redefine his life goals in light of limitations imposed by hemodialysis. The first goal after addressing the client's emotional needs arising from the diagnosis of renal disease is to ensure that the client is educated in all the treatment alternatives. Since Mr. Jones was immediately placed on dialysis, I actually focused on educating him on what hemodialysis involved. Once his medical condition stabilized, we were able to discuss other treatment alternatives and their ramifications.

Mr. Jones, like many patients, tended to inflate his expectations about transplantation. He viewed a transplant as a panacea — an opportunity to regain his independence, return to his previous lifestyle, and forget he had ever been afflicted with renal disease. In such cases, it is the social worker's task to bring the client to an understanding of the possible risks and complications that accompany transplantation (Carrosella, 1984). It should be pointed out, however, that clients tend to view transplant as such a salvation from the negative aspects of dialysis that they often tune out its drawbacks. Although this segment of the educational process is almost inevitably a failure, the social worker must nevertheless attempt to prepare the patient for the stresses which accompany life on the transplant floor and beyond.

Another early goal was to aid Mr. Jones in making a positive adjustment to life on dialysis. Although dialysis was literally all that was keeping him alive, Mr. Jones found it a decidedly mixed blessing. Dialysis imposes very stringent limitations on the patient's lifestyle, because it involves time commitments, travel restrictions and frustration of such basic drives as food, water, and sex (Fortner-Frazier, 1981). Mr. Jones, like most patients, deeply resented the restrictions and impositions dialysis entails.

In Mrs. Jones's case I was called upon to help his family adjust to his life on dialysis and redefine their roles within the family unit. Since Mr. Jones's grandmother tended to reinforce his dependency needs, I recognized a need to involve her in an effort to reinforce the independent behavior we attempted to foster in the dialysis unit. An adjunct to the goal of fostering independence was helping Mr. Jones assume an active role in his own treatment and rehabilitation. Specifically, it is desirable for the patient on dialysis to assume responsibility for his own medical and dietary compliance. Because he needed to deny his illness and his dependence on the machine, Mr. Jones did not take care of himself. Since such behavior was maladaptive and interfered with his treatment I resolved to help Mr. Jones to recognize the reasons for his noncompliance and assist him in channeling his denial and need for control into more positive directions, including employment and handling as much of his own medical care as possible.

In the early stages of our worker-client relationship, I left the terms of my relationship with Mr. Jones fairly open-ended and undefined. I initially let him know that I would be available and would meet with him weekly to discuss issues of concern and problems, for which we would jointly formulate goals and strategies. It soon became apparent, however, that such a broad definition of the roles within our relationship would not be sufficient. Instead, I came to recognize he would benefit more from an explicit, task-oriented, verbal contract of our respective roles and goals. We formulated a contract, which identified specific tasks to be worked on and set a time frame within which we hoped to accomplish these tasks. Mr. Jones had a tendency to be overwhelmed when faced with broad, nonspecific objectives, so we divided these general goals and plans into more defined, achievable components. We found utilizing such a step-by-step approach gave Mr. Jones a sense of accomplishment which provided him with the motivation to work on other identified goals. As specific tasks (e.g., to compose a job resumé within three weeks) were completed in accordance with our agreement, Mr. Jones and I would formulate additional specific tasks and goals. Hence we were continually entering into new contracts with varying terms, but all were within the same general format.

Meeting Place

Meetings between Mr. Jones and myself occurred in several different settings. During the periods of his hospitalization, we met in his hospital room. If he were physically able, I would encourage Mr. Jones to get out of bed and sit in a chair during our meetings in order to minimize his feelings of illness and to make our interviews as normal as possible. On other occasions I met with Mr. Jones while he was dialyzing. Physically, of course, this entailed my sitting next to his bed. I preferred to avoid, if possible, meeting with clients in the dialysis unit, because of the patient's being connected to the machine tends to reinforce feelings of powerlessness on his part and negatively highlights the differences between the social worker and client. In a real sense, the client is a "captive audience"; he lacks the option simply to get up and leave should he desire to do so.

The negative aspects of the dialysis setting may be ameliorated somewhat by, for example, drawing curtains around the patient's station for privacy; but the most desirable setting for patient meetings is a small, private conference room located off the dialysis unit. The room is furnished with several chairs, but there is no desk or table to create any barrier between the worker and patient. In this setting, the meeting may be carried on in as normal and as private a setting as possible, and the worker and patient can relate to each other more as equals.

In any of these settings there are possibilities, when it becomes necessary, for physical contact between worker and client. This contact generally takes the form of holding the client's hand or putting a hand on the patient's shoulder when he is experiencing physical or emotional pain.

Use of Time

As a general rule, the social worker-client relationship continues in one form or another for as long as the patient remains in the renal program at HUP. Since neither dialysis nor transplant patients are ever discharged in the sense that they no longer need medical treatment, I, as the social worker, remain available to them. The intensity of the relationship of course varies with the psychosocial factors, medical condition and treatment phase of the patient and family.

In Mr. Jones's case, I saw him and his family quite frequently when the diagnosis of ESRD was made and he was having considerable difficulty adjusting to dialysis. In most cases, the frequency of contacts declines as the patient stabilizes and adjusts to dialysis or transplant. Mr. Jones, however, experienced many emotional and medical crises such as loss of self-esteem secondary to changes in body image, learning his family would not act as donors for his transplant, followed by cadaver transplant, rejection of the transplanted kidney, readjustment to dialysis, and a cardiac arrest which led to debilitation requiring extensive rehabilitation services. Obviously, the number of crises and losses Mr. Jones suffered necessitated more frequent and intensive intervention.

The duration of my meetings with him, as with any patient, were usually dictated by his psychological or his medical condition. When his course was progressing badly, our meetings tended to last longer, as they did when he was hospitalized for transplant and when he faced losing the transplanted kidney. During this time it was necessary to help Mr. Jones deal with disappointment and feelings of hopelessness in losing the kidney and returning to dialysis.

Generally speaking, the only time constraints within the power of Mr. Jones and me to set were those contained in the contract discussed previously. The medical condition of the patient ultimately governs most time considerations. If, for example, the patient has agreed to complete a job resumé within three weeks, but a cadaver kidney becomes available for a transplant, the agreement deadline is discarded in favor of attending to the client's more immediate needs.

Treatment Modality

Crisis intervention was a frequently utilized treatment modality in Mr. Jones's case, since many crises developed during the course of his illness causing disequilibrium and interference with his emotional functioning. The first crisis, of course, was the sudden onset of his renal disease and his need for dialysis treatments. The goals of social work crisis intervention at the initial stage matched those of the dialysis staff: relief of symptoms and restoration to the fullest extent possible of pre-crisis functioning. Utilizing anticipatory guidance, I helped Mr. Jones to anticipate future crises that might develop and to plan effective coping strategies based on problem solving skills learned during preceding crises. The most relevant strategies were: analyzing sources of distress, accrediting successful efforts in coping with past crisis situations, anticipating needs, identifying and utilizing support systems and formulating and implementing tasks (Hepworth and Larson, 1986). When each succeeding crisis occurred, I utilized the same treatment approach to help Mr. Jones achieve a maximum level of functioning.

Another modality of treatment was, for lack of a better term, the educational approach. Renal patients are usually frightened of the prospect of dialysis, because it is a medical treatment with which they are by and large unfamiliar. On the theory that gaining knowledge about something hitherto unknown may reduce anxiety, I immediately attempted to expand Mr. Jones's understanding of his illness and his treatment alternatives. As mentioned before, much of the information initially imparted at the outset of treatment is not successfully integrated, because at that stage the client is overwhelmed physically and emotionally by his disease, and tends to deny his long-term need for treatment. Therefore, this educational process continues throughout the course of my relationship with the client (Gorman and Anderson, 1982).

Furthermore, since by definition renal disease affects all members of the family, the Jones family was seen several times in an effort to determine the nature of their emotional involvement and the degree of stress Mr. Jones's disease caused. I attempted to identify dysfunctional interactional patterns and replace them with more facilitative ways of relating to one another. Mr. Jones needed positive feedback from his family. This was particularly important after he learned that he would not have a family donor for transplant. The involvement of his grandmother, parents and siblings provided Mr. Jones with reassurance and encouragement. The family sessions seemed to particularly enhance the relationship between Mr. Jones and his father.

Mr. Jones conformed to the model of the patient who, while aware intellectually that medication and dietary compliance are critical to successful treatment, nevertheless refuses to adhere to medication and dietary requirements because of his high level of denial regarding his illness. Mr. Jones above all else desired a transplant. It was not until extensive counseling identified his reason for noncompliance that he came to realize his desire for transplant could only be fulfilled if he demonstrated an ability to assume responsibility for his treatment.

A technique that was also used successfully with Mr. Jones was task-oriented counseling. In order to enhance his self-esteem, motivation and ability to deal with his medical and emotional problems, Mr. Jones and I concentrated on setting those successively attainable goals discussed earlier. Finally, I used supportive therapy on several occasions during Mr. Jones's treatment. Different forms of support were offered to meet Mr. Jones' needs, including protection, acceptance, validation and education (Nelson, 1980). I found it particularly useful in helping him adjust to dialysis initially and cope with returning to dialysis after his transplanted kidney was rejected.

Stance of the Social Worker

My stance as a social worker in relation to Mr. Jones was necessarily variable. I adopted different roles depending upon, for instance, whether he was in a crisis or was stabilized medically and emotionally, or whether he was making progress toward his goals or was stymied. At the outset of Mr. Jones's renal disease, he was so overwhelmed by his medical problems and his introduction to dialysis that it would have been futile to try to get him to participate actively in a social worker-client relationship. At that stage, it was necessary for me to adopt a directive, active stance with Mr. Jones. I "took him by the hand" in almost a literal sense, trying to impress upon him the meaning and ramifications of dialysis and treatment options. Once Mr. Jones had achieved a fairly complete, rational understanding of what lay ahead for him, I was able to reduce the directive aspect of my role and relate to Mr. Jones as more of a partner, as we discussed and mapped out both medical and life goals for him.

The choice between a supportive or confrontational technique was also largely determined by Mr. Jones's emotional and medical condition at any given time. For instance, when Mr. Jones rejected his transplanted kidney, he was at first so devastated that he lacked the emotional, and possibly the physical, resources to cope with a confrontational approach. During such stages, I found it more effective to assume a supportive stance, providing Mr. Jones a shoulder to lean on and a friendly ear to hear him voice his concerns, his fears, his bitterness and his feelings of hopelessness. I had to be wary, however, of taking the supportive stance too far and reinforcing Mr. Jones's dependence and self-pity. He had a tendency to adopt a passive role, manipulating others, including me, in an attempt to get them to handle his problems and achieve his goals for him. Such manipulative behavior signaled to me a need to prod Mr. Jones, by confrontational tactics if necessary, to take more control over his life and participate more meaningfully in his treatment and life decisions. I also found a direct approach to be more effective with Mr. Jones than an indirect one. Since he often denied his illness, it was difficult to get him to arrive at conclusions about appropriate courses of action in an inductive manner. We made considerably more progress when we discussed the problems he faced and reviewed potential options which might increase coping and problem solving skills. We would then, as discussed earlier, divide and make concrete the various steps necessary to achieve his goals.

Outside Resources

In three instances, I was called upon to provide and make decisions about concrete services for Mr. Jones. As it was elsewhere, my overriding concern here was to maximize Mr. Jones's participation in his own care.

The first instance occurred when Mr. Jones and I agreed that a desirable goal for him was to obtain a job. Towards that end, I made the initial contact with Pennsylvania Office of Vocational Rehabilitation and conferred with the counselor assigned to the hospital, explaining Mr. Jones's medical condition and his desire for counseling which might lead to employment. From that point on, I attempted to assist Mr. Jones in following through with the referral, giving him the counselor's name and telephone number so he could set up an appointment. Later in the process I gave Mr. Jones an article detailing preparation of a resumé. After we discussed the format and what points to emphasize, he prepared a rough draft which we then refined for typing and submission. Throughout the process, I attempted to support Mr. Jones's progress toward independence by providing positive reinforcement for tasks he performed.

The next instance of concrete services occurred after Mr. Jones suffered a cardiac arrest that resulted in brain damage, making it impossible for him to return to his previous independent lifestyle. Although his brain damage was felt to be reversible, home care services were necessary until he fully recovered. Because of Mr. Jones's serious, albeit temporary, physical and mental handicaps, it was necessary for me to take an active role in arranging for necessary services, including home physical therapy, visiting nurses and home health aides. Additionally, a family meeting was convened to review Mr. Jones's emotional and physical needs, discuss family concerns and make arrangements for family members to assist with

Mr. Jones's care since he could not be left alone during the period immediately following his discharge.

The final instance of rendering concrete services was arranging for Mr. Jones's transportation to dialysis following his discharge from the hospital after his unsuccessful transplant. When Mr. Jones was physically able, he travelled to dialysis by public transportation. However, when his physical condition precluded this, I made arrangements for a volunteer organization to transport him. When he improved to the point where the special transportation arrangements were no longer necessary, he would nevertheless attempt to persuade me to continue them. Recognizing that cooperating with Mr. Jones's manipulative behavior would only reinforce his dependent sick role, as well a abuse the volunteer system, I resumed working with him towards the goal of reassuming responsibility for his own transportation arrangements.

Reassessment

Reassessment of the social worker-client relationship in Mr. Jones's case occurred regularly on two levels. First each month his condition, progress, health care needs, and treatment plans were discussed at the patient care conference. At these conferences, the entire treatment team, including doctors, nurses, technicians, social worker, dietician and pharmacist, discussed the full range of issues affecting Mr. Jones and his care. They included his analgesic abuse, demanding behavior, rehabilitation potential, high fluid gains between treatments, and medication noncompliance. By identifying and discussing the issues and problems I was confronted with at any particular time and by soliciting the suggestions of the other members of the treatment team I was exposed to possible alternative strategies applicable to Mr. Jones's case. These multidisciplinary conferences also offered valuable opportunities for me to update the other members of the team regarding the treatment plan I had formulated for Mr. Jones. Kress states "the goal of the treatment plan is to offer care in a way the patient can tolerate and to provide a regimen within the context of the client's personality structure and family life" (p. 43).

The second type of reassessment took place between the client and me. This took the form of a periodic renegotiation of our contract concerning Mr. Jones's goals and subsidiary tasks to be accomplished.

Transfer or Termination

As stated before, only death absolutely terminates the relationship between the social worker and the renal patient. In some cases, the patient may make a sufficiently satisfactory adjustment and be sufficiently stabilized so the relationship will become active again only if a specific problem arises requiring additional social work intervention.

The only instance other than the patient's death which might end my relationship with a particular client would be transfer of the client to another dialysis unit. This occurs, for example when a patient unsuccessfully transplanted at HUP is transferred back to the referring dialysis unit for continued treatment. In these cases, it is essential to maintain contact with the social worker at the referring unit so he or she is able to prepare for the client's return.

In Mr. Jones's case, a similar type of transfer occurred. HUP established an outpatient hemodialysis unit located several blocks from the hospital. The renal program set a goal of transferring medically stable patients who are able to participate in their own care to this outpatient unit, reserving the inpatient unit for medically unstable patients and pre- and post-transplant patients. Mr. Jones viewed his impending transfer with trepidation. The prospect of facing a new facility and entirely new staff (with the exception of the physicians) created feelings of anxiety in Mr. Jones. He, like many patients, had a substantial emotional investment in the people and surroundings that had sustained him through a crisis-ridden period in his life. It was my task to make Mr. Jones's transition to the outpatient unit as smooth and free of problems as possible, and this included establishing a relationship between him and the new social worker. To facilitate this transfer, I scheduled a series of conferences for Mr. Jones, the new worker, and myself to familiarize Mr. Jones and the new worker with each other, to review his progress and remaining goals, and to orient him to the new unit. In an effort to reduce his anxiety over his transfer, I attempted to impress upon

Mr. Jones that the move represented significant progress in his overall adjustment to dialysis. I believed that getting Mr. Jones to view in a positive light his transfer to the outpatient unit, where he would take a more active role in his dialysis treatment by performing limited self-care, would boost his self-esteem and feelings of independence. From then on, although Mr. Jones might have been referred to me if the outpatient worker were unavailable, my relationship with Mr. Jones as his social worker was effectively at an end.

Case Conclusion

Mr. Jones was transferred to the outpatient dialysis unit and, as anticipated, he experienced significant anxiety which manifested itself in manipulative behavior with the staff, increased requests for pain medication, and regression in goal attainment. As he began to settle into the routine of the outpatient dialysis unit and developed relationships with fellow patients and staff, his demanding behavior decreased, as did his requests for pain medication.

Mr. Jones is currently hemodialyzed three times weekly on the evening shift. His main problem continues to be noncompliance with the medication regimen and periodic high fluid gains between treatments. Despite his noncompliance, Mr. Jones has not required hospitalization in the past two years. His noncompliance is a symptom of denial of his disease and in some ways can be viewed as functional, in that it allows him to maintain a fairly high level of functioning. Unfortunately, the dysfunctional element of the noncompliance will become apparent over the long term as Mr. Jones develops complications (e.g., bone disease) associated with long-term medication noncompliance.

Despite an initial setback in goal attainment upon transfer to the outpatient unit, Mr. Jones developed a good relationship with the social worker there. Prior to his transfer Mr. Jones and I agreed that it might be beneficial for him to do volunteer work in an effort to prepare himself for other types of employment. He began volunteering at a local pediatric hospital and his experience not only increased his self-esteem but helped Mr. Jones become more responsible, which was an essential element of obtaining employment.

Mr. Jones has since gone on to a series of jobs, including security guard and taxi driver, and most recently went into business with his father.

When Mr. Jones realized he would require dialysis on a long-term basis he felt anxious about his ability to form and sustain a relationship with a woman because of the limitations imposed by his disease. However, as he began to accomplish goals which boosted his self-esteem, he became more willing to engage in relationships. After his transfer to the outpatient unit, Mr. Jones became involved with the local church and began dating a young woman. They are now married and Mr. Jones helps raise his wife's daughter from a previous relationship. He is quite devoted to the daughter; he thinks of her as "his daughter" and assists with her care since his wife works.

Mr. Jones has demonstrated a significant amount of growth. He has become increasingly responsible, as evidenced by his employment, his commitment to his marital relationship and the responsibility he has assumed for "his daughter." Despite his recurrent noncompliance, he has greatly improved from the time he began dialysis, when he refused to take any medications, demanded analgesics prior to needle sticks and had excessive weight gains between every treatment. Mr. Jones's noncompliance is not surprising in light of his desire to deny his illness when he is not in the unit. In the past, he saw the cause and effect of his noncompliant behavior and modified it appropriately. Now, however, given the absence of immediate impact of his failure to follow his prescribed regimen, he does not perceive any problems associated with his compliance and is thus less motivated to modify his behavior. Given Mr. Jones's personality, his current behavior is to be expected.

Differential Diagnosis

In general, I feel the relationship between myself and Mr. Jones was a positive one. Many of the goals we established were accomplished and Mr. Jones was able to utilize problem solving skills successfully in subsequent crises. I realized that there were times when I became very frustrated with his noncompliance and manipulative behavior and I know this interfered with my effectiveness in the therapeutic relationship. Furthermore, since Mr. Jones often alienated the staff with his demanding behavior I sometimes allowed the staff's opinion to influence my assessment and evaluation of him. Obviously, this led to incorrect assumptions on occasion, and I had to redefine the assessment to ensure relevant interventions. Additionally, I had to guard against focusing on the pathology or negative aspects of Mr. Jones's behavior. Unfortunately, the problem approach is part of the medical model. In team meetings the emphasis is on problems. Consequently, I found it necessary to emphasize the positive and functional aspects of Mr. Jones's personality and behavior, not only to enhance his self-esteem and motivation but to help the staff to see the incremental improvements in a positive light.

Although there were several family sessions, in retrospect it would probably have been more beneficial for Mr. Jones if I had been more aggressive about consistently including his family in the treatment program. I tended to push for family involvement during periods of crisis, and allowed them to disengage once the disequilibrium had resolved. Perhaps their consistent involvement would have further eased Mr. Jones's adjustment to chronic dialysis and minimized some of the problems he experienced.

PRACTICE IN CONTEXT

The treatment of patients in dialysis and transplant programs is, to a greater extent than is the case with other diseases, profoundly affected by social policy and technology. As discussed earlier, the targeting of renal disease for special legislative attention and appropriations has obviated the need for the sort of life and death decisions that were common fifteen to twenty years ago. Fifteen years ago, Robert Jones would very likely have succumbed to his illness within a few weeks of reaching end-stage renal disease; considering his socioeconomic situation and his multiple medical problems, he may well not have been selected by the admissions/uremia committee to receive treatment. Today, however, virtually any patient suffering from chronic renal failure can be afforded the opportunity for treatment, regardless of socioeconomic or medical considerations. But, in the future, finite resources and other pressures may restrict the ability to treat all individuals with end-stage renal disease and the quality of care provided.

Hand-in-hand with policy issues go the technological advances which have so affected the treatment of renal disease. The increased number of treatment options available in recent years not only gives the staff a greater variety of medical alternatives but also creates many more opportunities and challenges for social work intervention. For instance the choice and success of a given treatment (the decision made largely by the patient and family with staff advice) dictate whether the patient will spend a great deal or relatively little time in the unit; whether his family will actively participate or merely provide emotional support in his treatment; and whether he will lead a relatively normal or severely restrictive life. These and similar issues provide fertile ground for positive help by the social worker.

Perhaps the most perplexing aspect for the individual who is on dialysis or who has received a transplant is the expectation that he should not think of himself as ill and should get on with his life. This is often difficult when the patient is receiving mixed messages from the staff. Because of the physical location of the dialysis and transplant unit, the patient must come to the hospital for his treatment. He may be an outpatient, but he is aware that a hospital is a place where people go when they are sick and where other people do everything for them. However, the philosophy of both the dialysis and transplant programs is to expect the patient to participate fully in his care and to perform tasks independently. We encourage patients to return to their pre-illness lifestyles and to function as independently as their condition allows. On the other hand, we reinforce dependency needs and the concept of illness by having patients come to the hospital, where they are constantly reminded of their illness by medications and care given them and by dietary restrictions (Landsman, 1975). This almost schizophrenic existence tends to confuse the patient and often makes social work intervention frustrating. In Mr. Jones's case, he became quite comfortable with the sick role and was reluctant to take over for me and perform tasks independently. Therefore, conceptualizing the individual as part of several systems allows me to define my role and work with the patient towards goals which are realistic and achievable.

The main point about social work practice in a renal program is that patients and their families are confronting a serious, often life-threatening disease. There is no escaping that fact, although patients and their families often deny it in order to return to some semblance of a normal lifestyle. The role of the social worker is to educate the patient and family in the treatment alternatives available for renal failure and to help the people affected by the disease make a positive adjustment, redefine their life goals in terms of the limitations imposed and rehabilitate themselves to their fullest potential. Legislative aid, improving technology and a supportive staff all contribute in a meaningful way to that social work effort.

REFERENCES

Adams, L. Medicare Coverage for Chronic Renal Disease: Policy and Implications. *Health and Social Work*, 3(4): 41-53, 1978.

Atcherson, E. The Quality of Life: A Study of Hemodialysis Patients. *Health and Social Work*, 3(4): 54-69, 1978.

Blackburn, S., Piper, K., Wooldridge, T., Hoag, J., & Hanan, F. Diabetic Patients on Hemodialysis. *Health and Social Work*, 3(3): 91-104, 1978.

Brey, H. and Jarvis, J. Life Change: Adjusting to Continuous Ambulatory Peritoneal Dialysis. *Health and Social Work*, 8(3): 203-209, 1983.

Brown, C. and Ryersbach, V. Vocational Rehabilitation for Dialysis and Transplant Patients. *Health and Social Work*, 5(2): 22-26, 1980.

Cain, L. Casework with Kidney Transplant Patients. *Social Work*, 18: 76-83, 1973.

Carosella, J. Picking Up the Pieces: The Unsuccessful Kidney Transplant. *Health and Social Work*, 9(2): 142-152, 1984.

Council of Nephrology Social Workers. Bibliography: Topics 1-13, Volume 1. National Kidney Foundation.

Czaczkes, J. W. and Kaplan-DeNour, A. *Chronic Hemodialysis as a Way of Life*. New York: Brunner-Mazel, 1978.

Fortner-Frazier, C. *Social Work and Dialysis: The Medical and Psychosocial Aspects of Kidney Disease*. Berkeley: University of California Press, 1981.

Fox, R. and Swazey, J. *The Courage to Fail*. Chicago: University of Chicago Press, 1974.

Frazier, C. Renal Disease. *Health and Social Work*, 6(Supplement): 75S-82S, 1981.

Gorman, D. and Anderson, J. Initial Shock: Impact of a Life-Threatening Disease and Ways to Deal with It. *Social Work in Health Care*, 7(3): 37-46, 1982.

Hepworth, D. and Larsen, J. *Direct Social Work Practice Theory and Skills.* Chicago: Dorsey Press, 1986.

Hickey, K. Impact of Kidney Disease on Patient, Family and Society. *Social Casework*, 53: 391-398, 1972.

Holden, N. Dialysis or Death: The Ethical Alternative. *Health and Social Work*, 5(2): 18-21, 1980.

Kaplan-DeNour, A. and Czaczkes, J. Personality Factors in Chronic Hemodialysis Patients Causing Noncompliance with Medical Regimen. *Psychosomatic Medicine*, 34(4): 333-344, 1972.

Kress, H. Adaptation to Chronic Dialysis: A Two-Way Street. *Social Work in Health Care*, 1(1): 41-46, 1975.

Landsman, M. The Patient with Chronic Renal Failure: A Marginal Man. *Annals of Internal Medicine*, 82: 268-270, 1975.

Levy, N., ed. Living or Dying: *Adaptation to Hemodialysis*. Springfield, Ill: Charles C Thomas, 1974.

McKevitt, P. Treating Sexual Dysfunction in Dialysis and Transplant Patients. *Health and Social Work*, 1(3): 132-157, 1976.

Macklin, R. Ethical Issues in Treatment of Patients with End-Stage Renal Disease. *Social Work in Health Care*, 9(4): 11-20, 1984.

Mailic, M. and Ullman, A. A Social Work Perspective on Ethical Practice in End-Stage Renal Disease. *Social Work in Health Care*, 9(4): 21-31, 1984.

Nelson, J. Support: A Necessary Condition for Change. *Social Work*, 25: 388-392, 1980.

Oberly, E. and Oberly, T. *Understanding Your New Life with Dialysis.* Springfield, Ill: Charles C Thomas, 1979.

Palmer, S., Canzona, L. & Wai, L. Helping Families Respond Effectively to Chronic Illness: Home Dialysis as a Case Example. *Social Work in Health Care*, 8(1): 1-14, 1982.

Peterson, K. Integration of Medical and Psychosocial Needs of the Home Hemodialysis Patient: Implications for Nephrology Social Worker. *Social Work in Health Care*, 9(4): 33-44, 1984.

Perspectives: *The Journal of the Council of Nephrology Social Workers* (published quarterly).

Piening, S. Family Stress in Diabetic Renal Failure. *Health and Social Work*, 9(2): 134-141, 1984.

Ruchlin, H. The Public Cost of Kidney Disease. *Social Work in Health Care*, 9(4): 1-9, 1984.

Sheridan, M. Renal Disease and the Social Worker: A Review. *Health and Social Work*, 2(2): 132-157, 1977.

Simmons, R., Hickey, K., Kjellstrand, C. & Simmons, R. Family Tension in the Search for a Kidney Donor. *Journal of American Medical Association*, 215(6): 909-912. 1971.

Whatley, L. *Social Work with Potential Donors for Renal Transplant*, 53: 399-403, 1972.

Pediatric Oncology:
Open Communication in the Family
of a Child with Leukemia

Janet L. Taksa

DESCRIPTION OF THE SETTING

The pediatric unit of Thomas Jefferson University Hospital is a twenty-eight bed facility in a general teaching hospital in center city Philadelphia. The hospital itself has a capacity of 687 beds.

Some children suspected of having leukemia are admitted to Jefferson from local community hospitals; others are referred directly by their local physicians and have not been hospitalized. These children need the services of a specialist in pediatric hematology as well as the more sophisticated laboratories and diagnostic equipment available in a large teaching hospital. Once the diagnosis of leukemia is established, a child remains in the hospital for an average of two weeks. There is a foldout cot in each private room where a parent may stay, and there are also rooms in another section of the unit for parents and other family members.

When children are well enough to be discharged, they begin attending the pediatric hematology clinic. This clinic meets one day a week in a small area in another part of the hospital. It is a self-contained unit with its own laboratory. There are currently eighteen children with leukemia who attend the clinic. The youngest is two; the oldest is nineteen. Most of the patients are white, as the incidence of leukemia is much higher in white children than in black. Approximately one half of the families receive public assistance, while the other half have private insurance. Families are also encouraged to apply for assistance from the Leukemia Society of America and from the American Cancer Society.

One social worker, whose responsibilities include the entire pediatric unit, is assigned all children with leukemia. She is introduced to the family by the pediatric hematologist during the first family conference, when the diagnosis is explained, and generally sees the child and the family every day during the child's hospitalization. She attends clinic every week and maintains a close relationship with children and families throughout their outpatient therapy.

Policy

The major policies which affect the work of the pediatric hematology program are those which involve financial matters. Particularly important is the supplemental security income program (SSI), a federally funded income maintenance program for the aged, the blind, and the disabled. It became effective in January 1974 and was the first federally administered cash assistance program in the United States. Disabled children are covered by this program, which provides payments directly to their parents or legal guardians. Basic eligibility is determined by medical as well as financial criteria. Several families in Jefferson's pediatric hematology clinic population were accepted for SSI when their children were first diagnosed with leukemia. However, in each case, when the child had been in remission for some time, the benefits were terminated. The family was informed that a child in remission no longer met the necessary criteria for benefits: the child's condition was not deteriorating, and it was not certain the child would die. The pediatric hematologist wrote to the Social Security Administration to confirm that the disease was still present, serious, and that treatment was still necessary. However, the benefits were never reinstated. Policies like these present an additional burden to the parents of a child with a chronic illness.

Technology

Leukemia is a primary malignancy of the bone marrow characterized by a proliferation of abnormal cells called "leukemia blasts" (for an excellent overview of leukemia, see Cohen, Duval, Arnold and Olson, 1984; Weinberg and Siegel, 1986). This proliferation results in a lack of production of the normal cellular elements which compose the blood: white cells which fight infection; red cells, which transport oxygen; and platelets, which are essential for clotting. Acute leukemia is the most common malignancy in children, with approximately 2500 cases reported every year.

Today, improved methods of treating childhood leukemia have produced marked increases in survival times. It is estimated that at least 50 percent of children with acute lymphocytic leukemia have a potential for "cure" (disease-free, long-term survival without drugs) and the survival rate for certain low-risk patients is even higher.

The first step in treatment is induction: chemotherapy is administered to destroy the abnormal cells so that the normal ones can proliferate properly. When this is achieved, the child is said to be in remission: There is no evidence of the disease on physical examination nor on examination of the blood and bone marrow.

Induction is a critical phase in treatment because the drugs used cannot discriminate between abnormal and normal cells, and destroy both. The child being given these drugs thus risks overwhelming infection and bleeding. He is usually placed in isolation, where all staff and visitors must wear sterile gowns, masks, and gloves, and he is given antibiotics and transfusions of blood products, as needed. Weight loss and hair loss are very common.

Since leukemia originates in the bone marrow, periodic evaluation of this tissue is necessary. This is performed by bone marrow aspiration, a process which entails inserting a needle into the bone to withdraw a specimen of marrow. In addition, leukemia cells frequently infiltrate the central nervous system, and spinal taps, procedures in which spinal fluid is withdrawn through a needle inserted between the vertebrae, are required. In the most common form of leukemia in childhood, prophylactic drugs are injected into the spinal fluid during this procedure. Radiation therapy is also often administered to the brain to prevent this complication.

Once remission is achieved, the child is put on maintenance therapy, which is administered primarily on an outpatient basis. The child is seen, at regular intervals, in clinic visits during which he receives complete blood counts, physical examinations, and intravenous medicines. Instructions are also given pertaining to the appropriate dosages of oral medicines to be taken at home. Bone marrow aspirations and spinal taps are performed if a need is indicated by suspicious blood counts or symptoms. Some maintenance protocols also require brief hospitalizations, usually about 5 days, for more intensive chemotherapy.

If leukemia cells reappear in the bone marrow, the child is said to have relapsed. When this occurs, the prognosis for long-term survival becomes poor. The physician attempts to induce a second remission, but statistics show that second remissions tend to be shorter than first remissions. For this reason, once a second remission is obtained, it is the present policy to send the child for a bone marrow transplant if a suitable donor is available. This procedure has improved the outlook for children who suffer relapses.

Bone marrow transplantations are currently being performed primarily on patients who have a brother or sister who matches the various known transplantation types. The procedure involves the removal from the donor, under anesthesia, of fluid taken from the bone marrow, and the intravenous injection of that fluid into the recipient. The recipient is prepared to receive the transplant by undergoing extensive chemotherapy and radiation to destroy his own bone marrow. Before the new marrow begins to produce cells, the patient risks developing extensive infection or bleeding and so requires supportive care with antibiotics, and transfusions of various blood components from family members. The recipient may reject the graft, or the graft may reject the recipient. If the latter occurs, it is referred to as "graft versus host disease" (GVH). Following successful engraphment, if GVH does not occur, the greatest risk to the child is recurrence of leukemia in the transplanted marrow. For this reason, the child is followed in a manner similar to patients off chemotherapy, with periodic blood counts, physical examinations, and bone marrow aspirations and spinal taps when necessary.

In some cases where a suitable donor is not available, patients are sent to appropriate centers for transplantation of their own treated remission marrow. These autologous transplantations do not carry the risks of graft rejection or GVH, but patients are still subject to overwhelming infections, and recurrence of leukemia.

According to the present protocols used at Thomas Jefferson University Hospital, a child remains on chemotherapy for 26 to 36 months after remission. After chemotherapy, he continues to attend clinic for periodic counts and examinations. These visits become less frequent if the child remains well.

Organization

The department of pediatrics is part of a large teaching hospital governed by a vice-president for health services, who is responsible to the president of the university and an appointed board of trustees. There are twenty-five full-time staff physicians in the department.

The pediatric hematology clinic is directed by a pediatric hematologist who is an associate professor in the department of pediatrics and a member of the Cardeza Foundation for Hematologic Research. The clinic is staffed by a nurse, two medical technologists, and an office manager. When necessary, children with leukemia are hospitalized on the general pediatric floor under the direction of the pediatric hematologist. The unit employs nineteen registered nurses, four licensed practical nurses, three nursing assistants, two child-life specialists, and a unit clerk. Since Jefferson is a teaching hospital, medical students, pediatric residents, and hematology fellows are involved in both inpatient and outpatient care of the children.

The hospital's social work department has a professional staff of twenty-three, who are assigned to all of the clinical services. The director of the department is responsible to the associate hospital director for professional and support services.

Although Thomas Jefferson University Hospital is a large institution, the pediatric population makes up a small percentage of the total number of patients. For this reason, both the clinic and the pediatric floor tend to be self-contained units which enjoy may of the benefits of a smaller organization. Communication is open and informal, and rules are flexible.

The pediatric hematologist at Thomas Jefferson University Hospital is a dedicated physician who involves herself in all aspects of the child's care. Her goal in treating a child with leukemia is not just quantity of time but also a high quality of life. Other staff members are aware of this, and of her expectation that they share this goal. Thus, the children under her care tend to receive special attention.

Case Description

Lisa Reynolds is an eight-year-old girl who was admitted to Jefferson's pediatric floor with symptoms of fatigue, pallor, and bruises on her arms and legs. Her local pediatrician had examined Lisa in his office earlier that day and had referred her to the pediatric hematologist at Jefferson, who arranged for her immediate admission. A bone marrow aspiration was performed soon after admission, and the diagnosis of acute lymphocytic leukemia was confirmed. The pediatric hematologist met with Lisa's parents later that evening, and the diagnosis and treatment plan were discussed. Treatment was begun immediately.

Lisa is the younger of two children; a brother, Adam, is aged eleven. Mr. Reynolds is a mechanical engineer, and Mrs. Reynolds is a homemaker. The family lives approximately sixty miles from Philadelphia, and both children attend parochial schools.

DECISIONS ABOUT PRACTICE

Definition of the Client

A potentially fatal illness in a child is a devastating experience for the entire family. At the time the ill child most needs his parents to function supportively and well, the parents feel overwhelmed by the tasks confronting them, and, in particular, by the anticipatory loss of the child (Fischoff and O'Brien, 1976; Buckingham, 1983). Siblings may experience guilt and frustration and often feel abandoned by their parents (Lewis and Lewis, 1983; Coleman, 1984). Thus, parents and siblings, as well as the ill child, are seen as the identified client. In the Reynolds case, Adam was encouraged to visit Lisa in the hospital and interviews often included him as well as his parents and his sister.

Goals and Contract

The social worker's initial task is to help the family function at an optimal level during the crisis of the child's hospitalization. Parents undergoing this experience often find themselves cut off from their usual sources of support. Friends avoid them; relatives seek comfort from them; and they often feel isolated from each other because each may grieve in a different way (Zimmerman, 1985). The social worker becomes the objective person who is aware of what is going on in the child or the family.

In the beginning of the relationship, the social worker is often seen as a link to the physician and, thus as a source of daily information about the child. Like most parents in this situation, Mr. and Mrs. Reynolds focused almost entirely on Lisa's physical condition, asking concrete questions about blood counts and bone marrow (McCallum and Schwartz, 1972). They were terrified that she would die "any minute" and spent almost all their time in her room.

As the hospitalization continues, particularly if the child improves, parents begin to lose some of their fears of an immediate death and begin to realize that they are confronting a chronic problem (Waechter, 1984). At this point, the social worker becomes more of a counselor, distinct from the physician and from the physical care of the child.

At this time, the goals of the social worker and those of the family may clash. The social worker wants to be sure the child understands everything that is happening, and seeks to open communication among family members. The family, on the other hand, often seek to protect each other, and may begin playing games which can be destructive (Bluebond-Langner, 1973; Adams, 1984). Mr. Reynolds, for example, accepted having everything explained to Lisa, but he was very reluctant to share either information or feelings with Mrs. Reynolds. Having always encouraged her to be dependent on him in their marriage, he now felt that she was not strong enough to cope with Lisa's illness, nor with his own doubts and fears about Lisa's possible course. Mrs. Reynolds began to feel isolated from her husband and accused him of not caring about Lisa because he showed no emotion, and even went back to work. From their individual complaints to me, I realized that joint interviews were necessary. Eventually, Mr. and Mrs. Reynolds were able to express their feelings directly to each other, and their relationship was strengthened to a point where they were both able to relate better to Lisa.

Another major goal of the social worker is to help the parents treat the child as normally as possible. Here again, although the goal of a psychologically healthy child is the same for both social worker and parents, the means to that goal are perceived very differently. During the initial part of her hospitalization, Lisa was overwhelmed with presents and soon had both her parents answering her every whim. My attempts to intervene were met with anger and resistance. When I was able to convince Mr. and Mrs. Reynolds that their sudden change of behavior was actually very frightening to Lisa, they began to see that disciplining her was something they could do to make her hospitalization less traumatic. Lisa's improved behavior and acceptance of medical treatment reinforced this principle.

In making these kinds of decisions, the social worker must always remember that the child may die and the parents have to survive. To help them survive well, it is best to reduce any guilt that may ultimately affect the grieving process (Lewis and Lewis, 1983). Thus, although I agreed with the nursing staff that Mrs. Reynolds spent too much time in Lisa's room, we decided that if Lisa eventually died, Mrs. Reynolds would feel she had abandoned her if not allowed to be in the room this often.

Families are not given a choice as to whether they want to see a social worker. However, since the pediatric hematologist introduces the social worker as an integral team member from the beginning, acceptance is rarely a problem (Kupst et al., 1982). At this time, parents and child feel helpless and dependent, and the social worker usually initiates contact. A contract is not formalized, but grows to encompass all aspects of the child's illness and often other factors in the family's life.

Once remission is achieved and the child becomes an outpatient, the intensity of the relationship between the family and the social worker gradually diminishes. Parents begin to initiate contact only when they have specific concerns. The child often asks the social worker to be in the room during procedures. The social worker thus assumes a somewhat more passive role. If the child remains in remission, this pattern continues. The family gets more involved in its daily life and the child's leukemia becomes more accepted as a part of this daily life. If a relapse occurs, the relationship usually goes back to the intensity of the first admission.

Meeting Place

Finding an appropriate place in the pediatric inpatient unit for the social worker and the family to talk is always a problem. Space is very limited, and hence so is privacy. Often, parents are reluctant to go to the social worker's office because they feel it is too far away from their child's room. Crises can arise at any time and precipitate a need for immediate discussion. (Many unplanned interviews with Mr. and Mrs. Reynolds began in the hospital corridor.) Certain meeting places can take on particular significance for parents. Mrs. Reynolds, for example, found it very uncomfortable to talk in the conference room where she had first been told about Lisa's diagnosis.

In the pediatric hematology clinic, space is even more limited and interviews often take place in an examining room or in the nurse's office. Parents and children sit too close to each other in the small waiting room to remain isolated for very long; group discussions and conversation with the social worker both flourish. Many relationships between families being in this waiting room.

Use of Time

Because a child with leukemia is connected with the treatment facility for an indefinite period, the duration of the relationship between the social worker and the family cannot be predetermined. In the beginning of the child's hospitalization, the social worker conveys to the family her availability at all times during the difficult period ahead. Interviews are frequent and often lengthy. At times the duration of the contact may be decided by such factors as the parents' anxiety to return to the child, or by the child's treatment schedule.

The social worker remains available to the family when the child begins to attend clinic. Interviews are usually shorter, often depending on how well the child is doing. Clinic hours are not rigid, and both parents and children are encouraged by all team members to take the time they feel they need.

Treatment Modality

During the social worker's initial work with the hospitalized child and family, the most relevant treatment modality is crisis intervention. As the family later begins to realize that the child's leukemia is a chronic problem, the social worker uses the method of ego-oriented casework to enable the family to use its strengths to meet this reality.

Arranging for the parents of a child undergoing the induction process to meet the parents of a child already attending clinic can be quite effective in the treatment process. It is very important that the social worker not do this too soon, however, as the parents of the hospitalized child need time to absorb the impact of what has happened to them before they can benefit from relating to other families. Within this limit, the use of groups has also proved very beneficial to parents of children with leukemia.

Community groups are available to all parents of children with leukemia hospitalized at Jefferson or attending Jefferson's pediatric hematology clinic. Within the group, a parent can receive emotional support from other parents who have often experienced similar fears, anxieties, and "unacceptable" thoughts about their children (Heffron, Bommelaere and Masters, 1973; Northen, 1983). The very fact that other parents are coping, and thus "surviving," can be beneficial, especially to the parents of a recently diagnosed child.

Formal biweekly groups were organized at Jefferson several years ago, with the participation of the pediatric hematologist and the social worker. It has since been decided by the team that informal group interaction during weekly clinic hours is more successful (Hoffman and Futterman, 1971). This is probably due to the small population of children with leukemia here as compared with that of a children's hospital, and the resultant close relationship between parents, as well as the easy accessibility of clinic staff to children and families.

Stance of the Social Worker

In the beginning of the child's illness, when parents are overwhelmed by the diagnosis and stripped of their defenses, the social worker is very supportive. Parents are encouraged to express their feelings and are often more comfortable in revealing what they consider to be unacceptable thoughts to the social worker, who is not directly responsible for their child's medical care. Mrs. Reynolds, for example, felt very guilty when she experienced anger at Lisa for being ill. She was afraid she was a bad mother and did not want to be "found out" by the physician whom she considered to be Lisa's only hope.

As parents are reintegrated and begin to understand the chronic nature of the child's illness, the social worker can be more confrontational. Decisions of this nature must depend on the social worker's assessment of the family's coping mechanism at any given time.

The social worker may be indirect when counseling the parents on many aspects of the child's care. Inviting parents' opinions based on their knowledge of the child not only benefits the child but helps the parents to feel less helpless. Certain issues, however, must be handled very directly. For example, the social worker must insist that the child be told his diagnosis (if he is old enough to understand it) and be informed of such traumatic side effects of the treatment drugs as hair loss. Parents may object, as did Mrs. Reynolds when I insisted that Lisa be told about all procedures ahead of time. Experience has shown, however, that truthful communication with the child about all aspects of his illness results in optimal adjustment (Adams, 1984).

The social worker and the family of a child with leukemia usually share a close relationship which may last for years (Bergman, Lewiston and West, 1979). Within this relationship, it is important for the social worker to maintain objectivity without losing caring. This may become difficult when the child is very ill or dies. Parents welcome sincere interest in their child and see the social worker's sadness at this time as evidence of her caring. It is, however, never acceptable for the social worker to lose control of her feelings and thereby convey to the parents the impression that they must comfort her.

Outside Resources

In providing concrete services, the social worker usually encourages parents to take as active a role as possible. Because parents feel helpless in so many other areas of their child's care, this kind of responsibility is often perceived as something they can do for their child (Chester and Barbarin, 1984). Families are encouraged to apply to their local chapter of the Leukemia Society of America (LSA), which is a private foundation dependent upon contributions. Services vary among chapters, but LSA usually provides financial aid for drugs not already covered by protocols and in some cases, for transportation to outpatient facilities.

Taking responsibility in this way can also be part of the acceptance process. In Lisa's case, Mr. and Mrs. Reynolds became very upset when Lisa began to lose her hair. However, the whole family participated in getting a wig for Lisa when she decided she wanted one. Mrs. Reynolds cut a strand of Lisa's hair to take with her while shopping for the wig. Mr. Reynolds and Adam were asked for their opinions as to style and length, with Lisa having the final say. I then gave Mr. and Mrs. Reynolds directions to several stores most often used by previous families, and Mr. and Mrs. Reynolds brought back a wig.

Reassessment and Transfer or Termination

Because the course of the child's illness is unpredictable, reassessment of the relationship between the family and the social worker is frequently necessary. It often goes along with the physician's reassessment of the child's physical condition. When the child has been well for a long time, the social worker and family tend to have a more relaxed, friendly relationship. If the child relapses, it often becomes necessary to reactivate the relationship to a more directly therapeutic one.

A particularly complex reassessment of the relationship is necessary if the child dies. Some parents choose to terminate the relationship at this time because any contact with the hospital is too painful for them. More often, however, parents respond to the social worker's continued interest in them. The relationship then becomes a source of help for the parents as they mourn (Kupst et al., 1982).

Gradually, the parents are encouraged to become less dependent on the relationship with the social worker and to return to their previous support systems in the community. When this has been accomplished, the relationship between the parents and the social worker can be terminated.

Case Conclusion

Since improved technology has resulted in marked increases in survival times and even the potential of cure for children with leukemia, parents of these children face a unique, overwhelming task. Throughout the child's illness, they must care for the child and meet his needs. They must treat him as normally as possible and prepare him for adult life. At the same time, because they know their child may die, they must also prepare themselves to give him up (Eiser, 1979; Solnit, 1983). Within the setting of a modern teaching hospital and clinic, the social worker helps the parents to accomplish this task and enables the child to function as well as possible.

Lisa was discharged from the hospital three weeks after her admission and began to attend clinic. At first, Lisa's mother was very overprotective of her. Lisa was rarely allowed out of the house, and anyone who entered was scrutinized for signs of illness. Lisa became very demanding and was not disciplined. Gradually, through discussions with me and other parents, Mrs. Reynolds began to resume her original role as mother of an eight-year-old, normal child. Lisa's behavior improved. Adam came in for his share of attention, and Mr. and Mrs. Reynolds began seeing friends and enjoying activities again.

At the present time, Lisa has been in remission for two years and is doing well. She completed the 4th grade with no problems and is now on a swimming team with several of her friends. In addition, Mr. and Mrs. Reynolds's marriage seems to have benefited from the open communication initiated during Lisa's hospitalization, as has their relationship with Lisa and Adam.

Differential Discussion

The diagnosis of leukemia in a child usually places stress on the parents' marriage (Knapp, 1986), and this was certainly true in the Reynolds case. If open communication had not been emphasized through joint interviews with me, the relationship between Mr. and Mrs. Reynolds might have deteriorated.

I might, however, have put more emphasis on encouraging Mr.

and Mrs. Reynolds to participate in group interaction. Mrs. Reynolds, in particular experienced guilt about many of her thoughts and feelings. If she had discussed these with other parents, it is likely that she would have found comfort in the realization that these thoughts and feelings were shared by others parents in similar situations.

Adam felt his parents had deserted him, and he was angry at them and at Lisa for this. At the same time, he felt guilty because he did not have leukemia and Lisa did. If Adam had not been encouraged to discuss these feelings with me and with his parents, he might have been left with emotional scars.

Lisa began testing her parents soon after her admission to the hospital and again following her discharge. She became very frightened when Mr. and Mrs. Reynolds put no limits on her, overprotected her, and in general became very different from the parents she had known before her diagnosis (Eiser, 1979). If there had been no intervention by a social worker, Lisa's ability to lead a normal life might have been impaired.

Although our society has become somewhat more open on the subject of death, cancer is still a social stigma (Waechter, 1984). As part of a continuing effort to help Lisa and her family adjust to the "real world," I tried to prepare them for possible negative reactions to Lisa as a child with cancer. ("My mothers says I can't play with you; you're going to die.") Now, in looking back, I think I could have reinforced this preparation in several ways. I might have encouraged Lisa to invite friends to accompany her in clinic. I might also have visited Lisa's school, and conducted an open discussion of leukemia with her teacher and classmates (Spinetta and Spinetta, 1983). These interventions might have helped dispel the myths about leukemia and made social interaction more comfortable for Lisa and her family.

REFERENCES

Adams, D.W. Helping The Dying Child: Practical Approaches for Non-Physicians, in *Childhood and Death*. Edited by Wass, and Corr, C.A., Washington: Hemisphere Publishing Corporation, 1984.

Baker, L., Roland, C., and Gilchrist, G. *You and Leukemia: A Day at a Time*. Rochester, Minn.: Mayo Comprehensive Cancer Center, 1976.

Bergman, A.S., Lewiston, N.J., and West, A.M. Social Work Practice and Chronic Pediatric Illness, *Social Work in Health Care*, 4: 265-274, 1979.

Binger, C.M., Albin, A.R., Feuersteen, R.C., Kushner, J.H., Zoger, S., Mikkelsen, C. Childhood Leukemia: Emotional Impact on Patient and Family, *New England Journal of Medicine*, 280, 1969.

Bluebond-Langner, M. *The Private Worlds of Dying Children*. Princeton, N.J.: Princeton University Press, 1978.

Buckingham, R.W. *A Special Kind of Love*. New York: The Continuum Publishing Company, 1983.

Chesler, M.A., and Barbarin, O.A. Relating to the Medical Staff: How Parents of Children with Cancer See the Issues, *Health and Social Work*, 9: 49-65, 1984.

Cohen, D., Duval-Arnold, B., and Olson, A. Acute Lymphoblastic Leukemia of Childhood, *American Family Physician*, 30: 236-245, 1984.

Coleman, F. and Coleman, W.S. Helping Siblings and Other Peers Cope with Dying, in *Childhood and Death*. Wass, H. and Corr, A., eds. Washington: Hemisphere Publishing Corporation, 1984.

Eiser, C. Psychological Development of The Child with Leukemia: A Review, *Journal of Behavioral Medicine*, 2: 141-157, 1979.

Fischoff, J., and O'Brien, N. After The Child Dies, *The Journal of Pediatrics*, 88: 140-146, 1976.

Heffron, W.A., Bommelaere, K., and Masters, R. Group Discussions with The Parents of Leukemic Children, *Pediatrics*, 52: 831-840, 1973.

Hoffman, I. and Futterman, E. Coping With Waiting: Psychiatric Intervention and Study in The Waiting Room of a Pediatric Oncology Clinic, *Comprehensive Psychiatry*. 12: 67-81, 1971.

Knapp, R.J. *Beyond Endurance: When a Child Dies*. New York: Schocken Books, 1986.

Kupst, M.J., Tylke, L., Thomas, L., Mudd, M.E., Richardson, C.R., and Schulman, J.L. Strategies of Intervention with Families of Pediatric Leukemia Patients: A Longitudinal Perspective, *Social Work In Health Care*, 8: 31-47, 1982.

Lewis, M., and Lewis, D.O. Dying Children and Their Families, in *The Child and Death*. Schowalter, J.E., Patterson, P.R., Tallmer, M., Kutscher, A.H., Gullo, S.V., and Peretz, D., eds. New York: Columbia University Press, 1983.

McCallum, A.T., and Schwartz, A.H. Social Work and the Mourning Parent, *Social Work*, 17: 25-36, 1972.

Rudolph, L.A., Pendergrass, T.W., Clark, J.K., Josness, M. and Hartmann, J.R. Development of an Education Program for Parents of Children with Cancer, *Social Work in Health Care*, 6: 43-54, 1981.

Solnit, A.J. Changing Perspectives: Preparing for Life or Death, in *The Child and Death*, op cit.

Spinetta, P.D., and Spinetta, J.J. The Child With Cancer Returns to School: Preparing the Teacher, in *The Child and Death*, op cit.

Timmons, A.L. Leukemia, Is It So Awful? *The Journal of Pediatric Oncology*, 88: 147-148, 1976.

Waechter, E.H. Dying Children: Patterns of Coping, in *Childhood and Death*, op cit.

Weinberg, K.I., and Seigel, S.E. Acute Lymphoblastic Leukemia in Children, in *Leukemia Therapy*. Gale, R.P. Boston: Blackwell Scientific Publications, Inc., 1986.

Zimmerman, J. Some Insights From Counseling Bereaved Parents, in *Death and Children: A Guide For Educators, Parents and Caregivers*. Gullo, S.V., Patterson, P.R., Schowalter, J.E., Tallmer, M., Kutscher, A.H., and Buschman, P., eds. Dobbs Ferry, New York: Tappan Press, 1985.

Epilepsy in Childhood: Pediatric Neurology Clinic

Carol Appolone Ford

DESCRIPTION OF THE SETTING

The pediatric neurology clinic is an outpatient clinic at North Carolina Baptist Hospital, the teaching hospital for Bowman Gray School of Medicine. This medical complex is a referral center for the western third of North Carolina as well as parts of Virginia and Tennessee; some patients drive up to three hours to reach it. Clinic is held one morning a week, with approximately eighteen children with epilepsy scheduled. One social worker attends the clinic regularly and interviews families to gather psychosocial data and to assess the family's understanding of the disorder. If problems are identified, the family may be referred to an agency within their community or be scheduled for follow-up interviews with the clinic social worker, depending on the family's distance from the medical center and the nature of the problem. A packet of information on epilepsy is given to each family at the initial visit. The families are seen briefly on follow-up visits to check the status of the child and the family's adjustment.

All patients must be referred to this clinic by a physician or by their county Public Health Department. Most patients come from rural North Carolina and are low income. For these, medical care is provided by Medicaid or the Crippled Childrens Program. All doctor's visits, medications and tests are paid for by these programs. The patient population is racially mixed with the majority being white, and they range in age from infancy to twenty-one years. The frequently of clinic visits depends upon the child's degree of seizure control.

Childhood epilepsy often causes more psychosocial problems

than the medical condition would warrant. The majority of children are seizure-free when on medication, and most will eventually come off the medication and have no further problems with seizures (Middleton, Attwell and Walsh, 1981). However, the family's reaction to the disorder can greatly hamper the child's psychosocial development (Gardner, 1968; Lechtenberg, 1984; Ford, Gibson and Dreifuss, 1983). Underexpectation by parents and teachers may cause school underachievement (Holdsworth and Whitmore, 1974). Many parents are fearful and anxious after witnessing a seizure and this anxiety permeates their interaction with the child. The parental overprotection which often accompanies such anxiety can stifle a child's natural drive toward independence. Too often we see young adults whose spirit has been squelched by years of parental admonishment (Lerman, 1977). Parental guilt seems to be ever present even when there is no family history of epilepsy and no known cause for the child's seizures. This may contribute to dysfunctional parenting patterns (Voeller and Rothenberg, 1973). Some patients quickly learn that they can manipulate the family by threatening to have a seizure or by feigning seizures. Siblings may be instructed to give in to the "sick" child, not to upset him lest they cause a seizure.

It is important to intervene at the outset to educate parents about all aspects of epilepsy so that much of this can be avoided (Appolone, 1978). Truly, an ounce of prevention is worth a pound of cure. Those completely controlled by medication are seen annually; those still having seizures may be seen every few weeks or months for medication adjustments with the goal being complete seizure control.

Policy

Since this is a teaching hospital, patients coming to the outpatient clinics are examined by residents and medical students, who, in consultation with the staff physician, make the diagnostic and treatment decisions. The nature of medical education is such that these student doctors rotate between services, and patients usually see a different one each time they come. This results in less than optimum continuity of care. Patients often do not know who to contact if problems arise between visits. In the pediatric neurology clinic the social worker provides a sense of continuity of care and serves as a person to contact if problems, medical or otherwise, arise (Caroff, 1985).

There is a tollfree statewide Epilepsy Information Service which is a component of the Department of Neurology at Bowman Gray School of Medicine. Its purpose is to answer questions about all aspects of epilepsy which patients, professionals or the general public may have. It operates daily during business hours and is manned by trained professionals. The director of this service is also the social worker who attends pediatric neurology clinic. Patients in the clinic are advised of the availability of this resource. Not only may they use it for general information about epilepsy, but also to get in touch with the clinic doctor if problems should arise. These clinic patients often cannot afford a long distance call, frequently do not recall the name of the doctor they saw and would not know how to locate that doctor in the medical center. When a patient's family calls the tollfree number, the social worker is given the call. She has usually seen the family in clinic. She can order the chart and discuss the case with the appropriate staff doctor. In this manner clinic patients can receive much better access to medical care between visits than would otherwise be available.

Epilepsy is a collective term for a group of disorders caused by abnormal brain cell electrical activity. Each disorder of the group involves some sort of seizure associated with either loss or disturbance of consciousness, an abnormal psychic experience or behavior, or abnormal motor or sensory phenomena. Usually, but not always, epilepsy involves convulsive movements of the body. Sometimes it involves uncontrolled hyperactivity or only momentary inattention. In fact, epilepsy is not a disease but a set of symptoms (Kerson, 1985, p. 126).

Technology

The medical treatment for epilepsy is a drug therapy (Delgardo-Escueta, Treiman and Walsh, 1983). Complete seizure control is achieved in over half the patients (Lechtenberg, 1984; Emerson, D'Souza and Freeman, 1981). More than a dozen medicines are currently available, and research continues to investigate new drugs. Blood level tests are used to determine exactly how much medicine is in the blood. This test involves drawing blood from the patient, a task which is particularly difficult with children.

The electroencephalogram (EEG) is the main diagnostic test for epilepsy. It measures electrical activity in the brain through electrodes placed on the scalp. Since this electrical activity may be normal between seizures, a normal EEG does not rule out epilepsy. However, an abnormal EEG may confirm the diagnosis and may give the doctor important diagnostic information on the type of seizures and the drugs to be used. Another test often used is computerized tomography, the CT scan. In this procedure a beam of x-rays images cross sections of the brain, allowing the doctor to diagnose structural brain abnormalities that might otherwise not be detectable. Nuclear Magnetic Resonance is a relatively new test being used to detect structural abnormalities by the use of magnetic fields. It is expensive but often insurance and public programs cover the cost (Kerson, 1985).

Organization

The pediatric neurology clinic is staffed by two or more pediatric neurologists, a nurse, one social worker and about six residents and medical students. Two receptionists check in patients and file forms for medical coverage. They also gather financial information, as the family stands in the waiting room, so unfortunately one's private affairs are made public.

This is one of thirteen pediatric specialty clinics operated by North Carolina Baptist Hospital. One other clinic, pediatric hemophilia, has social work services available for patients. That position is funded by a federal grant through the Department of Pediatrics at the medical school.

Epilepsy is historically a very misunderstood disorder (Caveness, 1980; Temkin, 1971). Parents are often frightened and confused about this diagnosis. In this fast-paced clinic the doctor is responsive to questions the family may have, but he does not probe for areas of concern. Often the family is so overwhelmed by the diagnosis that they do not know what to ask. The social worker spends time with these families to cover common problem areas (Pomerantz, 1984).

There is actually no funding to pay for social work services to pediatric neurology clinic. A research grant to design a program of comprehensive care for epilepsy patients provided funding initially but this money ran out years ago. Small grants and some state money have continued to support various aspects of the program. Because the need for social work services is so great in this clinic, the social worker continues to provide it. Originally two social workers attended the clinic but only one is there now. Patients in the greatest need of social work services are seen. It is less than ideal but better than nothing.

The hospital might be expected to provide social work services to the pediatric neurology clinic, since it is one of their outpatient clinics and they do have a social work department. However, they employ only four social workers for a 675 bed facility; they cannot begin to meet all of the inpatient needs and thus do not attempt to service any of the outpatient clinics.

Community agencies, especially Public Health, are frequently involved in follow-up for medical as well as social and educational aspects of the treatment plan. Many patients have no phone and have chronic transportation problems so assistance by community agencies is often our only means of determining how the patient is getting along between visits, or of contacting them when they fail to keep appointments.

There is no department of social work at the medical school. Currently nine masters level social workers are employed by various departments, but each answers to the department chairman, a physician. Most are supported by federal grants. Some years ago social workers made an effort to keep in touch by meeting informally for lunch from time to time. New social workers were taken around to various departments by one of the veteran social workers to meet their social work colleagues. However, the medical center has grown rapidly. Social workers come and go without ever meeting one another now. They are much more isolated today than they were five years ago. It is the unfortunate but inevitable consequence of having no department of social work.

Case Description

Jeffrey Stone is an eleven-year-old boy who began having generalized tonic-clonic seizures (grand mal) eight months ago. After having unexpected difficulty in getting good seizure control, Jeffrey's pediatrician referred him to the pediatric neurologist who then hospitalized Jeffrey for further tests. Routine blood level tests found no trace of the prescribed seizure medicine in his blood. This indicated that the mother was probably not giving Jeffrey the medicine. The doctor found her to be defensive, but she offered no explanation for not complying with treatment. She was referred for social work evaluation (Heisler and Friedman, 1981).

Jeffrey is the younger of two children in a white, middle-class, urban home. His sister is fourteen-years-old and in good health. His mother is a thirty-six-year-old homemaker who seems to enjoy that role. His father is a thirty-eight-year-old manager of a hardware store, who works long hours but spends his free time with his family. Both parents are in good health. The maternal grandmother lives a few hours away and has frequent contact with the family.

The initial social work contact occurred while Jeffrey was still hospitalized. Mrs. Stone was interviewed in my office. She was defensive and reticent, although no mention had been made of the medication or the compliance problem. I took a patient education approach, saying that most patients know nothing about epilepsy and that I would like to explain some things about it. Although tense throughout the interview, Mrs. Stone appeared to relax somewhat as she listened. In simple terms I explained what occurs physiologically during a seizure, the appropriate first aid and the role of medication. Mrs. Stone had a few questions and I praised each one saying that many parents asked that very same question. Because the parent's account of the child's physical problems is usually quite useful in assessing their emotional reaction to it, I asked Mrs. Stone to tell me about Jeffrey's seizure history. By the end of the interview Mrs. Stone had warmed up noticeably. After giving her pamphlets about epilepsy, I scheduled another interview with her, this time in Jeffrey's room later that afternoon.

At this point there were several possible causes for Mrs. Stone's noncompliance. It was possible that she had her own ideas about the cause or nature of these seizures and that medicine did not fit into her understanding of what was going on. This is a common problem in situations of noncompliance (Tavriger, 1966; Voeller and Rothenberg, 1973). Another possibility was that the grandmother had been feeding misinformation to her daughter about this disorder and that Mrs. Stone was following her mother's dictates rather than the physician's. The influence of the grandparents on these situations cannot be overestimated. Still another possibility was that the mother had fears about giving daily medication, fears that it would have long term side effects or lead to drug addiction. Mrs. Stone seemed neither hostile nor rejecting toward the child, nor was she a negligent mother in any other aspect of her care. There was no indication of major psychiatric problems. I had no doubt that she understood the instructions on how to give the medicine.

The purpose of this next interview was to determine why medication was not being given. Rapport had been established during the initial interview and it seemed important to follow up quickly on this. Jeffrey was out having tests when I met with Mrs. Stone in his hospital room. I opened the interview by asking whether the pamphlets had been helpful. They had. She brought up some concerns about Jeffrey getting dependent on seizure medicine and not being able to get off it. Mrs. Stone's concern seemed mild and was obviously not the main problem. Other issues discussed were people's reactions to those with epilepsy, their misconceptions and how to handle them and the stigma associated with epilepsy (Taylor, 1987). After about thirty minutes Mrs. Stone seemed to feel relaxed and I posed the question "I know you have thought a lot about these seizures and you must have some idea about what causes them. What do you think it is?" Mrs. Stone responded in a confidential manner and seemed embarrassed at times as she explained: "I do. You see his favorite program on TV is 'The Hulk' and sometimes he gets to imitating the Hulk turning into that monster. You know how the Hulk does when he gets angry. I think he got to doing that and could not stop, and it just went into one of those seizures. I did not let him watch 'The Hulk' for months, but he begged and begged, so I finally gave in one Friday night. And do you know he had a seizure the very next day?'' Now it was understandable why medicine was forgotten so often. Medicine made little sense in the context of her unique understanding of Jeffrey's epilepsy.

Next I focused on how frightening the seizures are, and for the first time Mrs. Stone was able to verbalize the terror she felt when they occurred. She discussed the first seizure in detail, her thoughts, fears, and actions. She was tearful as she revealed that she thought he was dying each time he had a seizure. She was embarrassed that she had gotten so hysterical during the first seizure. I encouraged her to express her sense of helplessness and lack of control during these episodes. The goal of this interview was to uncover all of the fears that this mother kept hidden. Some information and reassurance were given about major misconceptions. I explained that behavior could not induce a seizure, that if a child voluntarily shook or jerked it could not cause him to go into a seizure. I again explained in simple terms the physiological phenomena and the role which medicine played. I reiterated that adequate blood levels of seizure medication should reduce the frequency of the seizures.

It was important to find out about the grandmother's and the father's reactions to Jeffrey's condition. What kinds of things did they say about it? By Mrs. Stone's account both were concerned, but neither seemed to be contributing to Mrs. Stone's fears and misinformation. The father had not seen a seizure and was rather matter-of-fact about the whole thing. At this point I felt confident that there were no other major issues and brought the interview to a close making an appointment to talk with Mrs. Stone again in the morning before Jeffrey was discharged.

Later I talked with the doctor about the case, and subsequently he was able to communicate much better with Mrs. Stone. He reinforced much of what I had said, stressing the good prognosis for Jeffrey's epilepsy with the use of seizure medication. Mrs. Stone's parenting techniques and Jeffrey's school situation needed to be discussed with the mother because there was some indication that she had become quite permissive and overprotective following the onset of seizures (Philbert et al., 1982). I also wanted to discuss drug treatment to make sure that Mrs. Stone was committed to following through with it.

The next morning Mrs. Stone came to my office; when I asked about the school situation she said that Jeffrey's teacher was fairly nervous about his condition. He had one seizure in school and that caused an uproar. She gave permission for me to contact the school. I discussed with Mrs. Stone the importance of treating Jeffrey like a normal child and continuing with the expectations and discipline she had always imposed. Mrs. Stone realized that she set few limits now because she feared that making Jeffrey angry would cause him to have a seizure. I explained that anger did not cause Jeffrey's seizures and that it was important to treat him just as before. I warned Mrs. Stone that behavioral problems which resulted from pampering these children were difficult to correct and could create serious adjustment problems later. Although she admitted she was still fearful, Mrs. Stone agreed that she needed to be stricter with Jeffrey. I asked whether she felt comfortable about the prospect of giving medicine to Jeffrey every day for the next several years. She replied that if it would prevent seizures, she would do anything. I again explained blood levels and the importance of keeping his in the necessary range, and gave her a pill organizer to help her remember. She was instructed what to do if she should forget a dose. I explained that blood levels would be checked when Jeffrey returned to the clinic in two weeks and that I would see her again then. I gave her my phone number in case problems or questions arose. Once more we went over first aid. I said I would contact the school and talk with Mrs. Stone about that at the clinic visit (Beniak, 1982). Mrs. Stone seemed genuinely grateful as she thanked me for my help.

Talking with Jeffrey's teacher, I found that she was indeed nervous about his condition. His seizure in school had panicked everyone, especially her. She had no previous contact with epilepsy and knew nothing about it. She now watched him closely because she worried he would have another seizure. His peers were a little stand-offish immediately after the seizure, but after two months had passed, things had returned to normal. I elicited questions about the disorder and talked about first aid. I also offered to send pamphlets on epilepsy, and the teacher gratefully accepted that. She agreed to call me after reading the material. Approximately a week later she did call and said she had enjoyed the information and had shared it with another teacher who also had a student with epilepsy. She asked whether I could present a brief talk about epilepsy at the next teacher's meeting, and I arranged to do so.

When Jeffrey and his mother returned to clinic in two weeks, she reported that he had done well, had had no seizures and no problems. She seemed fairly relaxed and said that she trusted the medicine. She said that she was better at setting limits but still hesitated at times. I again encouraged her to return to her normal parenting. She had shared the written information with her husband and with her mother. Her mother found it particularly helpful. I told Mrs. Stone that the school contact had gone so well that all the teachers wanted more information about epilepsy. I also told her that there were other children in the school with this disorder. The mother seemed pleased. Jeffrey was present throughout this interview. I decided to talk alone with him, and the mother stepped outside. I asked Jeffrey whether he had any questions about his epilepsy; he said not really. I asked whether he knew anyone else who had seizures. He knew such a boy in school, and he wondered whether it was true that one could catch epilepsy. I responded that one could not, and elaborated on that. He was quiet. I asked whether seizures scared him when he thought about them. He said that they scared his mother, that he had stopped breathing once and almost died. I explained that his mother had been so frightened that she misunderstood the situation. He had not nearly died. Seizures were not as dangerous as they looked. I said that I had told his mother what to do during a seizure and that his mother seemed to feel more relaxed now. I asked whether seizures had made any difference in school. He said that his teacher looked at him more now; he sensed her nervousness. I told him that his teacher had not known anything about epilepsy and that was why she had been nervous. Now that she was better informed, she should be more relaxed. I then told Jeffrey about a popular athlete from his state who had epilepsy, took medication, and was doing fine. Jeffrey looked pleased. I gave him my number in the event he should have any questions or problems about his epilepsy in the future. A return appointment was scheduled in three months, and I told Jeffrey and his mother that unless problems arose, I would not need to talk with the family before then. The blood level results showed his medication to be in the therapeutic range, and both Mrs. Stone and I were pleased with that.

The mother called me one time before the next appointment to ask whether it would be harmful to Jeffrey if she took a part-time job. She wanted to sell Avon products but needed assurance that it would not jeopardize his good progress. I encouraged her to pursue this.

When Jeffrey and his mother returned to the clinic in three months, he was doing quite well. He had no seizures. The mother was smiling and relaxed and looked unusually stylish and well groomed. She was pleased with her job, which allowed her to meet many people as well as to have her own spending money. She was not preoccupied with his seizures any longer. In fact, she did not think of them very often. He no longer got special treatment, and things had "settled back to normal." He wanted to go to summer camp, and she wondered whether that would be all right. I asked her what she would tell the camp officials about his condition, and Mrs. Stone gave a very good explanation of his disorder and his treatment. The doctor filled out the camp medical form she had brought and gave his consent for Jeffrey to do. Jeffrey was scheduled to be seen again in a year.

DECISIONS ABOUT PRACTICE

Definition of the Client

The primary client in this case was Jeffrey's mother. It was necessary to assess the reason for her noncompliance and to treat those problems before Jeffrey could come under good medical control.

His poor seizure control created secondary problems in school. His peers had shunned him for a while after the seizure; his teacher was apprehensive and overly attentive, and he was aware of this. Jeffrey's teacher was therefore also a client. Her anxiety and lack of information needed to be addressed. The other teachers in Jeffrey's school were clients. Through in-service training, they became better prepared to deal with his problem and with other children in the school who had epilepsy. This may prevent future problems.

Of course, Jeffrey was also a client. Attention needed to be given to his perception of the situation and to the problems which he identified. His awareness of the feelings of those around him is typical. Parental fears about the child's condition are usually incorporated by the patient. When parents understand and accept this disorder, the child generally does likewise (Middleton, Attwell, and Walsh, 1981; Ziegler, 1982).

There were several potential clients in this case who never actually became clients. The grandmother and the father might have been clients if the mother's information had indicated problems with either of them. Jeffrey's sister was also a potential client. Sibling reactions can be very important to the patient's adjustment (Goldin and Margolin, 1975). Jeffrey's classmates might have become clients if they had continued to isolate or stigmatize him. In that case an educational program in the classroom could be helpful.

Goals

The goals of this social work intervention were that Jeffrey achieve the best possible seizure control through medication, that his mother understand and accept his disorder, and that the emotional climate of the home and the school return to normal. Jeffrey's compliance was measured through the blood level testing. His mother's understanding and acceptance of the disorder was reflected in her willingness to give medication as well as in her openness in discussing his condition. She was cognizant of her overprotection and recognized when she began to improve and return to normal. It was relatively easy to evaluate the school situation because the teacher was cooperative and honest about feelings.

Besides the worker-client relationship, achievement of these goals depended in part on Jeffrey's physician. He was aware of what was transpiring between the mother and the social worker and was cooperative in reinforcing social work efforts rather than being overbearing or judgmental with Mrs. Stone.

Contract

Although the client worker contract was never clearly outlined, my initial statement that I wanted to help the mother understand her child's disorder was an honest basis for all that ensued. It was not necessary to verbalize that one of the main goals was to have the mother cooperate with medical treatment. Doing so might further have alienated this mother who was already feeling threatened. It is not always best to discuss all aspects of the contract. It is important that the client have a basic understanding of why he or she is seeing a worker but the worker may have a hidden agenda.

Meeting Place

The meeting place was of some importance in this particular case. The initial meeting should have taken place in the child's room at a time when he was not there rather than in my office. This would have been a less threatening setting since it was Mrs. Stone's turf. Parents on the pediatric ward spend their nights and days in the child's room, so it becomes a temporary home for them. Bringing the mother down to my office might have seemed to her a bit more like coming to the principal's office for a scolding, considering the circumstances. I sat behind a desk in a somewhat authoritarian arrangement. When we met later in the hospital room, we sat in identical chairs facing one another in a more equal and relaxed atmosphere.

Use of Time

Although this client will be followed periodically over a long period of time, the social work contact was essentially short-term. The exact number of interviews with the mother could not be predetermined, but I expected to have no more than six, provided all went well. If the mother had continued to be resistant, the father would have been brought into the situation and probably the grandmother too. The time frame for each interview was not preplanned. Each lasted 1 to 1-1/2 hours. An interview longer than that would be too fatiguing. There were goals for each interview, and I remained cognizant of them as time elapsed.

Treatment Modality

In this case the treatment modality was crisis intervention. The crisis precipitating social work intervention was the discovery that Jeffrey's mother was not compliant with treatment for a fairly serious medical disorder. The crisis which had overwhelmed Mrs. Stone was the onset of Jeffrey's seizures, which were terrifying and seemed life-threatening to her. The focus was on the immediate problem, and little in-depth attention was given to the social background. No attempt was made to explore or deal with problems the mother might have about specific issues, such as her need to control her anger, or her husband's aloofness. No attempt was made to interpret the symbolic nature of her Hulk fantasy. In the initial interview, I decided that Mrs. Stone had no psychopathology and that the family's functioning before the onset of the seizures seemed fairly normal. The treatment was limited to restoring that level of functioning.

Stance of the Social Worker

Because of the short-term nature of this intervention, I was direct, focusing on the immediate problem area and actively directing the course of the interviews. Initially I took a teaching approach, carefully avoided confrontation, and supported the few concerns Mrs. Stone expressed. During the second interview I wanted to draw Mrs. Stone out and did so with leading questions. It was important to listen during this interview, to express understanding and support for the mother's ordeal, and to universalize her feelings. Often parents of epileptic children feel isolated and think that no one can understand their fears and experiences. It can be helpful to let them know that the worker has talked with many parents of children with epilepsy and that their fears are universally shared. This must be done carefully so as not to discount the parent's feelings but rather to lend a base of support. There was some teaching during the second interview, but I was careful not to dominate with that since the main goal was to allow this mother to express her feelings (Fraser, 1983).

The third interview consisted of much confrontation and giving of advice. Giving advice is generally shunned as a social work task, but it is a valid task at times. Mrs. Stone needed to know that if she did not change her parenting pattern, trouble lay ahead. When Mrs. Stone protested that she was scared to be firm, I confronted. Did she want a spoiled child who was a problem in the classroom, could not get along with peers, and was impossible to live with at home? What kind of adult would such a boy grow up to be? Confrontation at this point was essential to change behavior so problems could be prevented.

In the fourth interview, I used praise for Mrs. Stone, who was coping much better and whose efforts needed to be rewarded. I further reinforced important points covered in previous interviews. By expressing confidence in Mrs. Stone's ability to continue to handle the situation, I attempted to bolster her self-esteem. By reminding Mrs. Stone that I was available if further problems arose, I offered her a sense of continued support. Giving permission to the mother to behave in certain ways provided the support she needed in the face of self-doubt. She needed the doctor's and my permission to treat Jeffrey normally. She also needed permission to pursue her job interest.

Use of Resources

In this case I provided educational pamphlets and a pill organizer to the family. Educational materials were given to the school as well. No other concrete services were needed.

Reassessment

This case was reassessed each time the patient returned to clinic, which was once a year after the first few visits. The physician and I agreed that Jeffrey and his mother continued to do well. She never had a need to contact us between scheduled appointments but that always remained an option.

Transfer or Termination

Active social work intervention terminated naturally at the time of the fourth interview. By that time the crisis was resolved. Mrs. Stone was giving the medication. Jeffrey's blood level was therapeutic and he was seizure free. The household was returning to a more normal state. The school had responded well to a minimum of intervention. I continued to check on this family but there were no problems which required reopening the case.

Case Conclusion

Jeffrey remained on medication for four years. Since he had been seizure free for that period of time and since his EEG was normal the physician decided to gradually discontinue the medication. Mrs. Stone was anxious but agreed to try this. He has had no further seizures. He seems to be a normal adolescent and Mrs. Stone continues to parent in an appropriate manner. Occasionally her concern about his seizure history does surface, as when he went to apply for a drivers license (Silber, 1983). However, she is able to quell her fears, and allows him to function normally.

Differential Discussion

It might have been a good idea to bring the father in for an interview to assess his response to Jeffrey's epilepsy. However, this might have presented problems. More than likely he was unaware that his wife was not administering the medication, and he might have been angry or accusing over that. It is possible that problems between the parents may have surfaced. There were indications that Mrs. Stone did not like her husband's long work hours and felt neglected and alone in handling the children's problems. A referral for marital counseling may have resulted. Instead, Mrs. Stone was left to cope with the seizure problem alone, and she did quite well. The successful mastering of a crisis situation can leave the person stronger than before. Mrs. Stone subsequently became more independent of her family by getting a part-time job which afforded her an occupation outside the home and an income of her own.

The importance of parents being open with their children about epilepsy has been stressed in the literature (Schneider and Conrad, 1983). If I were to treat this family today I would have discussed this with Mrs. Stone at the time of the final interview. I would make sure she used the terms seizures and epilepsy instead of "those" and "it" as if the condition were too horrible to call by name. While it is important not to dwell on Jeffrey's epilepsy, this topic should not be avoided if there is a need to discuss it with him or as a family.

PRACTICE IN CONTEXT

The nature of epilepsy dictates that a variety of interventions be utilized in the psychosocial treatment of epilepsy patients. Epilepsy can be a chronic, poorly-controlled seizure disorder in which the social worker provides long-term emotional support, guidance to resources, and a thread of continuity in the midst of ever-changing medical personnel involved in the treatment. Epilepsy may result in the occurrence of several seizures which are easily controlled by medication but which leave the family in a state of confusion, emotionally overwhelmed, and helpless. Crisis intervention can restore the family to a state of equilibrium, as in Jeffrey's case. Although epilepsy is a chronic disorder, patients are usually normal and healthy between seizures. Social work intervention may enable the parents and patients to deal with this dichotomy and to establish appropriate expectations, limits, and goals (Lechtenberg, 1984).

Poor seizure control makes good social adjustment more difficult. Especially over the past few decades, technology has been important in the psychosocial treatment of epilepsy by making better seizure control possible. Tests which indicate the level of anti-convulsant medication in the blood are important for accurate adjustment. These can also make noncompliance evident, as in Jeffrey's case. Without blood level tests, doctors would have engaged in lengthy and fruitless efforts to adjust Jeffrey's drugs without realizing that the problem was with the mother, not with the medicine. Technology has also provided improved diagnostic tests, further refining the diagnostic process so that treatable causes for epilepsy will not go undetected. However, even if technology achieved complete seizure control for all patients, this would not eliminate the psychosocial problems which sometimes accompany epilepsy. This disorder has been associated with shame, misunderstanding, and fear for so long that many families cannot accept it simply as a medical problem.

Since there is no formal organization of social work services in the medical school, Jeffrey was fortunate that this service was available to patients with his disorder. If Jeffrey had come in with orthopedic problems, for example, no medical social work services would have been available to help with his family problems. Because there is no department of social work, there is no coordinated effort to secure social work services in all areas.

In Jeffrey's case, technology was the key to further exploration of his family situation. It is ironic that the results of a chemical test were cause for social work referral. The policy of using a team approach in the pediatric neurology clinic made this referral a natural consequence of the compliance problem. In cases such as Jeffrey's, social work intervention itself may be fairly straightforward. It is the identification of the problem and referral for social work help which are crucial to achieving good medical and social adjustment.

REFERENCES

Appolone, C.A. "Preventive social work intervention with families of children with epilepsy." *Social Work in Health Care*, 4, 1978, pp. 139-148.

Beniak, J. "Patient education in epilepsy." *Journal of Neurological Nursing*, 14(1), Feb. 1982, pp. 19-22.

Caroff, P. and Mailick, M.D. "The patient has a family: Reaffirming social work's domain." *Social Work in Health Care*, 10(4), 1985, pp. 17-34.

Caveness, W.F. and Gallup, G., Jr. "A survey of public opinion toward epilepsy in 1979 with an indication of trends over the past 30 years." *Epilepsia*, 21, 1980, pp. 509-518.

Delgardo-Escueta, A.V., Treiman, D.M. and Walsh, G.O. "Treatable epilepsies." *New England Journal of Medicine*, 306, June 1983, pp. 1508-1514, 1576-1584.

Dodrill, C.B., Butzel, L.W. and Queisser, H.R. "An objective method for the assessment of psychological and social problems among epileptics." *Epilepsia*, 21, 1980, pp. 123-135.

Drotar, D. "Psychological perspectives in chronic childhood illness." *Journal of Pediatric Psychology*, 6(3), 1981, pp. 211-228.

Emerson, R., D'Souza, B.J. and Freeman, J.M. "Stopping medication in children with epilepsy." *New England Journal of Medicine*, 304(19), May 1981, p. 1125.

Ford, C.A., Gibson, P. and Dreifuss, F.E. "Psychosocial considerations in childhood epilepsy." In *Pediatric Epileptology*, F.E. Dreifuss (ed.). Boston, Bristol and London: John Wright, 1983.

Fraser, R.T. "A needs review in epilepsy rehabilitation: Toward solutions in the '80's." *Rehabilitation Literature*, 44(9/10), 1983, pp. 264-269.

Gardner, R.A. "Psychogenic problems of brain-injured children." *Journal of the American Academy of Child Psychiatry*, 7, 1968, pp. 471-491.

Goldin, G. and Margolin, R. "The psychosocial aspects of epilepsy." In *Epilepsy Rehabilitation*, G.N. Wright (ed.). Boston: Little Brown and Co., 1975.

Holdsworth, L. and Whitmore, K. "A study of children with epilepsy attending ordinary schools, II: Information and attitudes held by their teachers." *Developmental Medicine and Child Neurology*, 16, 1974, pp. 759-765.

Heisler, A.B. and Friedman, B. "Social and psychological considerations in chronic disease: With particular reference to the management of seizure disorders." *Journal of Pediatric Psychology*, 6(3), 1981, pp. 239-250.

Hermann, B.P. *A multidisciplinary handbook of epilepsy*. Springfield, Il.: Charles C Thomas, 1980.

Hobbs, N. et al. "Chronically ill children in America." *Rehabilitation Literature*, 45(7/8), July/Aug. 1984, pp. 206-213.

Hopkins, A. *Epilepsy: The facts*. N.Y.: Oxford University Press, 1981.

Jan, J.E., Ziegler, R.G. and Erba, G. *Does your child have epilepsy?* Baltimore, Md.: University Park Press, 1983.

Kerson, T.S. with Kerson, L.A. "The epilepsies." In *Understanding chronic illness*. N.Y.: Free Press, 1985, pp. 126-148.

Lechtenberg, R. *Epilepsy and the family*. Cambridge, Massachusetts and London, England: Harvard University Press, 1984.

Lerman, P. "The concept of preventive rehabilitation in childhood epilepsy: A plea against overprotection and overindulgence." In *Epilepsy: The eighth international symposium*, J.K. Penry (ed.). N.Y.: Raven Press, 1977.

Middleton, A.H., Attwell, A.A. and Walsh, G.O. *Epilepsy: A handbook for patients, parents, families, teachers, health and social workers*. Boston and Toronto: Little Brown and Company, 1981.

Philbert, A. et al. "The epileptic mother and child." *Epilepsia*, 23(1), Feb. 1982, pp. 85-99.

Pomerantz, B.R. "Collaborative interviewing: A family-centered approach to pediatric care." *Health and Social Work*, 9(1), 1984, pp. 66-73.

Schneider, J.R. and Conrad, P. *Having epilepsy: The experience and control of illness*. Philadelphia, Pa.: Temple University Press, 1983.

Silber, T.J. "Chronic illness in adolescents: A sociological perspective." *Adolescence*, 18(7), 1983, pp. 675-677.

Tavriger, R. "Some parental theories about the causes of epilepsy." *Epilepsia*, 7, 1966, pp. 339-343.

Taylor, D.C. "Epilepsy and prejudice." *Arch. Dis. Child*, 62(2), Feb. 1987, pp. 209-211.

Temkin, Q. *The falling sickness*, 2nd. ed. Baltimore and London: Johns Hopkins Press, 1971.

Tobel, H.V. and Lambert, L. *Introduction to developmental disability: Characteristics and psychosocial needs*, Vol. 1. Lexington: University of Kentucky, Human Development Program, 1981.

United States Department of Health and Human Services. "Medicine for the laymen: Epilepsy." Pub. No. 82-2369. Bethesda, Md.: National Institute of Health, June 1982.

Voeller, K. and Rothenberg, M. "Psychosocial aspects of the management of seizures in children." *Pediatrics* 51, 1973, pp. 1072-1082.

Ziegler, R.G. "Epilepsy: Individual illness, human predicament and family dilemma." *Family Relations*, July 1982, pp. 435-444.

Rehabilitation of a Quadriplegic Adolescent: Regional Spinal Cord Injury Center

Judith F. Hirschwald

DESCRIPTION OF THE SETTING

Magee Rehabilitation Hospital is a 96 bed, free-standing, not-for-profit physical rehabilitation center, offering comprehensive inpatient, outpatient, and follow-up services to individuals with physical disability. The origin and history of the hospital parallel the creation and growth of physical medicine as a branch of medical practice. Patients are evaluated and admitted to the hospital based on their ability to benefit physically from the services offered and on their potential to utilize these physical gains within the home and community setting. Thus, the criteria for admission are both medical and social. The average length of stay at Magee is approximately 30-35 days. The majority of patients are newly disabled and will return home with some degree of permanent disability.

In 1978, in conjunction with two other facilities, Magee received federal designation as the Regional Spinal Cord Injury Center of Delaware Valley. This designation altered the general complexion of the patient population at Magee. Since statistically, the 18 to 23 year-old male is at highest risk for spinal cord injury, the overall population has become younger. In addition, while all categories of disability continue to receive services, considerable additional expertise has been developed in the treatment of paraplegics and quadriplegics. New programs have been and are being created, especially in the psycho-social-vocational area, to better serve the needs of a younger population with severe physical disability.

Throughout the history of Magee, social workers have functioned as integral and crucial members of the treatment team. For inpatients, the ratio on the general rehabilitation services is one social worker to 12-14 patients and families; or, on the spinal cord and brain injury service, one social worker to 8-10 patients and families. These social workers also provide extensive service to patients and families in the outpatient and follow-up areas.

Policy

Policies affecting delivery of service in physical rehabilitation originate in both internal and external sources.

Internally, the primary policies derive from the Board of Trustees and the hospital administration. Such policies affect the scope of hospital services, admission policies, and overall hospital mission.

External forces which influence delivery of care include, primarily, third party payers, accrediting agencies, and general governmental and societal sanctions. Lengths of stay in rehabilitation are not dictated by third party providers, but as in all medical settings, they are influenced by them. In general, the field of rehabilitation is poorly understood by the major carriers, and standards applied to rehabilitation often parallel those for acute care hospitals. In addition, because there is no uniform health insurance, coverage varies and inequities in service exist. For instance, an individual who sustains a spinal cord injury in an automobile accident will, under existing conditions, be entitled to a variety of benefits which are not available to one who sustains the identical injury in a diving accident and who is covered under Blue Cross-Blue Shield.

In general, national policy in relation to health care and social services has been based on the premise that an enormous dollar expenditure in a program can be justified only if the result is the restoration of the individual to "normal, productive functioning." These policies have tended to release funding for care of individuals who are younger, perhaps less severely disabled, and who demonstrate a potential for return to competitive employment. However, more recent legislation, most notably Title VII of P.L. 95-602 (1978 Amendments to the Rehabilitation Act of 1973), makes provision for the development of independent living centers for the severely physically disabled (Amendments, 1978). While this legislation represents a significant attitudinal change, appropriations for both Part A and Part B of Title VII have been inadequate to fully meet the needs of severely disabled individuals. In short, policy-makers continue to debate the scope of governmental responsibility in meeting the long-term needs of individuals with severe physical disability.

Finally, Magee's commitment to lifelong follow-up care for individuals with catastrophic injury (specifically spinal cord injury) has been influenced at least in part by the stance of CARF (Standards, 1987) Commission on Accreditation of Rehabilitation Facilities) and by the former Department of Health, Education, and Welfare, who originally designed and implemented the Model Systems concept for spinal cord injury. Both these organizations placed emphasis on the outcome of rehabilitation and required the collection of follow-up data in order to evaluate patient outcome. The need to collect outcome data dictates the need for a system to track patients post-discharge to determine their current status in a number of defined areas. Around this data system evolved a commitment to a service system and consequently, a lifetime follow-up clinic was designed by Magee to meet the long-term needs of spinal cord injured persons within the community. From the spinal cord model, a similar system has evolved to address the needs of other severely disabled individuals in the community.

Technology

Recently, the technology available for treating individuals with severe physical disability has improved in two ways. First, increased medical sophistication has significantly lowered the mortality rate for many individuals with traumatic injuries and severe medical insults. The result of this new medical technology is that an increased number of individuals with severe residual disabilities survive and return to the community. Second, there has been a tremendous advance in making equipment available that allows even the most severely physically disabled individual some independent functioning. Elaborate environmental control systems, for example, now allow a severely disabled person to open, close, or lock doors, turn lights on or off, start or stop appliances, etc. These systems may be operated by verbal cues, a shoulder shrug, or often a mouth stick, the only motion that may be available to an extremely disabled person. Wheelchairs may be driven with "breath control," and specially equipped vans entered by hydraulic lifts are driven with the aid of elaborately adapted devices (Lange and Smith, 1978; Furlow, 1978).

Organization

Magee Rehabilitation Hospital is governed by a Board of Directors who represent a variety of community and hospital interests. The Chief Executive Officer is also the President of the Medical Staff, so that the primary decision-making power, both medical and administrative, rests in one office. The Director of Social Service reports directly to the Assistant Administrator for Clinical Services. Including the Director, the department consists of 14 social work staff, all with Masters Degrees, and two clerical staff.

As a relatively small institution, Magee lends itself to an informal atmosphere and to easy staff communication on all levels. Administrative staff are quite visible, the staff is generally close-knit, and planning occurs informally as well as formally.

Case Description

Jeffrey Bauer was admitted to Magee in September following an automobile accident in late July. He was nineteen years old, had graduated from high school the previous June, and had worked as a maintenance engineer in his local school district. He was one of six passengers in a car, all friends, returning from a weekend at the shore. Jeff was the only one injured in the accident; he sustained a complete fracture of his sixth cervical vertebrae that left him paralyzed below the neck. While drugs and alcohol were suspected to have been factors in the accident, Jeff was not heavily into either, prior to his injury. Following acute medical treatment at a local community hospital, Jeff was transferred to Magee for physical rehabilitation services. Although a "complete bed patient" on admission, he could be expected to attain mobility at a wheelchair level, learn to feed himself, transfer to and from the wheelchair, and dress himself with minimal assistance. Jeff's own goal on admission was to return to his "normal" level of physical functioning.

Although he was technically living at home prior to his injury, Jeff rarely spent any time there except to sleep. His major activity centered around his friends from high school. He was not an outstanding student in high school, although whether his low achievement was a result of lack of ability or lack of application was unknown. He had not chosen a career goal for himself but was planning to enter the armed services to secure training in some area. Generally, his life at this time consisted of having a good time with his friends and using the money from his employment for his own enjoyment.

He was a good-looking, personable young man but was not especially verbal except with his own peer group. He clearly valued his beginning independence from his family and, throughout the time in the general hospital, communicated with them as little as possible regarding his feelings and plans made with him for his ongoing care. His mother and father were feeling shut out by him, angry at his unwillingness to communicate with them, and guilty that they were not performing appropriately in their role as parents of a severely injured son (Wheeler, 1977).

DECISIONS ABOUT PRACTICE

Definition of the Client

The primary client as defined by a physical rehabilitation center is the individual patient. He is the key person who needs to gain an understanding of and ability to cope with his disability, and is therefore the primary target for all education efforts regarding his care and needs. To treat him alone, however, would be to assume that he will live in a vacuum. The definition of client, therefore, expands to include significant other persons within the client's environment (Crewe et al., 1979; David et al., 1978; Zola, 1981).

The delineation of significant other persons often changes during the course of rehabilitation as the patient and the family or friends begin to recognize the effects of severe disability and the implications for the future. For example, at times an employer or an attendant becomes part of the definition of the client. Jeff's significant others changed over time. Initially, his parents were most significant. As he began to go out for weekends, his younger brother became important. The brother's ability to cope emotionally and physically with Jeff's care was critical. In later stages of rehabilitation, Jeff's friends became important. Throughout, the representative from the insurance company was a key person to whom Jeff related. In the broadest sense, she too became part of the client group.

Goals

The broadest goal set by the social worker and the patient is to enable the patient to participate fully in the rehabilitation program and to return home at the highest level of possible function. Initially, the patient's goals are usually physical, most often complete recovery, and are not realistic to the limits of the disability. It is the social worker's first task then to enable the patient to begin the long process of coping with the reality of the disability (Athelstan, 1978). Obviously, the sudden onset of a physical disability is an overwhelming experience. To deal with the totality of the disability usually immobilizes the patient. Consequently, the joint setting of small, manageable goals helps the patient begin to cope. At an early stage of treatment, a shift must occur in the patient's perception of himself. He must change from viewing himself as a "sick person" who is the passive recipient of care to a "disabled person" who has the ability and the right to participate actively in his own program (Orbaan, 1986; Lane, 1976). In order to assert himself in this role, the patient must be given choices within the setting. For instance, he may not realistically have a choice of treatment, but he may be able to decide when it is begun.

For the most part, goals set by the social worker and client are measurable in terms of changes in the patient's behavior and feelings toward himself, his disability, and his rehabilitation program. As the patient begins to be able to assume more responsibility for himself, he will become more active in setting goals within the social work relationship and within his program as a whole. Ideally, he will begin to demand what he wants from the social worker and assume the initiative in setting appropriate goals.

Many outside factors impinge on the kinds of goals which social worker and client can set. One obvious and consistent reality is the physical disability itself. Goals cannot be set which do not account for the limitations that that imposes. Another critical factor is that the accomplishment of certain goals may be limited by the structure of the institution, the plans of another staff person, or a patient's family or significant others. The lack of resources within the community or within the institution may also alter the ability to accomplish certain goals.

Contract

In working with Jeff, a written contract was never utilized. An oral contract was established at the beginning of our relationship; but only during a four-to-six week period, when he was having a particularly rough time, was the contract really used to define our relationship. Typically in a rehabilitation setting, the need for intensive working together varies for the patient, depending on his ability to cope with his situation. For this reason a relationship can vary tremendously in intensity at various point in the rehabilitation process.

Meeting Place

Within a physical rehabilitation setting, there is a wide range of meeting places. Choices include the social worker's office, the patient's room, therapy areas, the dining room, the patient lounge, or, at times, a place outside the institution. Each place selected by the social worker or the client reflects the intent of the meeting, the amount of control each can exert, and the opportunity available for an extended, intensive meeting. The most structured, formal, and private atmosphere is the social worker's office. Other meeting places are informal and generally unstructured. They do not promise privacy or uninterrupted time, but they do demonstrate an interest in the patient's daily activities. The informal areas tend to be regarded more as the patient's turf, and his control over the content and length of the interview is greater.

With Jeff, as with many of my younger patients, my style of working tends to include the very conscious use of meeting place as a dynamic in building a relationship and in sustaining certain aspects of it. In general, my feeling is that our young patients in particular are wary of a structured, formal setting in which they feel they have limited physical control. In fact, as with Jeff initially, they do have limited physical control and cannot independently remove themselves from a situation in which they do not wish to participate. Many of the younger patients also initially view a request to see a social worker or psychologist in her or his office as an indication that they now have an emotional as well as physical problem. Therefore my initial meetings with Jeff were deliberately structured to occur on "his turf" and in as unthreatening an atmosphere as possible. These meetings occurred in either occupational therapy, physical therapy, or his room. Since my intention was to build a relationship with Jeff through an interest in his activities and his adaptation to the center, the meetings were frequent and deliberately brief. Little pressure was put on him to discuss his feelings. Instead, we discussed his current activities in the center, and I answered any specific questions he had regarding his program, passes from the center, etc. Once we had established a relationship, our meeting in the more formal atmosphere of my office was not threatening to him. Eventually, he reached the point where he set the meeting place. His choice was generally acceptable to me unless my goals for our meeting together differed from his. If so, we negotiated; but these negotiations were really about the purpose of our getting together at that time, and not the place itself.

If a patient has an especially difficult time forming a relationship and yet clearly has a need for it, several other alternatives are helpful in reducing the threat. Patients often participate in a structured therapeutic recreational program, both within and outside the center. Within, activities include volleyball, bingo, parties, etc.; trips outside can be to baseball games, restaurants, concerts, etc. Accompanying a patient on such a trip is often a useful dynamic in establishing a relationship when other efforts have failed. This meeting place is the least threatening, affords patient and social worker the opportunity to share a common experience, and provides a beginning with which to explore the patient's feelings about participating in an activity from a wheelchair perhaps for the first time.

Use of Time

In a physical rehabilitation setting, time is controlled by the relationship and by outside factors. The frequency and duration of interviews can generally be set by patient and social worker. As needs of patients tend to vary during the inpatient phase, the frequency and duration of meetings is continually renegotiated. While general points of high stress for the patient can be identified (e.g., admission, discharge, first visit home, goal-setting meetings with physician and staff), patients have their own patterns. Some do not really face their disability until after discharge, while others seem to be hit hardest upon admission. No typical pattern exists, nor does the timing of the point of greatest impact of the disability bear any real relationship to the eventual ability to cope. Therefore, the timing of interviews parallels the needs of the individual patient, his ability to cope, and his participation in treatment and in life outside the center.

The crucial factor in determining the relationship period is the patient's length of stay in the center. Discharge is determined primarily by the attainment of physical goals. This may dictate a premature ending to the relationship. Within reason, the length of stay can be extended for social or emotional causes, but certainly not for any prolonged period. The opportunity for continued patient-social worker contact after discharge is limited because of lack of transportation for the patient and lack of time to make home visits on the part of the social worker. Thus, the time period during which the relationship occurs is only minimally controllable by the patient or the social worker.

Stance of the Social Worker

From my experience, I have drawn three conclusions which affect my stance as a social worker. The first concerns a prominent treatment theory. Many articles in the literature adhere to a stage theory of adjustment to disability which identifies shock, denial, depression, anger, and then acceptance as the phases of disabled patients' attitudes (Cook, 1979; Hohmann, 1975; Kerr, 1972; Siller, 1969). In my experience, this theory has not been a useful construct. One can rarely discover distinct sequential stages, patients do not seem to follow consistent patterns, and in fact adjustment, or acceptance, as traditionally defined, may not be a realistic or desirable goal. A given patient may definitively state that he will never accept his disability. There is no need for a total acceptance. An individual must and does learn to live in spite of or with the disability, but probably never loses the hope that one day he will be able to return to "normalcy." Thus, the professional whose goal for the client is to hear him say "I know I will never walk again and I accept that as a fact" will in most cases never attain his treatment goal. The patient may in fact say "if I don't walk again" or "until I am able to walk," but those statements continue to imply hope that some day life will be different. In my opinion, that hope itself may be the essential thread allowing him to continue to go on living with or in spite of the disability. In general, the "markers" of the patient's feelings about himself as disabled are revealed through his adaptive or nonadaptive behaviors and rarely through actual words.

A second strong belief of mine is that understanding the interpsychic process may, for many patients, be in the long run a less important treatment goal than the need to manipulate the environment to the maximum extent possible to allow the disabled person to resume as much of his previous life style as he can. Depression may be more directly related to a patient's total physical dependence on a family member or inability to return to work and provide for his family than to the actual fact of his disability. Providing attendant care to help relieve a patient's feeling that he is a burden to his family, and reducing architectural and attitudinal barriers within the employment market, may be far more appropriate treatment goals than the interpsychic exploration of the patient's depression.

Third, the early attitudes of the able-bodied persons with whom a newly disabled individual comes in contact are crucial (Woodrich and Patterson, 1983). For most patients, the most consistently encountered able-bodied persons are close family members and hospital and rehabilitation personnel. Their attitudes are critical in beginning to help the individual form good initial opinions about himself as a disabled person. The individual needs to know that with the exception of now needing physical care, he is the same person he was before and should be treated the same way to the extent possible. The adolescent, in particular, needs to know that behaviors which were previously unacceptable are still unacceptable. The newly disabled person must assume responsibility for making decisions regarding his own life and for the consequences of those decisions.

Obviously, an individual brings to his disability the same problems and uses the same coping mechanisms that he had prior to the onset of the disability. For many, the support, understanding, acceptance, and willingness of the social worker to be with him and to believe in his continuing value and capabilities as a human being are the key elements in the helping relationship. For other patients, a total behavior modification approach is needed to help them change maladaptive, destructive forms of behavior. A psychoanalytic approach may be the treatment of choice for still others. For many, a combination of modalities will be needed at different times during the rehabilitation (Trieschmann, 1978).

Treatment Modality

The ability to cope with a severe disability develops over time, and intervention strategies must be employed with an acute sensitivity to this fact. The period a patient actually spends in the inpatient phase of rehabilitation is only a small beginning in learning to live with a disability. In fact, many patients say they did not begin really to deal with their disability until after they were discharged (Richards, 1986). The key decisions about modality are made according to the goals of the relationship and the assessment of the patient's ability to assume greater responsibility. In the very early stages following the onset of disability, the social worker will usually assume a more supportive role, accept some of the responsibility for certain decisions, and tolerate an expected level of maladaptive behavior. The role of the social worker changes, however, as the patient assumes more responsibility. If needed, confrontation is used to help the patient examine behaviors and attitudes.

Peer group therapy is frequently used because the peer group is a critical source of support in a physical rehabilitation center. With formal groups usually an integral part of the services offered, peer relationships can sometimes be influenced. This is important because peer influences are ever present and may be most crucial in determining a patient's attitudes. The status of each patient in the peer group and the impact of the group values on the goals of the individual patient also provide significant information to the social worker.

An individual with a disability must develop the behavioral skills necessary to survive in a society which will be generally hostile to him. He has to learn to manipulate his environment constructively and assertively. For these reasons, assertiveness is taught at Magee. It is a critical component in dealing successfully with different individuals and systems with which the disabled individual will now be forced to interact. For example, he may need to develop the skills to hire, supervise, and fire, if attendant care is to be a routine part of his life. He must also know how to handle agencies like Social Security and insurance companies.

Outside Resources

The provision of concrete services is obviously essential in a rehabilitation setting, as there are a myriad of services which need to be in place prior to a patient's discharge. In general, who assumes responsibility for obtaining needed services is determined by the goals of the relationship. Ultimately, the patient must be able on his own to secure services or, if not physically capable, to instruct another person in what must be done. At what point the patient is ready to begin to assume this responsibility is a professional decision. The sheer number of tasks to be accomplished often necessitates a sharing of responsibility by the patient and the social worker. The patient, however, ultimately needs to know exactly how to obtain needed services and what to do if services are not provided. This skill may be only partially or minimally acquired during the inpatient phase of rehabilitation, but eventually the responsibility must be totally assumed by either the patient or a family member. Ideally, the patient will assume the responsibility for knowing the resources available and how to obtain them, even if he remains physically incapable of securing them himself.

Reassessment

Reassessment occurs continually within the relationship; it is defined by either the social worker or the patient at different times. In general, in a rehabilitation setting, times for reassessment are not preset but occur at natural intervals as a dynamic part of the relationship itself.

The most crucial reassessment occurs at the point of discharge from the center. The time spent in anticipation of an eventual discharge is a period of high anxiety for the patient and family, and a reassessment of the relationship, goals, and plans for a continuing relationship, if any, occurs repeatedly as discharge becomes imminent.

Transfer or Termination

While planned transfers do occur within a physical rehabilitation setting, the most common causes of termination are external to the relationship and sometimes unplanned by either the social worker or the patient. For example, the most abrupt, disruptive termination during the rehabilitation phase occurs if the patient develops an acute medical problem and is transferred back to a general hospital. The patient may be readmitted later, depending on his medical status; but for the acute period, the relationship has been terminated and it is difficult to anticipate when it will be reestablished. Rarely does the social worker contact the patient in a general hospital except perhaps occasionally by telephone. A referral may be made to the social worker in the acute care hospital, but the opportunity for a planned, organized transfer does not exist.

Discharge from the rehabilitation center to return home is a less abrupt, more planned termination, but it too is usually determined by factors external to the social worker-patient relationship. Plans are often made for continuing the relationship after discharge, but the structure and the frequency of contact will probably be quite different. This type of termination serves as a dynamic to move the relationship to another level.

Case Conclusion

Jeff remained as an inpatient at Magee for roughly six months. Initially, he had some difficulty entering into a relationship with any "shrink type" because he did not see any need for such a relationship. However, the use of the informal, frequent contacts described earlier did eventually allow him to acknowledge some of his own need to talk about his feelings and to look at what had happened to him, what was happening in rehabilitation, and what would happen in the future. We were probably two months into the relationship before he was willing to come to my office.

Jeff eventually reached the point where he set the times and the structure of the interviews. As he began to feel the need, he came quite regularly to appointments. His major concerns revolved around relationships with his family and friends and the formulation of his own plans for discharge. Eventually he began to assume a greater sense of responsibility for his own care and his plans for the future. His plan for himself was to go directly from the rehabilitation center to his own apartment, using his money from the no-fault insurance carrier to pay his friends to be attendants. While this was not necessarily the safest or most ideal plan for a 19-year-old man with a newly acquired severe disability, I felt that he should have the opportunity to pursue his plans and to maintain his independence from his family. In time, he found the apartment, arranged for his friends to be attendants and had them trained by the center, and devised a method of payment for them acceptable to the insurance company.

By the time of discharge, Jeff was capable of managing all of his self-care with only minimal assistance. For instance, with dressing, he required help only with his shoes and socks and in starting his pants over his feet. With assistance, he was able to go from the bed to his wheelchair with his legs. He also required assistance with bowel and bladder care. In short, Jeff could manage independently with perhaps three hours of care during each day (two hours in getting up in the morning and one hour in the evening in going to bed). Once he was dressed and in his wheelchair, he appeared exactly as any 19-year-old man might and was capable of going by himself wherever he wanted to go, as long as he was not confronted with steps. The attendants did have to be available to provide the care he needed to get up and to go to bed. His alternative, of course, was to attempt to find someone else to "give him a hand," and in fact he often had to telephone friends, his brother, or others.

At the time of Jeff's discharge, I felt fairly optimistic about his eventual ability to survive and to gradually rebuild his life. The amount of difficulty he would encounter in the process seemed to me to depend heavily on the physical and emotional support system that he had to create (Goldiamond, 1973). His potential support system consisted of four major areas: his family, the center, his friends, both male and female, and his insurance company and its ability and willingness to provide the means for additional independence (i.e., a van). In addition, Magee had made plans for Jeff to return once a week to participate in a spinal cord group, see the physician, and receive the general support of the center. At one time or another, each of these support systems failed, and occasionally all systems failed at once.

Jeff essentially rejected two potential support systems, his family and the rehabilitation center. Shortly after discharge, he communicated to his parents in particular, but also to his brother, very specific guidelines for their involvement in his life: He made it clear that they were not welcome at his home on any regular basis, and if they appeared, he made his displeasure very clear. Eventually his family stopped trying to impose their presence on him and to offer assistance. Following discharge, Jeff returned to Magee once a week for only about a month, although he maintained close contact by telephone with some staff, including the social worker, for about three months. His primary contact after that period occurred when he was in a crisis, but even then he rejected coming to the center to talk. The opportunity to go to his home was extremely limited because of distance and because the hospital's defined mission does not include the provision of long-term, intensive counseling services.

The other two support systems, friends and insurance company, were intermittent in their support. His friends were not always able to provide the services required, although several demonstrated considerable sensitivity and maturity during extreme crisis. The insurance company continued to provide services but began to attach "strings" and, eventually, ultimatums to continued service, requiring such things as his enrollment in a local college or some other demonstration of his motivation to secure employment.

The times of major crisis for Jeff occurred when all support systems failed simultaneously or began to impose greater demands than he was able to meet. Since the four systems were separate and uncoordinated, the possibility of all pulling back simultaneously or of making parallel demands on him was increased.

The period since his discharge has been extremely difficult for Jeff, and for those of us even peripherally involved. It has been difficult at times to continue to support his need to manage on his own and to direct his own life. His friends were not always responsible as attendants, but although he did not always receive needed care, he has, in fact, remained relatively free of severe medical complications. He was given an eviction notice because of several late night, noisy parties, but he has gone to court on several occasions to appeal the eviction and so far remains in his apartment. On one occasion, he attempted suicide, precipitated, at least in part, by the rejection of a girlfriend (Seligmann, 1975). However, he finally has a van and is beginning to make plans to attend a community college. Obviously, he has matured considerably throughout this experience. He chose a very difficult route for himself and had to fight to be supported in that choice. He demonstrated the basic survival skills, however, so the plan had a chance of working.

PRACTICE IN CONTEXT

Two factors, which relate back to the policies of the institution and of this society, seem important to the outcome of working with Jeff. The first critical element is the fact that Jeff's original injury occurred as the result of an automobile accident. Although he had to work hard to accomplish it, he had a theoretical choice at least between returning to his parents or securing his own apartment. This choice was made possible through the benefits due him under his no-fault insurance policy. Those benefits include: eligibility for partial replacement of lost wages, which enabled him to share with the insurance company the cost of the apartment; total payment for medical expenses, which allowed him to secure needed medical/ nursing supplies without totally utilizing his social security disability payments; and coverage for attendant care services to provide the physical care which Jeff was unable to accomplish independently. This set of options would not have been available to another 19-year-old in exactly the same set of circumstances as Jeff, except for the fact that he broke his neck in a swimming pool. The inequities of insurance coverage for catastrophic illness in this country are clear from this example, and in many instances severely curtail the level of social and emotional independence which a disabled individual can attain.

The second key element is one which was not available to Jeff but which might have influenced his outcome had it been. This element is the greater availability of the rehabilitation center staff, particularly the social worker, during the first crucial six months to a year after discharge. Jeff's specific events would probably have occurred anyway, but the abruptness with which he lost the support of the entire center precipitated an additional crisis for him. His apartment is about an hour and a half away from the center, and home visits on a regular basis were not feasible. Contact was maintained by telephone but was irregular, occurring only in the midst of a crisis. Jeff did not have transportation available to him during this time, and so his potential for returning to the center with an regularity was limited. Magee has now made a commitment to lifetime follow-up services. Under current policy and practice, Jeff would have been scheduled for a regular comprehensive evaluation at one month, three months, six months, and a year following discharge.

However, the need for continuing intensive counseling would still be difficult to meet due to the limitations of the hospital and Jeff's transportation problems. While the city of Philadelphia now operates a door-to-door transportation service for individuals with disability, Jeff's apartment was located outside the city.

The need for educating the public about the individual with a severe disability is also crucial. The lack of understanding of physical disability by many community agencies is evident in Jeff's contact with the community mental health system. At the time of his suicide attempt, he was referred by the emergency service of his community hospital to the community mental health system for follow-up. The social worker assigned to him had no experience with physical disability and, by her own admission, was too overwhelmed by the disability to know how to begin to help him. Thus, while the elements of the relationship between patient and social worker need to be understood, the limitations and opportunities built into this relationship by outside forces are also crucial factors in determining the eventual outcome.

In summary, the field of physical rehabilitation has mirrored the general medical field. Historically, the primary resources and reimbursement have been deployed to inpatient services. In today's climate, increasing emphasis is placed on shorter lengths of inpatient stay and growth of outpatient and follow-up services. Improved technique and technology in emergency management and acute care has preserved and prolonged the lives of more individuals with more severe disability. The challenge for all rehabilitation professionals and for society in general is to ensure these people of the choice for an acceptable quality of life.

REFERENCES

Athelstan, G.T. et al. "Psychological, Sexual, Social, and Vocational Aspects of Spinal Cord Injury: A Selected Bibliography." *Rehabilitation Psychology*, XXV, No. 1 (1978), pp. 16-28.

Amendments to the Rehabilitation Act of 1973. Title VII. Part B, P.L. 95-102, 1978.

Bors, E. and A.E. Commar. "Neurological Disturbances of Sexual Function with Special References to 529 Patients with Spinal Cord Injury." *Urological Surgery*, X (1960), pp. 191-222.

Bracken, M.B., Shepard, M.P.H., and Webb, S.B. "Psychological Response to Acute Spinal Cord Injury: An Epidemiological Study." *Paraplegia* 19 (1981), pp. 271-283.

Bregman, S. *Sexuality and the Spinal Cord Injured Woman*. Minneapolis: Sister Kenny Institute, 1975.

Commar, A.E. "Sexual Classification and Expectations among Quadriplegic and Paraplegics." *Sexuality and Disability*, I, 4 (Winter 1978), pp. 252-59.

Commar, A.E., G.W. Hohmann, and C. Tempio. "The Sexual Function of the SCI Patient." A sourcebook: *Rehabilitating the Person with Spinal Cord Injury*. Washington, D.C.: U.S. Government Printing Office, 1972.

Cook, D. "Psychological Adjustment to Spinal Cord Injury: Incidence of Denial, Depression, and Anxiety." *Rehabilitation Psychology*, 26 (1979), pp. 97-104.

Coven, A.B., and Glazeroff. "The Rehabilitation of the Spinal Cord Person." *Rehabilitation Counseling Bulletin*, XXII, 1 (1978), pp. 22-29.

Crewe, N.M., G.T. Athelstan, and J. Krumberger. "Spinal Cord Injury: A Comparison of Pre-Injury and Post-Injury Marriages." *Archives of Physical Medicine and Rehabilitation*, LX (1979), pp. 252-56.

David, A., S. Gur, and R. Rozin. "Survival in Marriage in the Paraplegic Couple: Psychological Study." *Paraplegia* XV (1977-78), pp. 198-201.

Dembo, T., G. Leviton, and B. Wright. "Adjustment to Misfortune: A Problem of Social-Psychological Rehabilitation." *Rehabilitation Psychology*, XXII (1975), pp. 1-100.

Eisenberg, M.G. "Sex and Disability: A Selected Bibliography." *Rehabilitation Psychology*, XXV, 2 (1978), pp. 74-81.

Eisenberg, M.G. and J.A. Falconer. *Treatment of the Spinal Cord Injured*. Springfield, Ill.: Charles C Thomas, 1978.

Evans, R.L. "Multidisciplinary Approach to Sex Education of Spinal Cord Injured Patients." *Physical Therapy*, 16,5 (May 1976), pp. 541-45.

Furlow, W.L. "Surgical Treatment of Erectile Impotence Using the Inflatable Penile Prostheses." *Sexuality and Disability*, I, No. 4 (Winter 1978), pp. 299-306.

Goldiamond, I. "A Diary of Self-Modification." *Psychology Today*, I (1973), pp. 95-102.

Hohmann, G. "Psychological Aspects of Treatment and Rehabilitation of the Spinal Cord Injured Person." *Clinical Orthopedics*, CXII (1975), pp. 81-86.

Judd, F.K., Burrows, G.D. and Brown, D.J. "Depression following Acute Spinal Cord Injury." *Paraplegia*, 24 (1986), pp. 358-363.

Karacan, I. and I. Ilaria. "Nocturnal Penile Tumescence (NPT): The Phenomenon and Its Role in the Diagnosis of Impotence." *Sexuality and Disability*, I, 4 (Winter 1978), pp. 260-71.

Kerr, W., Thompson, M. "Acceptance of Disability of Sudden Onset in Paraplegia." *International Journal of Paraplegia*, 10:94-102, 1972.

Lane, Helen J. "Working with Problems of Assault to Self-Image and Life Style." *Social Work in Health Care*, I, No. 2 (1975), pp. 191-98.

Lange, P.H. and A.D. Smith. "A Comparison of the Two Types of Penile Prosthesis Used in the Surgical Treatment of Male Impotence." *Sexuality and Disability*, I, 4 (1978), pp. 307-11.

Lazarus, A.A. "A Learning Theory and the Treatment of Depression." *Behavior Research and Therapy*, VI (1968), pp. 83-89.

Lordyce, W. "Behavioral Methods in Rehabilitation." *Rehabilitation Psychology*. Ed. W. Neff. Washington, D.C.: American Psychological Association, 1971.

Masters, W.H. and V.E. Johnson. *Human Sexual Inadequacy*. Boston: Little, Brown, 1970.

Melman, A. "Development of Contemporary Surgical Management for Erectile Impotence." *Sexuality and Disability*, I, 4 (1978), pp. 272-81.

Mooney, T., T.M. Cole, and R.A. Chilgren. *Sexual Options for Paraplegics and Quadriplegics*. Boston: Little, Brown, 1975.

Orbaan, I.J.C. "Psychological Adjustment Problems in People with Traumatic Spinal Cord Lesions." *Acta Neurochirurgica*, 79 (1986), pp. 58-61.

Rabin, B.J. *The Sensuous Wheeler: Sexual Adjustment for the Spinal Cord Injured*. San Francisco: Multi Media Resource Center, 1980.

Richards, B. "An Evaluation of Home Care after Spinal Cord Injury." *Paraplegia*, XII, 4 (February 1975), pp. 263-67.

Richards, J.S. "Psychologic Adjustment to Spinal Cord Injury During First Postdischarge Year." *Archives of Physical Medicine and Rehabilitation*, 67 (June 1986), pp. 362-365.

Rotter, J. "Generalized Expectancies for Internal versus External Control of Reinforcement." *Psychological Monographs*: General and Applied, LXXX (1966), pp. 1-28.

Seligman, M. *Helplessness: On Depression, Development, and Death*. San Francisco: Freeman, 1975.

Shaul, S. et al. *Toward Intimacy: Family Planning and Sexuality Concerns of Physically Disabled Women*. Everett, Wash: Planned Parenthood of Snohomish County, 1977.

Shontz, F. "Physical Disability and Personality." *Rehabilitation Psychology*. Ed. W. Neff. Washington, D.C.: American Psychological Association, 1971, pp. 38-49.

Siller, J. "Psychological Situation of Disabled with Spinal Cord Injuries." *Rehabilitation Literature*, 30 (1969), pp. 290-296.

Small, M.P. "The Small-Carrion Penile Prosthesis: Surgical Implant for the Management of Impotence." *Sexuality and Disability*, I, 4 (1978), pp. 282-91.

Standards Manual for Organizations Serving People with Disabilities. Commission on Accreditation of Rehabilitation Facilities, 37, 1987, pp. 47-50.

Summary of Selected Legislation Relating to the Handicapped: 1974. Washington, D.C.: U.S. Department of Health, Education, and Welfare, May 1975.

Trieschmann, Roberta B. "The Psychological, Social, and Vocational Adjustment to Spinal Cord Injury: A Strategy for Future Research." Washington, D.C., Rehabilitation Services Administration Publication, 1978.

Wheeler, Doris et al. "Emotional Reactions of Patients, Family and Staff in Acute Care of Spinal Cord Injury." *Social Work in Health Care*, II, 4 (Summer 1977), pp. 369-78.

Woodrich, F. and Patterson, J.B. "Variables Related to Acceptance of Disability in Persons with Spinal Cord Injuries." *Journal of Rehabilitation* (July/August/ September 1983).

Young, J.S. and N.E. Northrup. "Statistical Information Pertaining to Some of the Most Commonly Asked Questions about SCI." *Model System's SCI Digest*, I (Spring 1979), pp. 11-32.

Zola, I.D. "Communication Barriers Between 'Able-Bodied' and 'The Handicapped'." *Archives of Physical Medicine and Rehabilitation*, 62 (August 1981), pp. 355-359.

Mutual Help Group for Emphysema Patients: Veterans Administration Medical Center

Zelda Foster

DESCRIPTION OF THE SETTING

The program for emphysema patients began at the Brooklyn Veterans Administration Medical Center in 1966. The medical center, a three site facility, offers veterans hospital admission to a variety of services, including Medicine, Surgery, Neurology, Rehabilitation, and Psychiatry for the treatment of acute illness on an inpatient and outpatient basis. The medical center also operates a 420 bed extended care facility at a second location and a large outpatient ambulatory care center at a third location. Medical treatment is offered by full-time physicians, interns, and residents. The interns and residents select the hospital for training in a particular specialty and remain for limited periods of time. The hospital has extensive programs in Nursing, Social Work, Dietetics, Psychology, and Speech Pathology.

The Veteran's Administration's medical centers and ambulatory care clinics serve veterans with honorable discharges. Eligibility requirements are based on a priority system: Service connected veterans, veterans exposed to Agent Orange, Prisoners of War and World War I veterans are highest; lower priority is given to non-service connected veterans with other VA pensions or who meet the established income criteria. There is a co-payment required if the income is above the established amount. Space availability determines whether lower priority veterans are accepted for treatment.

Currently the Veterans Administration is billing private health insurers for non-service connected patients who are accepted for treatment and have coverage.

The veterans population is aging, and increasing numbers are facing chronic and debilitating illness (Rothman and Becerra, 1987). Some veterans choose care at a VA hospital because they are not covered by private medical insurance and therefore cannot afford care in voluntary hospitals (Page, 1982). Outpatient services tend to be narrowly defined, limiting the availability of long-term, comprehensive care. Other significant programs offered by the Veterans Administration are domiciliaries, nursing homes, contract nursing homes, VA operated hospital-based home care programs, and several Adult Day Health Care Centers. Respite, Hospice Care and Geriatric Evaluation Units are offered in some VA facilities.

The emphysema program was developed in 1966. Emphysema patients previously assigned to various medical units were instead placed on one unit, and a physician specializing in respiratory care was hired. This resulted in an organizational change wherein these patients were now regarded as a group with common needs. The immediate assignment of a social worker contributed to addressing this population in medical and psychosocial terms. This provided a cohesive framework, unifying multiple aspects of patient need and patient care.

Patients were generally hospitalized for treatment of acute episodes of respiratory distress. A team composed of nurses, a social worker, respiratory care therapists, and dietitians had as its charge the development of an initial plan of care. The social worker, during the admission (often readmission), reached out to the patient to engage him in a ward mutual help group and to define and to work on multiple psychosocial concerns. (The same patients were seen in the emphysema outpatient clinic for follow-up care.) This organizational design changed in 1980 when patients were dispersed instead on various units, with the out-patient clinic becoming the major structure for unifying this population. This impacted programming and resulted in greater concentration of psychosocial services in ambulatory care allowing for specialized services.

Policy

Policies which support a comprehensive, coordinated approach to patient care always grow out of competing priorities, strains between forces, and ambivalent commitments and convictions. Many of the policies and struggles affecting this particular population can be traced to unresolved issues and practices affecting the very nature of medical care in the United States. Other policies have more local origins. The complex interaction between local and larger systems and spheres of influence has had continuous effect on our program and has been capable of drastically changing its growth and course over the years (Black, Durnan and Allegrante, 1986). A number of policy issues are relevant in tracing the direction which the mutual help group for emphysema patients took, how it changed, and in what ways it survived. Several of the larger forces impinging on it are worthy of discussion. Medical treatment in the United States continues to be oriented toward acute and episodic care. Management of long-term chronic illness is of significantly less interest except at the times the illness has a dramatic manifestation. Even then, if the patient has ongoing manifestations, these may become less dramatic and hence less interesting. This becomes stigmatizing to the patient and places him in a lesser position. Patients with emphysema require help with long-term management. There are no marvelous cures or advanced technology. There are professionals interested in this population; however, in our cure-oriented system, the resources available and the organization of health care services tend to devalue their contribution (Strauss, 1984).

Most hospitals have an enormous stake in physician training. The nature of this training emphasizes heavily the treatment of singular disease entities for which there is clear-cut knowledge and research regarding pathology, specific organicity, and linear treatment methods. When patient care needs come into conflict with medical training needs as currently defined, patient care often loses precedence. Medical training in the treatment of chronic disease is seen as having little desirability. Training in disease management supplants training in helping patients to manage complicated physical and psychosocial aspects of illness. Consequently, hospitals tend to restrict clinics, follow-up care, and other programs geared to long-term and continuous care. Health professionals connected to the needs of these patients are viewed as ancillary. That these health professions have not had enough of a voice in policy development and may not have fought forcefully enough for their imperatives is worth considering as one possible obstacle to policy change.

Current practice in some medical schools is moving toward training in general medicine rather than in specialized areas. This may have very positive implications for less fragmented training and for promoting generalists capable of treating multiple kinds of illnesses. Policies which move from enhancing general medicine training to specialty training and back again are bound to influence the kinds of services available to patients. In either approach, however, training tends to remain disease-rather than people-oriented.

Self-help and mutual help groups grow out of consumerism, patient education, and the capacity of patients to help one another (Gartner and Reissman, 1984). The role of the professional in these groups can be central or peripheral, depending on the purpose, formation, and auspice of the group. The availability of both professionals and interdisciplinary teams with a role and investment in the group depends on the support, resources, and conceptual orientation of the institution and the various disciplines. Each discipline has its own priorities and high status populations. This affects who gets service, in what form, and for how long. How well interdisciplinary teams carve out common goals, share in decision making, and invest in each other's contributions depends on complex issues of power, professional competitiveness, territorialism, and institutional sanction (Weiner, 1958).

For our emphysema patients who at the inception of the program were for the most part poor, chronically ill, mainly in their fifties, and marginally employed if at all the establishment of a special unit represented a marked shift in their care. One primary physician and a stable staff got to know them. Their breathing and functioning difficulties were responded to with acknowledgment and empathy and were regarded as capable of treatment and improvement. This hope, consistency of care and recognition enlisted patients into a more active role. Recognizing this dynamic, staff moved clearly and firmly. Yes, patients had common needs, could help one another, and could in their collective being participate in and influence their treatment. Patients who were passive, felt victimized, and found dependency comforting were both nurtured and challenged to assume a more contributory role (Foster, 1979).

By the very nature of the orientation to care and treatment, institutional practices were thrown into question. Physicians had mixed feelings about how much to encourage patients to raise questions about their illness and treatment. Some nurses were not geared toward patients assuming more self-care. Helping patients to express feelings of anger was threatening to some staff. The patients' eventual interest in promoting day treatment, in having a twenty-four hour respiratory center, in seeking ways to bypass admission procedures when in need of hospitalization, and in insisting on aftercare from physicians who know them, ran counter to current institutional practices, which reflect the prevailing notions of the times. The patients did, however, manage to get clinic care and a small respiratory care center and often were admitted to the hospital by the direct intervention of the respiratory care physician. Through their inpatient and outpatient groups, they proceeded to help one another, to have more say in their own care, to assume more responsibility for what happened to them, and to become more knowledgeable about their disease (Silverman and Smith, 1984).

Even though local policy constraints were overcome, other ramifications of larger health care policy issues continue to play a major role. The patients need a twenty-four hour respiratory care center and day hospital treatment where a consistent staff is attuned to them. Home care services are needed to provide for patients too ill to be transported back and forth to the hospital and who do not have the full and daily help required to keep them stable and comfortable. In 1983, the Medical Center initiated a Hospital Based Home Care Program and in 1984, an Adult Day Health Care Program. Emphysema patients have access to both. When good preventive and palliative services are not offered, hospitalization becomes a recourse. Cost-containment policies are shrinking resources available to patients with these kinds of needs.

As the emphysema program continued, the population served included many of the same patients. The inpatient group became less purposeful, but the outpatient group continued over a twenty year period (Silverman and Smith, 1984). More recently, a weekly service for severely disabled emphysema outpatients was instituted. These patients see the respiratory team physician, the nurse, the respiratory therapist, and the social worker. Each patient comes to the weekly clinic and also joins the group session led by the social worker. The physician and nurse also participate in the group sessions when indicated. This kind of clinic, group, and staffing represent the interests and commitment of specific health care professionals rather than institutional policy and backing. Therefore, it risks discontinuance if the interested professionals leave, if the hospital pulls out its already-limited resources, or if priorities are changed by competing forces. A program not in the mainstream risks not having a voice when resources shrink. In these cost-containment times, one must address the issues the acute sector will raise—whether a program is critical, the potential for cure, the value for physician training. The issue becomes whether we can afford to care for and maintain chronic patients requiring long-term care with minimal potential for recovery or productivity. Similar issues emerge out of the hospice movement in regard to the humanistic concerns of offering treatment which is non-cure oriented and which has lesser value in more aggressively oriented medical circles.

New reimbursements models are further impacting on care. Payment based on diagnostic related groupings (DRGs) are resulting in significant shifts from inpatient to ambulatory care. Emphasis on discharge planning with the thrust toward continuing care in the community often places social workers in the role of short term planners rather than as deliverers of ongoing services. Establishing the appropriate level of care and moving patients along the continuum has value and certainly meets an agreed-upon institutional purpose. Longer term case management and comprehensive treatment services encompass more than the referral to services and assurance that they are provided; it also offers an ongoing programmatic address of population needs. How these services will get paid for is unresolved. Presently there is a resource allocation model payment which covers ambulatory care. However, chronic patients needing continual and extensive ambulatory care create financial pressures. If a capitation form of payment is introduced, this population may be even less desirable since it is a large consumer of services. These concerns apply to non-veteran populations and users of other systems since payment for long term health care continues to be limited. Preventing further erosions of health by maintaining and improving levels of functioning is not yet viewed as offering long term economic and well-being benefits. Cost containment can be a desirable aim; but one must question shortsighted models of care and payment which diminish the access to and availability of long-term care and treatment.

Technology

Emphysema is a form of damage to the lungs in which some of the walls of the lung's air sacs have broken down, trapping stale air in them. Exhaling air puts a squeezing pressure on the air passages. If these are weakened, they may close up and trap more air. The damaged parts of the lungs cannot take the oxygen which the body needs out of the fresh air, and they cannot get rid of carbon dioxide by passing it from the blood into the air (Selecky, 1982).

Emphysema is generally irreversible, with increasing disability in pulmonary capacity. Relief obtained from medication, breathing apparatus, and respiratory care does not change the course of the disease, which varies in intensity from patient to patient (Kerson, 1985). The roles of pollution, climate, and stress in reducing the effect and the progress of the disease are considerations taken into account when treating it. Smoking is a definite prohibition, and obesity is a handicap because of the increased strain on the lungs and heart.

When medically indicated, patients are admitted to the hospital and followed in the clinic. They receive medication and respiratory therapy (Schuman and Cohen, 1982). Some outpatients attend a general monthly outpatient group. In addition, nine or ten patients with severe emphysema attend a weekly clinic and outpatient group. Both groups are led by a social worker assigned to the program (Hardiker and Tod, 1982). The weekly group has considerable participation from the nurse and the physician. This provides the patient with a framework of care which helps integrate his immediate medical treatment with his ability to cope with the illness. It also allows patients an opportunity to communicate their needs more directly to staff. This connection is not built into the structure of the general emphysema clinic or the monthly outpatient group, where services are offered in more separate and categorical ways. It has over the years become both a social and educational opportunity for patients and is seen by them as a source of support, attention and connection (Lock, 1986). The weekly group has an ongoing agenda which focuses on how patients are coping with severe breathing limitations. It offers its members opportunities to exchange information, share experiences, and discuss upsetting incidents which may have precipitated respiratory crises. There is a social element as patients communicate with others with similar symptoms and concerns. Many of these patients lead isolated lives and feel prevented from participating in many social activities. The group allows for participation and conviviality. In both groups, the agenda is usually developed by the group. The social worker provides an impetus for the raising of more crucial issues and encourages the kind of group process which will result in a real exchange — a sharing of feelings and experiences and a stake in giving help to (and receiving it from) others. The social worker acts as medicator, enabler, catalyst, and, reflector (Beck and Drachman, 1985). The aim is to help the group to work on real issues, to further their knowledge of the disease and their capacity to feel greater control and independence (Parry, 1975). It has been valuable to incorporate the views of other disciplines into this process so that there is a sense of unity, of shared purpose and goals.

Organization

The emphysema clinics operate out of the department of Medicine. Other disciplines assign staff who offer patients a variety of services. The Social Work Department assigns one of its sixty social workers to the program. Social work has a stake in the program and has offered staff at a somewhat higher ratio than on a number of other services to which social workers are assigned.

At present, emphysema patients are for the most part admitted to general medical wards. The physicians who specialize in its treatment may act as consultants or request that the patient be followed on a small inpatient unit or a specialty chest clinic. Social Work Service has had to adapt its program for offering specialized psychosocial services to this population now dispersed on more general medical wards. Defining unique needs, identifying patients and offering them a collective experience is harder to do.

The emphysema program currently has developed its own inner structure with several unique features (Weiner, 1984). The physician most closely tied to the emphysema patients has carved out a sustained personal and caring role. Because it is personal and individualistic, it also is unstructured at times and reflective of the particular stresses on the one major person. Not tied at this time to the residency training program, the program allows patients ongoing care from the same primary physician. Yet, the potential for his becoming overly taxed in offering this care clearly exists. The other disciplines assigned to the program share responsibility as colleagues in ways based, too, on preference and style. A more centralized and defined leadership pattern with clear goals and direction might allow for greater accountability and standardization.

DECISIONS ABOUT PRACTICE

Definition of the Client

The outpatient group was seen from the beginning as the major unit of service. Although various patients and families were seen individually and/or as couples, the group is a major focal point of service. This grew out of the conviction that the patients needed and could help one another. Many are dealing with similar adaptive tasks representing a range of coping abilities. It was expected that with skilled help, patients could experience other ways of responding and could broaden the alternatives available to them. Several common patterns are evident. Many patients tend to globalize their problems and patterns of reaction. Subdividing and examining intervening and incremental responses are key areas of work for the group. Extreme anger, fear of anger, and strong reactions of feeling victimized are prevalent themes. These patterns are amenable to change in a group-oriented service. There is enough difference in personal styles and emotional makeups to allow for the range of feelings and coping patterns needed for a solid group process. All patients are invited to the group. Patients have varying degrees of commitment to the group and differing lengths of involvement. Several take on patient-volunteer status; they contribute to greeting and orienting new patients, and participate in the teaching of dia-phragmatic breathing.

Goals

Goals change and at times conflict during the course of the group's existence. Originally tightly geared to offering patients help dealing with the management of the illness, medical treatment, family and interpersonal relationships, the hospital system, and vocational concerns, the focus shifted at one point to more social change kinds of issues. This posed a threat to the group. It polarized some patients who wanted to relate only to personal, coping issues, and others who did not want to hear or share problems but to struggle for change in delivery of hospital services. A common denominator, however, throughout this period was the role in helping patients look at typical response patterns — their tendency to feel helpless, their overwhelming anger and fear of reprisal. Patients learned to look at next steps, consider consequences, anticipate renewed efforts, and plan to further their own aims. It was essential to mediate between both pulls in the group, and to recognize the need for personal change and social action as an integrated process for people who have chronic illness and long-term dependencies on medical institutions (Sharma, 1985).

An important goal is to encourage group members develop more adequate communication and problem solving with other important people in their environments (McGrath, 1984). Group members clearly develop better communication and problem-solving skills. Aspects of relationship building are enhanced. Health education has become increasingly valued by group members who actively seek more substantial information.

Contract

Patients are identified as having the ongoing task of managing a chronic and stressful illness which affects every aspect of their lives. How they manage will determine to some extent the degree of their disability and the number of problematic respiratory episodes. The agreement is that, in a group context, they can share concerns, work on them in a mutual and reciprocal way, and identify together how each of them might cope with aspects of their illness with greater control and effectiveness. This broad promise of self-change and systems change is broken down into specific issues that patients are grappling with in their day-to-day lives.

An important aspect of the agreement is the affirmation of the social work role as helper, mediator, and enabler. The ongoing contract is redefined as the group process evolves so that it remains sharpened, continually significant, and mutually agreed upon (Toseland and Hacker, 1985).

Meeting Place

The meeting place has shifted from year to year. For the monthly group now in a large assembly room, it feels too empty and anonymous. Its separateness from where medical treatment is taking place creates a sense of isolation and disconnection. At the same time it might be supporting increased independence. As staff assess recent problems in assuring the vitality of the group, one question is the effect on the group of where it is meeting and whether the separation in spirit and location from the clinic is dulling the purpose and ongoing work of the group. The weekly group of more disabled and needy patients has a more intimate setting which has contributed to greater group cohesion.

Use of Time

Most group meetings last approximately one and a half hours. The patients move very slowly, making for longer beginnings and endings for each session.

Although open to changing membership, the group has maintained some members for many years. This has led to questions of how valid and helpful such an open-ended membership and an open-ended duration are for this population. One problem associated with a long-term group is the tendency to slide into ritual and away from content. As this group now is being called upon to examine its very existence, differing stakes in continuity become apparent and must be discussed and resolved (Luft, 1984).

TREATMENT MODALITY AND STANCE OF THE SOCIAL WORKER

The group approach is based on a mediating role for the social worker. Because of a strong systems orientation, the group is viewed as a system designed to encourage mutual help (Gitterman and Germain, 1980). This system interacts within itself and interacts as well with other systems. This interactional approach assumes that the patients together have real work to do in modifying their feelings, thinking, and actions. The social worker's primary concerns are a focus on the here-and-now orientation and on how the group process is unfolding to permit a deepening of the work. The social worker is attuned to issues of commonality and specificity, to feelings and their ambivalence, to content and affect, to challenging the group members to tune in, to speak, to hear, and to respond. The agenda and the work belong to the group, but the social worker is there as a catalyst, an integrator, and a reflector of the group process ready to encourage unspoken thoughts, to both narrow and deepen the content, to search for affect, and offer respect and protection. In this sense, the role is very active (Garvin, 1983).

Outside Resources

Emphysema patients require a vast array of services, from financial help to job counseling to changes in living arrangements. Although the Veterans Administration offers benefits counselors, there are state and city programs which social workers have the best knowledge of and access to. The social work role is one of helping patients to consider all available options and to enhance their ability to seek the kinds of assistance needed. How much the social worker directly intervenes depends on a judgment regarding the patient's and family's abilities to intervene on their own behalf, and how difficult it is to obtain a response from a particular agency or program.

Patients require different degrees of help with concrete planning. Skill is crucial in helping the patient assert himself without either making him feel impotent or abandoning him to forces beyond his ability to manage.

Reassessment and Transfer or Termination

Reassessment of the group is in process. As medical wards are more geared to general medical diagnoses, the specific identification of this population is harder. There is a need in the monthly group to reconnect the patient to his medical treatment to achieve a more dynamic interplay.

We have not yet sufficiently focused on the new emphysema patient, at the very beginning of what will be an ongoing, disabling process. As the program continued over the years, it emphasized perhaps too much the long-term patient or the very ill patient rather than the newly diagnosed one. The struggle over specific, time-limited, goal-oriented services continues as we feel pulled between the long-term, ongoing needs of patients and the demand on us to hone in on the critical issues with which we can be most effective. Various ongoing management issues will affect our practice as we are required more and more to address outcomes and goal achievement. The role of quality assurance programs and cost-containment pressures will increase and we will be compelled by our own profession and regulatory agencies to document, account for our work, and audit our outcomes. As we look at beginnings, middles, and endings in our services to patients, we find that these definitions require a constant assuring of meaningful purpose and process. As reassessment takes place, termination will be a necessary outgrowth, if not for the group itself, perhaps for some members. Termination for the group will be based on how well it is serving a real and needed purpose, whether its purpose can change to meet changing needs and whether its purpose meshes with agency goals and sanction. For some patients, the process of the group may not meet their ongoing needs and together those patients and staff will have to consider what service might be offered which would make sense for them. This will be a challenge to identify what is happening, what the remaining needs are and how we can respond to them.

DIFFERENTIAL DISCUSSION

In keeping with the view that social work practice and medical treatment in a hospital should be integrated, one might have reassessed the purpose and life of the ongoing monthly group when it became fragmented from the emphysema clinic. If the social work role is defined as mediating between systems, one might ask whether the internal system of the group began to spin off from the larger system of medical care for which the patient was presumably coming to the hospital. Maintaining connective links is very hard work and there is some wish at times to provide one's own separate service. This understandable wish needs to be addressed when it runs the risk of becoming dysfunctional.

Time-limited and goal-oriented services in the face of chronic and debilitating illness call for difficult decision making. Defining the immediate and more urgent problems within this population must be continually grappled with. Along the way, the needs of this population can be asserted in ways which will interest the institution and which will help define meaningful work for the patients.

More structured short-term goals might be considered which offer the newly diagnosed patient an opportunity to learn how to manage his illness and deal with adjustment concerns. Patient education for the more chronic patients might deal with needs for refresher courses and would be even more useful if coupled with a helping experience tied to concerns about reduced functioning. For the end-stage patient, close medical follow-up, the meeting of increased dependency needs and a socialization experience would be especially helpful (Mailick, 1979).

Patients also need opportunities to teach others, to volunteer their services, and to be more than consumers and passive recipients of services. This calls on the social worker not to be all things for all patients, not to accept the provision of a service because it is in place, but to imaginatively examine patients needs, agency purpose and scope, and perhaps, most important of all, to be open to expand the kinds of clinical and program skills which can enhance the work.

PRACTICE IN CONTEXT

Decisions hospital social work departments make about how to carve out and integrate social work practice are becoming increasingly more deliberate and connected to larger hospital goals. The demand in social work to play a vital role in the life of the institution places on the profession the responsibility to offer a focused, goal-oriented service capable of measurement and explicit articulation. The visibility of programs and the support they have from the administration and the medical services are crucial to our vitality within the institution. The creativity and challenge comes with translating patient needs in a context to which the institution can lend its sanction, feel a stake, and be encouraged to offer backing and commitment (Bergman, 1984).

REFERENCES

"Administration assault on VA benefits and services." *Disabled American Veterans News*, 1, Winter 1985.

Beck, R.B. and Drachman, D. "Hospital social workers and self-help groups." *Health and Social Work*, 10(2), Spring 1985, pp. 95-103.

Bergman, A.S., Contro, N. and Zivetz, N. "Clinical social work in a medical setting." *Social Work in Health Care*, 9(3), 1984, pp. 1-12.

Black, R.B., Durnan, D.H. and Allegrante, J.P. "Challenges in developing health promotion services for the chronically ill." *Social Work*, 31(4), 1986, pp. 287-293.

Foster, Z. and Mendel, S. "Mutual-help group for patients: Taking steps toward change." *Health and Social Work*, 4, 1979, pp. 82-98.

Gartner, A. and Reissman, F. (eds.). *The self-help revolution*. N.Y.: Human Sciences Press, 1984.

Garvin, C.D. "Theory of group approaches." In *Handbook of clinical social work*, A. Rosenblatt and D. Waldfogel (eds.). San Francisco: Jossey-Bass, 1983, pp. 155-175.

Gitterman, A. and Germain, C.B. *The life model of social work practice*. N.Y.: Columbia University Press, 1980.

Hardilar, P. and Tod, V. "Social work and chronic illness." *British Journal of Social Work*, 12(6), 1982, pp. 639-667.

Hundson, S. "The impact of illness on patients and families: Social workers teach medical students." *Social Work in Health Care*, 10(2), 1984, pp. 41-52.

Kerson, R.S. with Kerson, L.A. "Respiratory diseases. In *Understanding chronic illness*. N.Y.: Free Press, 1985, pp. 187-219.

Lange, M.E. and Wolf, A. *Promoting community health through innovative hospital-based programs*. Chicago: American Hospital Pub., Inc., 1984.

Lock, S. "Self-help groups: The fourth estate in medicine." *British Medical Journal* (Clinical Research), 293, Dec. 20-27, 1986, pp. 1596-1600.

Luft, J. *Group Processes: An introduction to group dynamics*, 3rd ed. Palo Alto: Mayfield Pub. Co., 1984.

Mailick, M. "The impact of severe illness on the individual and family: An overview." *Social Work in Health Care*, 5(2), 1979, pp. 117-125.

McGrath, J. *Groups: Interaction and performance*. Englewood Cliffs, N.J.: Prentice-Hall, 1984.

Page, W. F. "Why veterans choose VA hospitalization: A multivariate model." *Medical Care*, 20(3), 1982, pp. 308-320.

Pancoast, D., Parker, P. and Froland, C. (eds.). *Rediscovering self-help: Its role in social care*. Beverly Hills, CA: Sage Publications, 1983.

Parry, J. and Kahn, N. "Group work with emphysema patients." *Social Work in Health Care*, 1(1), 1975, pp. 55-64.

Petty, T.L. and Nett, L.M. *Enjoying life with emphysema*. Philadelphia: Lea & Febiger, 1984.

Reed, B.G. "Women leaders in small groups: Social-psychological perspectives and strategies." *Social Work with Groups*, 6(3/4), 1983, pp. 35-42.

Remine, D., Rice, R.M. and Ross, J. *Self-help groups and human service agencies: How they work together*. N.Y.: Family Service America, 1984.

Rossner, R. et al. "Breathlessness and psychiatric morbidity in chronic bronchitis and emphysema: A study of psychotherapeutic management." *Psychological Medicine*, 13(1), Feb. 1983, pp. 93-110.

Rothman, G. and Becerra, R.M. "Veterans and veterans' services." In *Encyclopedia of social work*, 18th ed., A. Minahan (ed.). Silver Spring, MD: NASW, 1987, pp. 809-817.

Schuman, E. and Cohen, A.B. "Effective therapy for chronic bronchitis and emphysema." *Geriatrics*, 37(9), Sept. 1982, pp. 74-76.

Selecky, P.A. (ed.). *Pulmonary disease*. N.Y.: John Wiley & Sons, 1982.

Sharma, S.K. " A study of chronic disease and family burden." Maryland, Ph.D. dissertation, January 1985.

Silverman, P.R. *Mutual help groups: Organization and development*. Beverly Hills, CA: Sage Publications, Inc., 1980.

Silverman, P.R. and Smith, D. "Helping in mutual help groups for the physically disabled." In *The self-help revolution*, A. Gartner and F. Reissman (eds.). N.Y.: Human Sciences Press, 1984, pp. 73-93.

Strauss, A. and Glaser, B.G. *Chronic illness and the quality of life*. St. Louis: C.V. Mosby, 1984.

Toseland, R. and Rivas, R. *An introduction to group work practice*. N.Y.: Mac-Millan Pub. Co., 1984.

Weiner, H. "An integrated model of health, illness, and disease." *Health and Social Work*, 9(4), 1984, pp. 253-260.

_____. "Group work and the interdisciplinary approach." *Social Work*, 3(7), 1958, pp. 76-82.

Discharge Planning:
Acute Medical Service

Toba Schwaber Kerson
Joan D. Zelinka

DESCRIPTION OF THE SETTING

The Service is a unit of the Francis Scott Key Medical Center, a private, non-profit, 339 bed teaching hospital within the Johns Hopkins Medical System. Sharing the grounds is a chronic hospital/nursing home with 222 beds. The hospital is located in an urban, industrialized section of the city whose population is predominantly white, blue-collar and ethnically identified.

Policy

In 1983, in order to halt the imminent bankruptcy of Medicare, the Health Care Financing Administration altered the basis for determining the ways in which hospitals are reimbursed for inpatient care. In the Tax Equity and Fiscal Responsibility Act, reimbursement changed from fee-for-service to a prospective payment system (Tax Equity and Responsibility Act, 1983). "Under this system a hospital is reimbursed a preestablished amount based on a series of calculations used to compute the average cost of care for patients with similar conditions and treatments. These conditions and treatments are defined as a set of mutually exclusive categories called diagnosis-related groups, or DRGs" (Graves, 1987; Caputi and Heiss, 1984; Vladeck, 1984a; Vladeck, 1984b; Haley, 1981).

"The primary objective in the construction of DRGs was a definition of case type, each of which could be expected to receive similar outputs or services from a hospital" (Fetter, R.B. et al., 1980). This approach to financing operates on the assumption that patients with similar medical conditions should receive similar care and use approximately the same resources. Even if there is variation in use of services within a diagnosis-related group, the variation is expected to balance out over the total range of patients.

Payment is calculated by a formula in which DRG weight multiplied by dollar rate equals prospective payment. Weights are statistically determined and based on the resource use of a particular illness. The highest weight is 6.8631 for DRG 457 (extensive burns); the lowest weight assigned for DRG 382, false labor, is 0.1842. The dollar rate is based in another formula related to hospital characteristics (Shanko, 1984; Shaffer, 1984). Prior to 1986, the rate was calculated based on regional rates and specific types of hospital costs. As of October 1, 1986, Medicare determined the reimbursement based only on geography and rural or urban location. The health characteristics of the area's patients and teaching status will no longer be included in the analysis (Dolenc and Dougherty, 1985; Mintzer, 1981). DRGs and the relative cost weights are subject to modification, and current DRGs and relative cost weights are published in the Federal Register.

Basically, the system indicates a prescribed length of stay and a monetary sum for each patient. If a hospital can discharge a patient in a shorter number of days than prescribed, the hospital makes money. If the patient stays in the hospital for additional days beyond the prescribed number, or if cost of care exceeds Medicare reimbursement, the hospital loses money; that is, it has to absorb the costs beyond Medicare payment.

Some have argued that patients are now being discharged "quicker and sicker" (Cahill, 1982; Kelly and Bankhead, 1985; Dolenc, and Dougherty, 1985). Others are concerned that diagnosis-related groups are too broad, imprecise, and do not account for the severity of the specific illness which can dramatically alter the cost of treatment (Kosterlitz, 1985). The system places tremendous strain on the social worker as discharge planner because it does not account for the patient's life situation or the availability of outside resources.

Since the enactment of Medicare (Title XVIII of the Social Security Act) and Medicaid (Title XIX), the federal contribution to hospital reimbursement had risen from 12.9% in 1966 to 41.2% in

1981. The contributions of state and local governments had remained under 15% (McCarthy, 1981). Previously, Medicare reimbursed hospitals for whatever inpatient costs accrued. Aggressive medical interventions, a multitude of tests and longer hospital stays were the norm, although there has been a steady decline in average length of stay in all regions of the country since 1970, with a more precipitous fall beginning in 1980 (Pokras, 1986). Congress hopes that the DRG system will provide the incentive for hospitals to review procedures, curtail costs, and become more efficient.

Medicare, itself, with its system of full day, co-payment day and lifetime reserve coverage is difficult to comprehend. Often, families think that Medicare or another form of insurance will pay the whole bill. Also, they do not understand a hospital's insistence that a patient be discharged because he is no longer covered (Health Care Financing Administration, 1984). This causes resentment, disillusionment and bitterness toward the insurance carrier, the government and especially the hospital and its staff.

If the patient must leave the hospital and cannot live independently, he can be discharged to the care of family members, and/or home care (pp. 373-390), hospice (pp. 449-474) or a nursing home (pp. 411-430, 431-448). Ironically, the Health Care Financing Administration has decreased spending for home care while instituting diagnosis-related groups. Policies effecting discharge to nursing home are becoming more stringent as well. Before 1980, the necessity for treatments such as placement of a feeding tube would automatically obtain a skilled level of care. Now, families can be taught to use feeding tubes so skilled nursing is no longer deemed necessary for those patients. Skilled nursing home beds may be covered for people who need physical therapy after a stroke or care for a sufficiently deep wound or decubitus.

Patients and families are horrified to learn that their insurance does not pay for nursing home care. Before a nursing home grant application can be made to Medical Assistance, the patient must essentially exhaust savings and have no assets. While dealing with disappointment and anger, the social worker must continue to assist the patient and/or family with the application so the best possible care can continue (Abramson, 1985; Roseland and Newan, 1982).

Technology

Most patients on the Service are emergency admissions for a broad spectrum of diagnoses. In addition to helping the patient and family to understand and manage an illness, the social worker is aware of ethical and moral ramifications of intervention (Kerson, 1985; Reamer, 1986). Also, in the last few years, a number of technological interventions such as IV antibiotic therapy, sleep apnea monitors and home ventilators have allowed patients who would have required inpatient care to return home. Each of these innovations requires astute planning and coordination of services (see pp. 373-390).

Organization

Like most hospitals, Key has designated service areas such as medicine, surgery or orthopedics. Each unit has its own permanent nursing staff and social worker and a medical staff comprised of four medical interns who are the primary physicians, two medical residents in supervisory/teaching roles, and one attending physician who rotates monthly through the medical units, coronary care unit and emergency room. If any of the medical areas are filled, a medical patient may "board" in another area. Consequently, although unit space bed capacity for medicine is seventy-four, the census of medical patients has been as high as ninety-five. Knowing the nurses on the "boarding" unit less well can affect discharge planning since often the social worker relies on nursing staff for opinions regarding mental status or other areas of functioning.

The social worker is responsible for discharge planning, some counseling of terminally ill patients and families and educating house staff about social work. Discharge planning has always been a keystone of social work in health care, yet social workers have often denigrated its importance and the skill and creativity which the task requires. In the early days of medical social work, "physicians were concerned about keeping patients on their course of treatment and being sure they had a place to go when they left the hospital. The first function was called follow-up and the second, discharge planning. Social workers became expert in both (Kerson, 1980). In 1952, Ida Cannon referred to discharge planning when she described one of the responsibilities of social work as "clearing the wards," the familiar phrase for keeping the patient population moving and ridding the wards of an accumulation of the sick (Cannon, 1952).

In 1955, Harriett Bartlett suggested,

"Another valuable project would be the re-definition of the concept now known as "discharge planning" which covers an important area of practice in medical social work. The concept itself does not appear adequate and may even have blocked us in a definition of our own role. It is an administrative concept which suggests to physicians and social worker a type of activity far removed from the essential social work approach. Actually, we know better than this from our experience. We are aware that patients referred for "discharge planning" may reveal any type of psychological problem related to their illness, from the simplest to the most complex." (Bartlett, 1955)

Although the profession has not replaced the words *discharge planning*, social work researchers have contributed to the enrichment of the concept and the function (Berkman and Rehr, 1972; 1973; Berkman, Rehr and Rosenberg, 1980; Boone, Coulton and Keller, 1981; Blumenfield and Lowe, 1987). In 1980, in an editorial in *Health and Social Work*, Rosalie Kane said, "those social workers who choose to do discharge planning as a clinical process have the opportunity to help persons make difficult decisions" (Kane, 1980). For me, the social worker's primary contribution to the discharge process is enhancing the participation of patient and family (Abramson, 1988; Cahill, 1982; Schlesinger and Wolock, 1982).

The Department of Social Work has a staff of thirteen full-time, seven part-time Master's Degree social workers, and one full-time Bachelor's Degree social worker, and two employees of the hospital department of transportation. There are also additional social workers assigned to specific programs in the hospital which have their own funding.

After discharge, each intern and resident see patients in the medical house staff clinic unless the patient returns to a private physician. Due to a heavy caseload, follow-up for a social worker on an inpatient medical floor is restricted to telephone contact to monitor community support. Often, post-discharge reports are available at weekly Discharge Planning Rounds attended by unit physicians, nurses, social workers and representatives of the visiting nurse program and other community agencies.

Case Description

Mrs. Moss is an eighty-year-old, widowed black woman, admitted to the inpatient service unit with venous stasis ulcers on her legs and decubiti on her lower back and buttocks. She was referred the day after admission as a possible nursing home candidate because of her perceived inability to care for herself (Kane, 1980; Coulton, 1980; Inui et al., 1981). She could not walk and her wounds needed extensive dressing. Prior to admission, she lived in a high-rise apartment complex for the elderly. Mrs. Moss has many siblings, nieces and nephews with whom she claimed close contact, although almost none visited her in the hospital (Goldberg, 1986).

She loves telling stories about a long work experience which provide insight into her view of life. One set of stories is about a "well-to-do" lady for whom she worked as a domestic who loved her and gave her cash bonuses and clothes. Mrs. Moss raised the lady's children and taught them "lessons of life." Some years later, the lady moved to the West Coast, but Mrs. Moss could not go with her because of family responsibilities. They still correspond, and Mrs. Moss could ask the lady for help at any time, but she would not do that because she didn't want to take advantage of her.

The second story is about Mrs. Moss's caring for her father. The family lived in a rural area, and the sheriff wanted to put her father in a nursing home. Mrs. Moss was adamantly opposed to this and even went to court to tell the judge she would take care of her father. Mrs. Moss's pride at accomplishing this task is mingled with anger at such a suggestion. In great detail, Mrs. Moss describes the way she kept her father clean and comfortable until his death.

Because she talks so much about the past and always steers conversation in that direction, she could appear demented, but she is, in fact, oriented and sharp. Part of the message she communicates in her stories is her independent nature and unwavering ability to accomplish her goals. Her determination gives her strength but could be frustrating for staff.

Until very recently, Mrs. Moss has tried to provide total care for one of her sisters who lives next door to her and is bedridden as the result of a series of strokes. Another sister had been placed in a nursing home by her daughter and subsequently died there. Mrs. Moss has never forgiven her niece for not letting her care for that sister as she did for her father and blames the nursing home for her sister's death. A friend, Mr. Frank, is an insurance agent and has helped the two sisters over the years. More reliable than the family, he arranged for home care when Mrs. Moss could not manage (Taylor and Chatters, 1986).

DECISIONS ABOUT PRACTICE

Definition of the Client

A childless widow, Mrs. Moss has none of the family members usually consulted in decision making (Proheska and McCauley, 1983). Alert, she communicates effectively. Her sister is too debilitated to participate, and although Mr. Frank was contacted frequently, Mrs. Moss made it clear that she would make her own decisions.

Goals

On the service, goals are established by various specialties and levels of authority (Schreiber, 1981; Granite, 1981). Sometimes, the goals set by one person can conflict with those set by another (Lindberg and Coulton, 1980; Simmons, 1986; Bennett and Beckerman, 1986). In Mrs. Moss's case, the physician referred Mrs. Moss for nursing home placement. Agreeing with the physician, the home health agency said Mrs. Moss needed more intensive care than they could provide. The physical therapist's goal was unassisted ambulation prior to discharge. Mrs. Moss's emphatic and persistent goal was to return home with assistance from the home health agency. My professional goal was ultimately incompatible with the organizational goal, creating an obvious value dilemma

(Abramson, 1981; Blumenfield and Lowe, 1987). As a representative of the hospital, I wanted to arrange the safest possible environment for Mrs. Moss. It was clear, as far as her physical health was concerned, that this would mean a nursing home. Professional ethics instill a belief in the patient's right to self-determination (Robinson and Barbaccia, 1982).

Initially, although I believed that Mrs. Moss would never consider even a temporary placement, I was sufficiently worried about her poor physical condition that I found myself advocating for the physician's goal. I spoke to her about the difference between an acute and chronic hospital, the temporary nature of the nursing home placement (until the ulcers healed), and the need to consider all of the alternatives to make the most informed decision (Abramson, 1985). Though Mrs. Moss listened politely and voiced appreciation for my time and concern, she never wavered in her decision.

Once I presented the information, and she remained adamant, I told her I would be her advocate. She was my client, and while it was my responsibility to help her understand alternatives, it was critical that I allow her to set the goal of my work with her. Our joint goal would be discharge back to her home (Sager, 1982; Kaye, 1985).

Contract

Divergent goals made contracting difficult. In the beginning of our relationship, I tried to establish a contract based on providing Mrs. Moss with alternatives so she could make the best decision. She "heard me out," but did not accept this contract. Only after I made it clear that I would support her desire to go home did we come to any active agreement.

Meeting Place

In hospitals, private space is at a premium so the choice of meeting place is limited. The social work offices which afford some privacy are far from the medical floors. Privacy is difficult to arrange in a four bed room. Though curtains can be drawn around a bed, they are designed to restrict vision, not hearing. If a patient has a hearing problem and is confined to bed, privacy is next to impossible. Consequently, the public nature of the social worker's visit sometimes affects the relationship. When I must work with a patient under those circumstances, I draw the curtains, focus entirely on my client and try to have the client do likewise. Even if we have to be overheard, we can create an important space for our work.

When family members or friends are involved, and I leave with them, I always tell my patient where I am going and what I am going to discuss. When the meeting with relatives is over, I go back to discuss that meeting with the patient. Without this attention, the patient feels she has no part in decision making (Abramson, 1985). With Mrs. Moss virtually every meeting occurred at bedside. She thrived on attention and loved being in a four bed room where people could see her visitors. To her, multiple visits from many hospital staff meant increased status. Although she left the unit for physical therapy, it never seemed necessary to either of us to have her travel from her room to my office, four floors and two wings away. When I acted to minimize the lack of privacy, Mrs. Moss gave me her attention. She and I discussed all my conversations with Mr. Frank and the home health nurse. She seemed pleased that nothing was being kept from her.

Use of Time

The duration of the relationship is determined by the length of hospital stay, which is determined by the patient's physical state and DRG. If the patient is quite ill or has had major surgery, general anaesthesia or particularly uncomfortable diagnostic tests or treatment, I do no more than greet her until she is able to participate in the relationship. In the same way, I am aware of the unit routine and try to avoid seeing patients during the nurses' morning work rounds or at mealtimes. Sometimes, attendants interrupt an interview to take the patient to physical therapy or radiology. It is often necessary to negotiate with other staff for time.

Time was an issue with Mrs. Moss because she wanted to talk so much. Her storytelling helped me to understand what was important to her, but later I had to structure each interview by stating the reason for my visit and how much time I could spend, without being rude and damaging the relationship. Once our goals had converged,

Mrs. Moss was less inclined to ramble. I realized she used this technique to control and assess people.

Treatment Modality

Drawing from the range of frequently cited treatment modalities, crisis intervention and problem solving best fit the constraints of my practice. Crisis intervention techniques help assess a patient's reaction to highly stressful situations (Burgess and Baldwin, 1981; Madonia, 1984; Golan, 1987). I generally ask my client what happened to her and why she was admitted to the hospital. A patient's description of her experience provides information about her way of handling stress, perception of illness and mental status. Mrs. Moss went into vivid detail about the size, shape, smell, and quality of drainage of her leg ulcers. While trying to control my stomach, I realized she was being very calm about a situation that would have made me hysterical. In a matter-of-fact way, Mrs. Moss explained the way in which she had been trying to keep her legs clean. As her condition worsened, she finally realized that she had to come to the hospital. The crisis intervention model provided me with a tool to evaluate the way Mrs. Moss negotiated between externalities and her self. Hearing about her present and past patterns helped me to predict how she would manage future events. The problem solving model emphasizes client responsibility and thus contributes to an understanding of issues regarding patient compliance with medical regimen (Reid, 1987). Because Mrs. Moss was unwilling or unable to define a problem on any but the most concrete level, we worked on that level only.

The primary treatment method is discharge planning. Discharge planning can be seen as a task or method. The Society for Hospital Social Work Directors defines it as follows:

> Successful discharge planning is a centralized, coordinated, interdisciplinary process that ensures a plan of continuing care for each patient. It reflects both the patient's and family's internal and external social, emotional, medical and psychological needs and assets. It recognizes that the transition from the hospital is often more threatening than the actual hospitalization and that a plan must be developed to both provide for a

continuum of care and address the patient's immediate needs following discharge. It is the clinical process by which health care professionals, patients and families collaborate to ensure that patients have access to services that enable them to regain, maintain, and even improve the level of functioning achieved in the hospital. (Society for Hospital Social Work Directors, 1980)

Here, the social worker engages the patient/family in considering available options, accounting for physical, social and emotional needs by collecting pertinent information about the patient's functional abilities, physical condition, social situation and emotional status. Options may include return to the prior situation, increased assistance from family/friends, development of formal home care, or a variety of institutional options such as nursing home, rehabilitation hospital, boarding home or hospice (Abramson, 1985).

The nursing home option requires the most profound alterations in the person's life (Hunt and Hunt, 1983; Mirotznik and Ruskin, 1984). For the last twenty years, studies have demonstrated that relocation of the elderly depends on the characteristics of the people moved, the reasons for the move, the process of determining how the move would be made and the ability of the people to predict and exercise control over events (Brody, 1975; Schulz and Brenner, 1977; Mirotznik and Ruskin, 1984; Hunt and Hunt, 1982). Enhanced control and predictability have made for more positive outcomes in other studies as well (Mercer and Kane, 1979; Slivinske and Fitch, 1984).

Stance of the Social Worker

In the beginning, an awareness of Mrs. Moss's need to control what was happening to her caused me to take a passive stance, to listen and ask questions as if we were having a conversation rather than an interview. As soon as Mrs. Moss was admitted to the hospital, her friend Mr. Frank made arrangements for her sister, Mrs. Rogers, to be placed in a nursing home. Mr. Frank discussed this with Mrs. Moss. When I talked to her about the placement, she explained that she had let her sister be put in a nursing home, and her sister would return home when she did. Then I became more active, pointing out the realities of Mrs. Moss's living alone, cooking for herself and caring for her sister (Dawson et al., 1984; McPhee et al., 1983). I reviewed every aspect of daily living that I could imagine, but Mrs. Moss had an answer for every possibility, usually involving the home health agency. Her final answer was, "It's better to die at home in your own bed than in a nursing home, and I'm ready when God calls me." Mrs. Moss also responded positively to my crediting her with being able to solve problems.

Outside Resources

The visiting nurse and home health aide were critical in Mrs. Moss's care. From the time of admission, agency personnel were clear that they could not manage Mrs. Moss's total needs and that, at least temporarily, she would have to go to a nursing home. Although the hospital understood and even supported the agency's point of view, we could neither force Mrs. Moss into a nursing home nor keep her in the hospital. Finally, we decided that if the agency could not provide service, and the agency retained that choice, we would be forced to refer Mrs. Moss to another home health agency. In the end, the agency agreed to continue providing her with such care as it could.

REASSESSMENT

The reassessment of goals has been discussed. The other area of reassessment relates to Mrs. Moss's additional admission diagnosis of dementia (Kerson, 1985). Although I believe that she is not demented, her unrealistic view of her physical state caused staff members to question her competence, and I have concluded that she was using denial to defend against her unacceptable reality.

Termination

Basically, Mrs. Moss and I terminated our relationship when she was discharged from the hospital. Her discharge date was set, Mr. Frank was notified in advance and arranged transportation, and the home health agency began visiting the next day. I made one follow-up phone call to Mrs. Moss to be sure the arrangements were in place and she knew the hospital was concerned about her well-being. If she is readmitted, I will again be her social worker (Zook, 1980; Gooding and Jette, 1985).

Case Conclusion

Mrs. Moss has remained at home approximately six weeks since discharge. Initially, a nurse visited five days a week to care for the dressings on her legs. An aide was trained to change the dressings, and she visits seven days a week. The ulcers and decubiti are remarkably improved, Mrs. Moss is walking unassisted with a walker, and her sister remains in a nursing home. Mr. Frank continues to provide some assistance, and Mrs. Moss's future in her own home is secure, at least for the present.

Differential Discussion

The process might have been smoother had I immediately accepted Mrs. Moss's goal of returning to her home and her view of the permanence of nursing home placement. It is also important to note that Mrs. Moss did not have any medical setbacks during her stay, such as a hospital-acquired (nosocomial) pneumonia or infection to her wounds. If she had, the outcome may have been different (Kane, Matthias, and Sampson, 1983).

PRACTICE IN CONTEXT

Policy has the greatest effect on Mrs. Moss's care. DRGs have placed staff and patient under enormous time constraints. The DRGs reaffirm the medical model in hospital-based social service delivery. Physiology and disease etiology are the basis of treatment, while the psychosocial components of health and illness are devalued or excluded (Caputi, 1984). The degree to which third-party payers cover community-based support services often severely limits choices (Marcus, 1987). Mrs. Moss was aware of the limits of her coverage. In fact, the burden of getting home before her coverage expired often interfered with her ability to plan realistically. At times, she could only think about her hospital bill. Anything was better than receiving a bill she could not pay.

Mrs. Moss's hospital course was also affected by the hospital's organization. Because she was admitted at the end of the month, she was in the hospital during a change in rotation. Although this did not seem to affect her medical care, it did interfere with discharge plans. The new team of physicians had to be convinced that Mrs. Moss was not demented. Since a physician is the only one who can order a date of discharge, and the hospital is legally bound to offer a sound discharge plan, the time it took me to convince the new team of Mrs. Moss's competence probably allowed her more time in the hospital and therefore more days of physical therapy than she might otherwise have had. For her, this proved to be advantageous.

Profession in Context

DRG policy and hospitals' resultant concern about discharge planning also presents a great opportunity for social work. Efficient, productive and well organized discharge planning can strengthen the role of social work and have a positive impact on care (Dinerman, Scater and Schlesinger, 1986). Social work must remain mindful of the patient's right to self-determination (Abramson, 1985), the criteria used to distribute services, and the possible tendency of hospitals to provide care for people solely on their ability to pay once DRG limits are reached (Reamer, 1985; Veatch, 1986). As hospitals continue in their endeavor to discharge patients quickly and effectively, it will be possible for social work departments to document their effectiveness in planning discharge and to increase their value in the eyes of the hospital (Coulton, 1984; Ranch and Schreiber, 1985; Packner and Wattenberg, 1985).

REFERENCES

Abramson, J. "Participation of Elderly Patients in Discharge Planning: Is Self-Determination a Reality?" *Social Work*, 33(5), September-October 1988, pp. 443-448.
Abramson, M. "Ethical dilemmas for social workers in discharge planning." *Social Work in Health Care*, 6(4), Fall 1981, pp. 33-42.
American Hospital Association. *Guidelines on discharge planning*. Chicago: Author, 1984.

Bartlett, H.M. "Fifty years of social work in a medical setting: Past significance and future outlook." *Fiftieth Anniversary Celebration: Social Service Department, Massachusetts General Hospital*. Boston: Social Service Department, Massachusetts General Hospital, 1955, p. 213.

Bennett, C. and Beckerman, N. "The drama of discharge: Worker/supervisor perspectives." *Social Work in Health Care*, 11(3), Spring 1986, pp. 1-8.

Berkman, B. "Social work and the challenge of the DRGs" (Editorial), *Health and Social Work*, 9(1), Winter 1984, pp. 2-3.

Berkman, B.G. and Rehr, H. "The 'sick role' cycle and the timing of social work intervention." *Social Work Review*, December 1972, pp. 567-580.

_____. "Early social service case finding for hospitalized patients: An experiment." *Social Service Review*, 47, June 1973, pp. 256-265.

_____ and Rosenberg, G. "A social work department develops a screening mechanism to identify high risk situations." *Social Work in Health Care*, 5, 1980, pp. 373-385.

Blazyk, S. and Caravan, G. "Therapeutic aspects of discharge planning." *Social Work*, 30(6), Nov./Dec. 1985, pp. 489-496.

Blumenfield, S. and Lowe, J.I. "A template for analyzing ethical dilemmas in discharge planning." *Health and Social Work*, 12(1), Winter 1987, pp. 47-56.

Bonander, E.E. "Comprehensive assessment: The heart of discharge planning: A social work perspective." *Discharge Planning Update*, 1(2), pp. 6-8.

Boone, C.R., Coulton, C.J. and Keller, S.M. "The impact of early and comprehensive social work services on length of stay." *Social Work in Health Care*, 7, Fall 1981, pp. 1-9.

Burgess, A.N. and Baldwin, B.A. *Crisis intervention theory and practice: A clinical handbook*. Englewood Cliffs, N.J.: Prentice Hall, 1981.

Cahill, T.I. "Prospective reimbursement: Its effect on discharge planning services." *Discharge Planning Update*, Fall 1982, pp. 14-16.

Caputi, M.A. and Heiss, W.A. " The DRG revolution." *Health and Social Work*, 9(1), Winter 1984, pp. 5-12.

Coulton, C. "Social worker in discharge planning." *Social Work*, 25(1), 1980, pp. 81-82.

_____. "Confronting perspective payment: Requirements for an information system." *Health and Social Work*, 9(1), Winter 1984, pp. 13-24.

_____ et al. "Discharge planning and decision-making." *Health and Social Work*, 7(4), Fall 1982, pp. 253-261.

Dawson, D., Hendershot, G. and Fulton, J. "Aging in the eighties: Functional limitations of individuals age 65 years and over." *Advance Data: Vital and Health Statistics*, 133, June 1987.

Dinerman, M., Seaton, R. and Schlesinger, E.G. "Surviving DRG's: New Jersey's social work experience with prospective payments." *Social Work in Health Care*, 12(1), Fall 1986, pp. 103-113.

Dolenc, D.A. and Dougherty, C.J. "Drugs: The counter-revolution in financing health care." *Hastings Center Report*, 15(3), June 1985, pp. 19-28.

Fromstern, R.M. and Churchill, J.G. *Psychosocial intervention for hospital discharge planning*. Springfield, IL: Chas. C Thomas, 1982.

Golan, N. "Crisis intervention." In *Encyclopedia of Social Work*, 18th ed., A. Minahan (ed.). Silver Spring, MD: NASW, 1987, pp. 360-372.

Goldberg, G.S. et al. "Spouseless, childless elderly women and their social supports." *Social Work*, 31(2), March/April 1986, pp. 104-112.

Gooding, J. and Jette, A. "Hospital readmissions among the elderly." *Journal of the American Geriatrics Society*, 33(9), 1985, pp. 595-601.

Granite, U. "Priorities in discharge planning." *Health and Social Work*, 6(4), 1981, p. 64.

Graves, E.J. "Diagnosis-related groups using data from the national hospital discharge survey: United States, 1985." *Advance Data: Vital and Health Statistics*, 137, July 1987.

Hunt, K. "DRGs: What it is, how it works, and why it will hurt." *Medical Economics*, 5, Sept. 1983, pp. 262-269.

Hunt, M. and Hunt, G. "Simulated site visits in the relocation of older people." *Health and Social Work*, 8(1), 1983, pp. 5-14.

Inui, T.S., Stevenson, K.M., Plorde, D. and Murphy, I. "Identifying hospital patients who need early discharge planning for special dispositions: A comparison of alternatives." *Medical Care*, 19(9), 1981, pp. 922-929.

Johnson, C.L. and Grant, L.A. *The nursing home in American society*. Baltimore: The Johns Hopkins University Press, 1985.

Joseph, E.D., Sandrick, K. and Shannon, K. *A DRG and prospective pricing action plan for social service/discharge planning*. Chicago: Care Communications, Inc., 1983.

Kane, R. "Discharge planning: An undischarged responsibility?" *Health and Social Work*, 5(1), 1980, pp. 2-3.

Kane, R.L., Matthias, R. and Sampson, S. "The risk of nursing home placement after acute hospitalization." *Medical Care*, 21, 1983, pp. 1055-1061.

Kaye, L.W. "Home care for the aged: A fragile partnership." *Social Work*, 30(4), July/Aug. 1985, pp. 312-317.

Kelly, J. and Bankhead, C.D. "DRG's: How are they stacking up?" *Medical World News*, March 1985, pp. 80-103.

Kerson, T.S. with Kerson, L.A. " The dementias." In *Understanding Chronic Illness*. NY: The Free Press, 1985, pp. 71-103.

Kosterlitz, J. "Factoring poverty into DRG formula is troublesome brainteaser for Congress." *National Journal*, 31, Aug. 1985, pp. 1940-1942.

Lindenberg, R. and C. Coulton. "Planning for post-hospital care: A follow-up study." *Health and Social Work*, 5(1), 1980, pp. 45-50.

McPhee, S.J. et al. "Influence of a discharge interview on patient knowledge, compliance, and function status after hospitalization." *Medical Care*, 21, Summer 1983, pp. 755-766.

Madonia, J.F. "Clinical and supervisory aspects of crisis intervention." *Social Casework*, 65(6), 1984, pp. 364-368.

Marcus, L.J. "Discharge planning: An organizational perspective." *Health and Social Work*, 12(1), Winter 1987, pp. 39-46.

Mercer, S. and Kane, R. "Helplessness and hopelessness among the institutionalized aged: An experiment." *Health and Social Work*, 4(1), 1979, pp. 91-115.

Mintzer, J. "Case mix reimbursement: DRG experiment in New Jersey." *Discharge Planning Update*, 1(4), 1981, pp. 5-6.

Mirotznik, J. and Ruskin, A. "Inter-institutional relocation and its effects on health." *The Gerontologist*, 24(3), 1984, pp. 286-291.

Patchner, M.A. and Wattenberg, S.H. "Impact of diagnosis-related groups on hospital social service departments." *Social Work*, 30(3), May/June 1985, pp. 259-261.

Prohaska, T. and McCauley, W. "Role of family care and living arrangements in acute care discharge recommendations." *Journal of Gerontological Social Work*, 5(4), 1983, pp. 67-80.

Rauch, J.B. and Hanita, S. "Discharge planning as a teaching mechanism." *Health and Social Work*, 10(3), Summer 1985, pp. 208-216.

Reamer, F.G. "Facing up to the challenge of DRGs." *Health and Social Work*, 10(2), Spring 1985, pp. 85-94.

———. "The use of modern technology in social work: Ethical dilemmas." *Social Work*, 31(6), Nov./Dec. 1986, pp. 469-472.

Reid, W.J. "Task-centered approach." In *Encyclopedia of Social Work*, 18th ed., A. Minahan (ed.). Silver Spring, MD: NASW, 1987, pp. 757-765.

Robinson, B. and Barbaccia, J. "Acute hospital discharge of older patients and external control." *Home Health Services Quarterly*, 3(1), 1982, pp. 34-57.

Ross, A., III. "Health spending trends in the 1980s: Adjusting to financial incentives." *Health Care Financing Review*, 6(3), 1985, pp. 1-26.

Sayer, A. "Evaluating the home care service needs of the elderly: A research note." *Home Health Care Services Quarterly*, 3(2), 1982, pp. 87-91.

Schilling, R.F. II and Schilling, R.F. "Social work medicine: shared interests." *Social Work*, 32(3), May/June 1987, pp. 231-234.

Schreiber, H. "Discharge-planning: Key to the future of hospital social work." *Health and Social Work*, May 1981, pp. 48-53.

Shanko, R. *Physician's guide to DRG's*. Chicago, IL: Pluribus Press, 1984.

Shaffer, F.A. (ed.). *DRG's charges and challenges*. New York: National League for Nursing, 1984.

Sheehan, S. *Kate Quinton's days*. Boston: Houghton Mifflin Company, 1984.

Simmons, J. "Planning for discharge with the elderly." *Quality Review Bulletin/ Journal of Quality Assurance*, 12(2), 1986.

Taylor, R.J. and Chatters, L.M. "Patterns of informal support to elderly black adults: Family, friends, and church members." *Social Work*, 31(6), Nov./Dec. 1986, pp. 432-438.

Toseland, R.W. and Newan, E. "Admitting applicants to skilled nursing facilities: Social workers' role." *Health and Social Work*, 7(4), Nov. 1982, pp. 262-274.

United States Health Care Financing Administration. *A guide to medicare* (booklet). Washington, D.C.: Government Printing Office, 1984.

Veatch, R.M. "DRGs and the ethical reallocation of resources." *Hastings Center Report*, 16(3), June 1986, pp. 32-40.

Zook, J., Savizkis, S.F. and Moore, F.D. "Repeated hospitalization for the same disease: A multiplier of national health costs." *Milbank Memorial Fund Quarterly*, 5(3), 1980, pp. 454-471.

Part 3

Public Health Services

Maternal and Child Health: Teen Mother-Well Baby Clinic

Toba Schwaber Kerson
Denise DuChainey
Wendy Wollwage Schmid

DESCRIPTION OF THE SETTING

The United States' teen birthrate is higher than most other industrialized countries. More than one million teenage girls, 11% of all adolescents and 30% of all black girls under 19, become pregnant each year. Forty percent of these teenagers have abortions and almost half will keep the baby. Research conducted by the Center for Population Options deduced that, in 1985, public spending on teenage parenthood equalled 16.7 billion dollars (Kosterlitz, 1986). Each year in Philadelphia, approximately 5,000 babies are born to adolescents. An estimated 3,300 of these are non-white births (Junior League, 1986).

In West Philadelphia, pregnant adolescents use the facilities of three interrelated medical institutions: Children's Hospital (CHOP), Hospital of the University of Pennsylvania (HUP) and the Philadelphia Child Guidance Center (CGC). Located in the midst of a large, sprawling, urban university, these institutions are in turn surrounded by a low-income community with some middle-income pockets. All three of the medical facilities are physically connected but fiscally and managerially separate. CHOP is a 238-bed hospital, and HUP, a 694-bed facility. The Philadelphia Child Guidance Clinic is a primarily outpatient facility which provides psychiatric services. The Hospital of the University of Pennsylvania offers comprehensive obstetric and gynecological services to women in the Philadelphia area. In 1967, HUP opened its obstetric teen clinic as the first teen pregnancy program in Philadelphia. In this specialized setting, family planning services and prenatal care are offered to teens aged eighteen and under. In 1979, CHOP, which had always offered general pediatric care to infants of these adolescents, began a special teen mother-well baby clinic, which offered comprehensive care to teen mothers aged eighteen and under.

The primary population served by these programs consists of black teens (90 percent) whose families are supported by grants from the Philadelphia Department of Public Assistance and who live in the southern and western sections of the city. Together, these two programs assist the never-pregnant and pregnant teen, the teen mother, her baby, partner and family. The joint programs offer services of physicians, nurses, social workers, family outreach workers, midwives, and nutritionists. In addition, pregnant adolescents and teen parents are referred to appropriate schools and community agencies for ongoing education, jobs and job training, day care, psychiatric help, financial assistance, and housing resources (Barth and Schinke, 1984).

Public funds allocated for women's health care are distributed through the Family Planning Council of Southeastern Pennsylvania which in turn contracts with numerous organizations throughout the city. In Philadelphia, twenty-four family planning/teen clinics serve approximately 8,000 adolescents a year. Nine of these clinics are located in city health centers; two, in community health centers, and others, at Planned Parenthood and teaching hospitals. Services which are free of charge for adolescents under eighteen are: sex education, contraceptive supplies, gynecological care, pregnancy testing and options counseling (Junior League, 1986).

Policy

In the United States, federal, state, and local public health authorities share responsibility for maternal and child health programs. In 1912, the U.S. Children's Bureau was created to investigate and report on the welfare of children throughout the United States. Infant and maternal mortality rates were found to be related significantly to social and economic factors: the poorer the family, the higher the risk of maternal and infant problems and death. The Maternal and Infancy Act of 1921 (Sheppard-Towner Act), administered by the Children's Bureau, was one of the first grant-in-aid programs in the health field. It laid the groundwork for national maternal and child health programs administered by the states, and set precedents for later federal-state relationships. In 1935, the Social Security Act created the maternal and child health program and the crippled children's program. Grants-in-aid were administered for both programs by the Children's Bureau until 1969, when the Maternal and Child Health Service in the Public Health Service became responsible. At present, administration is by the Bureau of Community Health Services within the Health Services Administration of the Public Health Service of the Department of Health and Human Services (Leukefeld, 1987).

Maternal and child health programs under state administration provide a wide range of services, including child health conferences, school health examinations, health education, sex education, poison control centers, and comprehensive services for teenage pregnancy, narcotics addiction, and child abuse. State maternal and child health staff also generally set standards for hospital maternity and newborn services. In 1952, the first statewide program to coordinate medical and social services for unwed mothers was developed. Now such comprehensive programs are mandated by Title V of the Social Security Act. The federal maternal and child health program relies on local (city and county) health departments to provide services. States focus on providing funds and technical support to local governments.

In 1963, federal legislation created a program of special projects for maternity and infant care. Adolescent pregnancy and early parenthood were considered to be precursors of welfare dependency and poverty (Gilchrist and Schinke, 1983). Hospital based programs and clinics sponsored by the Office of Economic Opportunity provided women in low-income areas with comprehensive maternity care and health care to their infants up to a year old. The projects usually include prenatal care, hospitalization for complications of pregnancy, hospital delivery, postpartum care, family planning, health care of infants, homemaker services, transportation to and from clinics and hospitals and the services of public health educators and other specialists. Linkage between maturity and infant care projects and other community services is encouraged in order to promote comprehensive family health care.

In 1978, Titles VI, VII, and VIII of the Health Services and Centers Amendment created the Office of Adolescent Pregnancy Programs (OAPP) which was responsible for programs related to teenage pregnancy. The goals of the APP were to provide comprehensive services including health, family planning, nutrition, sexual, educational and vocational counseling. Title VI established a grant program to provide comprehensive services for pregnant adolescent parents and to teenagers at risk of pregnancy. Emphasis is on school-aged teens seventeen and under, although projects may serve women up to the age of twenty-one (Moore, 1979). In 1981, the Adolescent Pregnancy Programs (APP) were consolidated into Maternal and Child Health block grant funds. A new Federal initiative, the Adolescent Family Life Program (AFL) was enacted as part of the Omnibus Budget Reconciliation Act of 1981 and incorporated as Title XX of the Public Health Service Act (Monroe, 1987). In 1985, the budget for demonstration projects was $11,243,974 with the range from $40,000 to $408,000, and the average award was $170,000. The 1985 budget for research awards was $1,495,782. Funding for all programs was to continue at the same levels for 1986 and 1987.

AFL legislation, expanding on goals set for Adolescent Pregnancy Programs is concerned with primary and secondary prevention. Primary prevention programs which receive the majority of the funding must provide designated services plus referral to resources for licensed residential care or maternity home services and mental health services. AFL's secondary prevention legislation mandates research toward understanding the causes and consequences of adolescent sexual relations, contraceptive use, pregnancy and child rearing. Research is designed to indicate services which will alleviate negative consequences (Mecklenberg and Thompson, 1983). Because 74% of unmarried adolescents who give birth continue to live with their families, both AFL programs include family members in research and/or treatment plans (U.S. Congress, 1985).

Technology

Adolescent pregnancy often has a poor prognosis. Teen mothers are the group least likely to receive prenatal care. Teenagers under fifteen are two and one-half times as likely as women aged twenty to twenty-four to forego medical attention in the first trimester of pregnancy and four times more likely to avoid prenatal care or wait until the final trimester (Guttmacher, 1981). Pregnant teenagers often experience hypertension, premature labor, and birth injury of their babies due to the mothers' smaller pelvises. They often have poor nutritional habits, smoke and drink, and comply poorly with prenatal health care recommendations. Mothers under fifteen years of age have the highest incidence of low birthweight babies, and a low birthweight places babies at high risk for many developmental problems (Naeye, 1981). Childhood mortality rates, congenital disease and handicaps are all notably higher than average for children of adolescent mothers. Despite an overwhelming amount of data, the primary cause of reproductive disadvantage experienced by teenage mothers and their babies has not yet been determined. At present, the cause appears to be a combination of biological and social factors (Zuckerman, 1983).

In the Philadelphia teen clinics, the pregnant adolescent is followed as a high-risk patient. At HUP, for example, clinic appointments are scheduled every two weeks for the first and second trimester and every week for the third. The patient is invited to attend classes taught by nurses and social workers. If she develops additional physical conditions such as hypertension, she is treated.

Organization

The Hospital of the University of Pennsylvania Obstetrics and Gynecology Department provides gynecological, obstetric, and family planning services. At Children's, the adolescent clinic is available to teens up to the age of nineteen for general medical follow-up, and the teen mother-well baby clinic cares for teen mothers and their babies (up to the age of three) for comprehensive medical care. Both clinics are funded by medical assistance, third-party insurance, and special grant monies.

The social worker in the teen mother-well baby clinic is responsible to the directors of the clinic and of social work. Dual accountability, rather than imposing conflicting standards and goals, actually broadens the social work perspective. The social worker counsels the mother, her family and the father of the baby regarding educational, vocational and financial concerns as well as referral for day care and psychotherapy.

At each clinic visit the teen talks to the social worker and the family nurse-clinician. Her baby is examined by a pediatrician for assessment, preventive health care counseling, and reinforcement of parenting skills. Group meetings scheduled during the visit focus on such topics as safety, growth and development, nutrition, management of episodic illnesses, family/life issues, and telephone and job/interview skills.

The smooth functioning of the teen mother-well baby clinic depends on role flexibility and professional teamwork. In addition to the clinic activity, social work, nursing and secretarial staff provide close supervision which includes reminder phone calls before clinic visits, follow-up phone contact after missed appointments, family and school involvement and community outreach.

Case Description

Ruth is a nineteen-year-old, black mother who was referred to the teen mother-well baby program by HUP's maternity ward clerk. Although Ruth was nineteen at the time of delivery, she was given an appointment because the program was new and uncrowded.

Born when her mother was eighteen, Ruth is the oldest of four children. Her mother and father live together, and the family was and is supported by mother's Aid to Dependent Children grant and father's disability grant. Ruth remembers her father as a heavy drinker who would come home drunk and beat her mother. Ruth's mother started drinking heavily when Ruth was nine, and as a result of mother's drunken scenes, the children were ridiculed in their neighborhood and at school. Consequently, they avoided school whenever possible. According to Ruth, the younger three children were placed in special education classes and still live with their alcoholic parents.

Ruth did well in school but described herself as "always nervous." At the age of twelve, she received Valium at a neighborhood health clinic. At sixteen, Ruth was admitted to the Philadelphia Child Guidance Clinic for depression. She had called the CHOP emergency room frightened that she would kill herself. A month prior to this she had been treated and released at CHOP's emergency room for an overdose of Darvon and penicillin. After a month in the Philadelphia Child Guidance Clinic, Ruth was transferred to a residential facility for emotionally disturbed adolescents where she lived for a year. From that facility, Ruth moved to a halfway house for teens and then back to her mother's home at the age of seventeen.

While attending high school, Ruth lived intermittently with her mother and with her grandfather. When she was in the eleventh grade, she met T.J. who lived in her neighborhood. T.J. was the first male with whom Ruth had a sexual relationship. She had some knowledge of birth control but made no attempt to use contraceptives. "I thought I would not get pregnant," said Ruth, as do many of the teens in the program. Three months after beginning their sexual relationship, Ruth became pregnant. She and T.J. agreed on a therapeutic abortion which was performed at HUP. Ruth claimed she was never counseled on birth control nor given an appointment for the family planning clinic. She did not see a social worker and terminated contact with the counselor at the Philadelphia Child Guidance Clinic. Feeling guilty about the abortion, Ruth became pregnant again within four months. Eight months later, Lee was born.

For the last year and a half, Ruth and T.J. have shared an apartment. T.J. works full-time as a telephone operator. Ruth receives an Aid to Dependent Children grant for herself and her baby and is registered as living at her grandfather's apartment in Philadelphia.

Ruth received prenatal obstetric care at HUP. Because she was eighteen at the time the baby was conceived, she did not participate in their teen prenatal clinic. Her high risk pregnancy was complicated by asthma, neurodermatitis, and pre-eclampsia. When she was twenty-eight weeks pregnant, she was admitted to the hospital for premature labor. After one week of bed rest with no further contractions, she was discharged on oral Vasodilan therapy to reduce premature contractions. At the time of discharge, Ruth was told to return to the high risk clinic every week for the remainder of her pregnancy.

Almost six weeks later, Ruth was admitted in active labor. After twenty-six hours, she delivered a normal, healthy, female infant weighing 6-1/2 pounds by Caesarean section using epidural anesthesia. Her delivery was complicated by pre-eclampsia, a genital tract infection, anemia, and postpartum eclampsia. One week later, Ruth and baby Lee were discharged together in stable condition. A postpartum hospital clinic visit for Ruth was scheduled for one month after delivery.

Ruth and her baby first came to the CHOP teen mother-well baby clinic when the baby was two months old. The delay in contact with the teen clinic was the result of the internal scheduling problems of the new clinic program. As with all teen mothers, Ruth and her baby were seen by a pediatrician, an adolescence nurse, and a social worker. Both the baby and the mother were described by the pediatrician as "hyperirritable." The baby was colicky and fussy. The mother was unusually nervous, talking incessantly and pressing us with her need. We were frankly worried that Ruth could abuse Lee because she repeatedly pointed out that she was stuck with this baby, had no one to help her, and she could not stand the baby's screaming anymore. Ruth's own sense of urgency compounded by her loveless, deprived, and troubled background identified her as "high risk."

Ruth sought help in raising her child. She said, "The worst thing that could happen is that the baby would not be loved enough or could be hurt or be wrongly influenced." In response to this plea, for that is what it was, the pediatrician, the nurse, and the social worker set to work. Ruth was taught swaddling and given ideas on infant care by the pediatrician. Both the nurse and I focused on the situation and the needs of the teen mother. The nurse dealt primarily with family planning and birth control. Ruth's blood pressure was too high (150/92) to allow the use of birth control pills, and she did not seem interested in other available methods. Ruth did intimate an interest in an interuterine device (IUD) but added that she was afraid that it "could hurt or puncture" her. With fears allayed, she kept her appointments at HUP's family planning clinic.

Ruth described herself as a girl who had had many problems in the past. She said her mother was an alcoholic, and she had found it best to stay away because home depressed her and she could do nothing to change it. She implied a past history of emotional problems but did not discuss this in detail. She smiled to express her positive feelings when she talked about T.J.

I was more impressed with Ruth's strength than with her deprivation. She is a fighter. Some staff became irritated with her barging into offices. What they had originally viewed as neediness came to be seen as manipulation. However, I liked the fact that she asked for help and knew how to use it. Ruth used our support to learn to care for herself and her baby. Her being a fighter made me stand beside her and fight along with her when she asked for help.

DECISIONS ABOUT PRACTICE

Definition of the Client

Despite her age, Ruth was accepted as a patient because of her interest in the program and our initial assessment of her as insecure and immature. Ruth as invited to bring her mother and/or T.J. with her to the clinic, but she chose to come alone because both worked during clinic hours. Therefore, services were provided only to Ruth and her baby.

Goals

In the teen mother-well baby clinic at CHOP, goals for each client are determined primarily by the teen mother with the participation of any extended family she wishes to include and of the professional team members (pediatrician, family nurse, clinician, and social worker). At Ruth's initial visit, the team decided to follow her and Lee for at least one year. After that interval, they would be reevaluated and referred for continued care.

To set goals, each professional in the team meets individually with the teen mother. Initial pediatric goals were to help Ruth adjust to motherhood and a fussy baby. The primary nursing goal was to have Ruth practice effective birth control and thereby avoid a third unplanned pregnancy. The social work goals were those to which Ruth had given highest priority: identification of resources for education, job training, day care, counseling, and support (Kraus, 1980). Ruth's first goal was to enroll in a nurse's aide program with supplemental education classes oriented toward a high school equivalency degree, and her second was adequate day-care.

Contract

The contract negotiated with each teen mother is fluid, informal and evolves as goals are met and needs change. Teens' usual lack of predictability also accounts for shifting priorities. In fact, it seems that the younger the teen, the more difficult it is to establish a working contract. Ruth and I contracted to work on her goals.

Meeting Place

The CHOP outpatient clinic area is the primary meeting place for teen mothers and their babies. A crowded corridor is used as a waiting area and, of necessity, as an area of group discussion. The corridor is disliked by staff who must stumble through it, but it encourages informal discussion throughout the afternoon. Individual and small group work occurs in consulting rooms which offer privacy but little else. Ruth was seen in clinic, in the emergency room when the need arose and on an inpatient floor during Lee's one brief hospitalization. When necessary, visits to the homes of our most difficult families are made by a family worker. Family workers can accompany teens to schools, hospitals, or other agencies and help with problem solving.

Use of Time

The teen mother-well baby clinic meets weekly, and routine appointments are scheduled at one to three month intervals for three years. Additional appointments are made as needed for medical, psychosocial, or parenting problems. The teen and the baby are seen by the social worker during any emergency room visits if the teen initiates the contact.

During Lee's first year, Ruth and Lee had six scheduled clinic visits, four emergency room visits for treatment of ear and acute viral infections, and five additional visits. For Ruth, as for many other teens, more visits were needed than originally anticipated by the team at the outset of the program in order to avoid emergency room visits. Frequent telephone contact also was necessary with Ruth until the situation stabilized.

Treatment Modality

The primary treatment modalities are case management and problem solving. Case management here means that the social worker both counsels the client and helps her negotiate other necessary services. The nature of the service means that I also incorporate techniques of crisis intervention, family therapy and behavior modification when such needs arise. Parenting skills are taught by the pediatrician and the social worker using a behavioral modification framework. Deep psychological problems remain and long-term therapy may be useful at some time, but attempts to refer Ruth for psychotherapy evoke a bristling response. Given Ruth's achievements, pressing her about psychotherapy may be deleterious to our relationship.

Stance of the Social Worker

Adolescents benefit most from a direct, honest approach that sets tasks which further the goals they have chosen. Decisions about intervention are difficult. The social worker's degree of activity depends on the teen's problems and variable emotional state. Developmentally, teens are moving from childhood to adulthood, and they vacillate between enjoying the safety of dependence and the pride of accepting adult responsibility. What intervention the teen requires depends on her level of maturity, past life experiences, and family support.

In order to determine the amount of responsibility a teen can assume, I establish a task which she can accomplish unassisted. If she does complete the task, further ones are assigned. Help is offered only when the teen is frustrated, resists, or fails. If the teen cannot complete the tasks, family members or a family worker can assist (Hulbert, 1984).

Self-Disclosure

Ruth and I discussed our parenting experiences and difficulties in coping with a complex medical system. Sharing some of the universal frustrations of parenthood allowed Ruth to describe more of her experiences with Lee. Since I am white, my talking about frustrations with doctors and hospitals empowered Ruth and made her feel less a victim of racial prejudice.

Outside Resources

Nearly all our teen parents need many support services (Barth and Schinke, 1984). Unfortunately, one of the greatest needs, adequate housing, is virtually unattainable for low-income teen parents. Ruth needed little more than a list of service-providing agencies. She could borrow a car and was able to arrange day care and job training herself. I was informed regularly about Lee's day care attendance and progress.

Reassessment

Younger teen parents are far less responsible and independent. Their goals and means of support often remain in flux. Thus, the majority of teen mothers need continuous reassessment. When most are asked, "How are things going?", they close the conversation by answering "Fine." Direct questions around specific issues such a birth control, finances and day care are more effective (O'Leary et al., 1984).

With Ruth, the need for reassessment came on Lee's first birthday. After Ruth received her high school diploma she questioned the necessity for continuing in the clinic. She was then twenty years old, her relationship with T.J. and her emotional state were stable, and she was applying for nurse's aide positions which would make it difficult for her to come in during clinic hours. Also, Ruth used social work and medical services but was uncomfortable in the educational groups because the other mothers were younger.

Transfer or Termination

The clinic commitment to teens is for three years of medical care. Occasionally, patients are transferred because teens request a facility closer to home, or because primary parenting responsibility has been relegated to another family member who wants to use a different facility. At present, Ruth is considering options, and I will remain available until she transfers to a new clinic.

Case Conclusion

After a full year of intensive medical, nursing, and social work intervention, Ruth has attained her educational, training and day-care goals. In addition, she continues a responsible birth control plan and has had no unplanned pregnancies. She has maintained a stable, loving relationship with T.J. and Lee. At age one, Lee is thriving. Ruth successfully coped with several stressful medical emergencies, including Lee's one hospitalization at four and a half months for reaction to pertussis vaccine. Considering her past psychiatric history and personal experience in CHOP's emergency room, these are significant accomplishments. Ruth made full use of clinic resources and in one year moved from tumultuous adolescence to responsible adulthood.

Differential Discussion

Now that the clinic is established, we would not accept someone as old as Ruth. I wonder whether the same investment would have been made elsewhere and whether Ruth would have met her goals. Specifically, in terms of my relationship with Ruth, I do not know what would have happened if I had followed the advice of the rest of the team and insisted that she be sent to a mental health facility for psychotherapy once she had been diagnosed at the Child Guidance Center as having "histrionic character disorder." She may have refused to relate to me or she may have had a positive experience. I think that I correctly focused on Ruth's own goals rather than the goals of the team. Finally, I might have found a way to work with T.J. as well as with Ruth.

PRACTICE IN CONTEXT

The care of low-income adolescent mothers and their children has been variously the responsibility of health care organizations, schools, community mental health workers and local welfare agencies. As more federal and state monies are made available specifically for adolescent mothers and their families, more services and, perhaps more importantly, the rational coordination of services between agencies can be initiated. Policy constraints determine the parameters of available programs, which individual patients must be helped to utilize effectively. Without federal and state supplements to local monies, there can be no programs for this rapidly increasing group of patients in urban America. Formal and informal organization is certainly as important as the constraints of policy in the delivery of patient care. Good care requires intra- and interorganizational professional networks. If individual professionals work in isolation, conflicting messages may confuse the teen mother, who often lacks experience and definitive goals.

As medical technology advances, more pregnant teens can be safely delivered of healthy babies. If advances in social policy were to keep step with those of technology, sex education and family planning concepts would be introduced to students at the grammar school level rather than the senior high school level. Young adolescents can be taught to understand the techniques of birth control and the personal benefits that result from delaying childbearing. Policy, organization, technology, and the individual treatment setting all affect the relationship between medical social worker and teen mother. Advances in medical technology allowed Ruth a safe pregnancy, and the teen mother-well baby clinic helped Ruth to cope with the complexities of contemporary urban hospital systems, to work through the early crises of motherhood, and to reach some important personal goals.

REFERENCES

Badger, E. *Effects of Parent Education Program on Teenage Mothers and Their Offspring*. Cincinnati: University of Cincinnati College of Medicine, 1980.

Barnett, P. and D.W. Balak. Unplanned Pregnancy in Young Women: Managing Treatment. *Social Casework*, 67:484-490, 1986.

Barth, R.P. and Schinke, S. Enhancing the Supports of Teenage Mothers. *Social Casework*, 65: 523-531, 1984.

Brindis, C., Barth, R.P., and A.B. Loomis. Continuous Counseling: Case Management with Teenage Parents. *Social Casework*, 68:164-172, 1987.

Cannon-Boventre, K. and Kahn, J. Interview with Adolescent Parents: Looking at Their Needs, *Children Today*, 17-19, 1979.

Elster, A. and McAnarrey, E.R. Medical and Psychological Risks of Pregnancy and Childbearing During Adolescence. *Pediatric Annals*, 12: 11-20, 1980.

Elster, A., McAnarrey, E.R., and Lamb, M.E. Parental Behavior of Adolescent Mothers. *Pediatrics*, 71:494-503, 1983.

Everett, M. Group Work in the Prenatal Unit. *Health and Social Work*, 5:71-74, 1980.

Furstenberg, F., Brooks-Gunn, J., and Morgan, S.P., *Adolescent Mothers in Later Life*, Cambridge, Cambridge University Press, 1987.

Giblin, P.J. et al. Pregnant Adolescents' Health Information Needs: Implications for Health, Education and Health Seeking. *Journal of Adolescent Health Care*, 7:168-172, 1986.

Gilchrist, L. and Schinke, S.P. Teenage Pregnancy and Public Policy. *Social Service Review*, 57:307-319, 1983.

Goodwin, N.J. Unplanned Adolescent Pregnancy: Challenge for the 1980's. *Journal of Community Health*, 11:6-9, 1986.

Greydanus, D.E. Contraception in Adolescence: An Overview for the Pediatrician. *Pediatrics Annals*, 12:52-66, 1980.

Hall, W.T. and Young, C.L., editors. *Proceedings Health and Social Needs of the Adolescent: Professional Responsibilities*. Pittsburgh: University of Pittsburgh Graduate School of Public Health, 1979.

Heald, F.P. and Jacobson, M.S. Nutritional Needs on the Pregnancy Adolescent, *Pediatric Annals*, 12: 21-31, 1980.

Hulbert, A. Children as Parents. *The New Republic*, 15-23, September 10, 1984.

Junior League of Philadelphia, *Adolescent Pregnancy Child Watch Project*, 1986.

Kosterlitz, J. Split Over Pregnancy. *National Journal*, 25: 1538-41, 1986.

Kraus, L.M. Therapeutic Strategies with Adolescents. *Social Casework*, 16: 313-16, 1980.

Lee, R.S. et al. Neonatal Mortality: An Analysis of the Recent Improvements in the U.S. *American Journal of Public Health*, 60:15-22, 1980.

Leukefeld, C.G. Public Health Services. *Encyclopedia of Social Work*. Minahan, A., ed. Silver Spring, Maryland: National Association of Social Workers, 1987.

Marsiglio, W. and Mott, F.L. The Impact of Sex Education on Sexual Activity, Contraceptive Use and Premarital Pregnancy Among American Teenagers. *Family Planning Perspectives*, 18:151-154, 1986.

Mecklenberg, M.E. and Thompson, P.G. The Adolescent Family Life Program as a Prevention Measure. *Public Health Reports*, 98:21-29, 1983.

Merritt, T.A., Laurence, R.A., and Naeye, R.L. The Infants of Adolescent Mothers. *Pediatric Annals*, 12:32-51, 1980.

Monroe, P.A. Adolescent Pregnancy Legislation: The Application of an Analytic Framework. *Family Relations*, 36:15-21, 1987.

Naeye, R. Causes of Fetal and Neonatal Mortality by Race in a Selected U.S. Population. *American Journal of Public Health*, 69: 857-863, 1979.

Naeye, R. Teenaged and Pre-teenaged Pregnancies: Consequences of the Fetal-Maternal Competition for Nutrients. *Pediatrics*, 67:146-150, 1981.

O'Leary, K.M., Shore, M.F., and Wieder, S. Contacting Pregnancy Adolescents: Are We Missing Cues? *Social Casework*, 64: 297-306, 1984.

U.S. Congress. Select Committee on Children, Youth, and Families. *Teen Pregnancy: What's Being Done?, A State by State Look*. 99th Congress, 1st session, Washington, D.C., Government Printing Office, 1985.

Zuckerberg, B. Neonatal Outcome: Is Adolescent Pregnancy a Risk Factor? *Pediatrics*, 71:489-493, 1983.

Family Planning Agency:
An Unsuccessful Contraceptor

Toba Schwaber Kerson
Helen Peachey

DESCRIPTION OF THE SETTING

Planned Parenthood of Southeastern Pennsylvania (PPSEP) is one of the 188 affiliates of Planned Parenthood Federation of America. One of the ten largest in the federation, it maintains clinics in Delaware, Montgomery, and Philadelphia Counties. PPSEP raises 84% of its $3.4 million annual budget from private funds (47%) and patient fees (37%), and 16% from government grants.

The agency provides medical services which include birth control counseling, pregnancy testing, first-trimester abortions, vasectomies, and infertility evaluations to approximately 49,000 family planning clients each year. Education and training programs are offered for a variety of audiences: health professionals, adolescents, school teachers and counselors, parents, and family planning volunteers. Program topics include such topics as sex education, services for the handicapped, human sexuality, and natural family planning. PPSEP has developed education projects for specific audiences such as "Parents and Teens Together" and "MARCH" ("Men Acting Responsibly for Contraception and Health"). A very active public affairs program publicizes family planning needs, pre-natal education and reproductive health issues.

Family planning services are provided by a team of physicians, nurses and family planning counselors whose goal is to involve the client in her own reproductive health care by providing her with information necessary for making informed decisions. Since many clients served by the agency have no other regular health care, services include some general health screening and education as well.

231

Planned Parenthood serves a relatively young patient population, with 76% of the clients under the age of 24. This population reflects trends in the United States, where two thirds of the twelve million single women who are sexually active are below age twenty-five, and the highest abortion rates are for unmarried, nonwhite women between the ages of eighteen and twenty-four (Henshaw, 1987). Many are postponing their first pregnancies until they have completed their education or until they have become more secure financially. In recent years the agency has made services to teenagers its first priority, and 39% of our clients are under age nineteen (Planned Parenthood, 1985). About half the clients pay a fee for service; the others are funded by Medicaid or by Title XX, a federal funding program which covers the cost of birth control services for any client under 18 years of age or anyone who meets the programs' definition of low income.

Policy

PPSEP is a pioneer in the field of sex education and reproductive health care. The agency opened in 1929 to become the first public resource for contraceptive services in the area. From that time until the present, its activities have often involved controversy.

During its early years, PPSEP provided family planning services despite legal and social deterrents. Sexual concerns were not discussed openly and there was much ignorance about human reproduction. The medical profession considered birth control a social rather than a medical issue and generally was not supportive. The Comstock Law of 1873, in effect until 1970, labeled all contraceptive information as "lewd and lascivious" and made anyone who provided such information liable to fine and imprisonment. The effect of the law was to inhibit the discussion or publication of anything pertaining to contraception.

Between 1929 and the mid-1960s PPSEP was the primary family planning resource in the Philadelphia area for those who could not afford or obtain services from private physicians. Not until 1965 did the federal government make a public commitment to family planning services by providing financial resources. The involvement of other health agencies in the provision of family planning information and services resulted in acceptance and respectability for the family planning movement.

Family planning services to minors without parental consent is another controversial service provided by Planned Parenthood. The startling increase in teenage pregnancy, along with the realization that teenagers have special service needs, resulted in the establishment of a clinic especially for high school and junior high students in 1972. Although parental consent is not required for any services at Planned Parenthood, adult involvement is encouraged. PPSEP's experience in this area of family planning care resulted in gradual involvement by other agencies. In spite of controversies and legal actions, the federal government has also made contraceptive education and birth control services to teenagers a high priority (Freeman, 1987). Since the beginning of the Reagan administration, Congress has continually rejected the proposal that Title X be repealed and family planning services be incorporated under state regulation into block grants along with community health centers, migrant health and black lung programs (AGI, 1985).

Federal funding for family planning services has four sources: Title X of the Public Health Service Act; Maternal and Child Health grants (also part of the Public Health Service); Social Services block grant programs (Titles V and XX of the Social Security Act); and Medicaid (Title XIX of the Social Security Act). Of these funding sources, Title X, administered by the Department of Health and Human Services, is the only federal program specifically directed toward the provision of family planning services. In fiscal year 1985, 333 million federal dollars were spent on contraceptive services and supplies. Medicaid and Title X provided the majority of funds ($137 million and $133 million respectively); $40 million were contributed by the Social Service block grants and $23 million from Maternal and Child Health (Gold and Macias, 1986).

While the provision of birth control services was greatly improved in the 1960s, the social and political climate was less accepting of abortion-related services. In 1970, abortion was legal in only a few states. Public funds could not be used to provide such services as pregnancy testing, problem pregnancy counseling, or abortion. PPSEP became one of the few resources in the area where a woman with an unwanted pregnancy could obtain pregnancy diagnosis and counseling. If she desired, she could be referred to New York City, where the procedure was legal, for a safe abortion at a reasonable cost. In 1973, in Roe vs. Wade, the United States Supreme Court affirmed a woman's constitutional right to choose, in consultation with her physician, whether or not to terminate an unwanted pregnancy. In 1975, the agency opened its own first-trimester abortion service. An important factor in that decision was the belief that involvement in one health setting, which provided abortion, effective birth control services and follow-up, would help the client prevent future unwanted pregnancies.

The Hyde Amendment, implemented in 1977, drastically limited federal assistance with abortion services for poor women. In fiscal year 1985, $66 million was spent on 188,000 subsidized abortions, of which only 1% was provided by the federal government. Federal funds are to be used only where the life of the woman would be endangered if the pregnancy were carried to term. Using their own criteria, a number of states fund abortion services for indigent women. In Pennsylvania, grounds for state funding are life endangerment, rape, and incest (Gold and Marius, 1986). In recent years, many of the agency's public affairs activities have been directed toward maintaining a woman's right to abortion, to resist the well-organized and well-financed attempts to make abortion illegal.

Technology

The development of modern methods of birth control has revolutionized contraceptive practice in the United States. The oral contraceptive, developed in the 1950s, remains a popular option used by more than ten million American women because it is almost 100 percent effective. Safe and simple surgical sterilization of women or their partners is the method used by many married couples in the United States who have the number of children they desire. The intrauterine device (IUD) used by over two million women is controversial because it can cause injury to the woman and fetus. In 1985, the Ortho Pharmaceutical Corporation stopped marketing and distributing their Lippes Loup IUD in the United States. Lippes Loup previously accounted for 31% of IUD sales. In 1986, G.D. Searle and Company also halted its United States distribution of two

IUDs, the Copper 7 and T Cu 200 which accounted for 66% of sales. Primarily, the two companies ceased production of the IUDs because of lawsuits (Forrest, 1986). Presently, the only IUD available to women in the United States is the Alza Progestasert, which previously accounted for only 3% of all IUDs in the U.S. Due to the dramatic fall in the use of the IUD, women have switched to other forms of contraception or remain unprotected (Forrest, 1987).

Although highly effective methods are available, the choice of a suitable contraceptive is difficult. Sterilization must be considered permanent, and many couples cannot be certain that they will want no more children. Although reversal techniques have been developed, they are successful in only a small percentage of cases and involve complicated and expensive surgery.

Research involving women using oral contraceptives indicate that serious side effects of the pill are more common than previously realized. Studies of the Research Council of Great Britain, reported in 1967, brought many of the concerns regarding cardiovascular effects into perspective. In addition, since the pill affects virtually every organ system, complications resulting from long-term use and cumulative effects of the pill could be potentially dangerous. Experience with the IUD has raised concerns regarding the development of pelvic inflammatory disease (PID), which may have much greater than expected incidence. PID can lead to serious health problems and has an effect on future fertility in a certain percentage of women. Many physicians do not consider this method advisable for women who desire future pregnancies (Ory, 1983). Questions regarding the safety and side effects of these methods have resulted in a trend toward older and less effective barrier methods, especially the diaphragm. At PPSEP, 7% of clients used the diaphragm in 1972 compared to 30% in 1979.

One important factor enabling women to rely on less effective contraceptive methods is the availability of abortion, an acceptable alternative for many women who experience a contraceptive failure. The rediscovery of vacuum aspiration in China in 1958 led to its adoption in the West by the late 1960s for terminating first-trimester pregnancies. This simpler method encouraged the development of centers providing outpatient abortions under local anesthesia with few complications or after-effects. The contrast between this procedure and a woman birthing and caring for an unwanted child, going to an illegal abortionist for what may be a dangerous, sometimes unsterile abortion, or trying to abort herself, is sharp and poignant. Such services became widely available in the United States after the 1973 Supreme Court decision (Petchesky, 1984).

Even with advances in technology, family planning workers in the '80s have no ideal method of birth control to offer their clients. Instead, they help each client choose the most suitable method for her present situation by providing information about the advantages and disadvantages of each. Since social and psychological factors require as much consideration as medical factors in that choice, counselors have become an important part of the family planning team (Boston Women's Health Book Collective, 1984).

Organization

Planned Parenthood, with a staff of approximately 160, is governed by a volunteer board of 60 members. New programs and policies must be reviewed and approved by the board prior to enactment. The size of the organization means that ideas for programs and policy decisions usually originate with the executive or management committee rather than with the board as a whole. The executive committee consists of board members who are officers or committee chairpersons. Four key agency staff members, the president, and directors for programs, development, and finance attend executive committee meetings and provide meaningful information and advice. The management committee is composed of a group of staff members who are program or department heads. Program and policy ideas are often referred to various other committees who prepare the working details. Medical programs are the responsibility of the affiliate medical committee, a group of about ten to fifteen board and staff members who are health professionals.

In theory, new programs and policies are determined by the board of directors. In practice, the board often reacts to programs and policies which have been determined by either the Planned Parenthood Federation or by state and federal guidelines. Policies and decisions emanating from these sources can result in conflicts with the agency's own planning. For example, the federation has proposed increasing medical services at a time when the agency's plans call for keeping medical services at a constant level and increasing education and public affairs activities. In addition, at a time when PPSEP has made the availability of abortion a high priority for public affairs activities as well as medical services, the public controversy surrounding the abortion issue has made the federal government hesitant to fund agencies providing these services. This has resulted in financial insecurity for the agency.

Due to the size of PPSEP, its departments (which include education, medicine, public affairs, development and two county divisions) tend to operate quite independently. The medical department at the main clinic consists of approximately thirty-five full- and part-time staff people. Most are female, in their twenties or early thirties, and have had some college or technical training. The staff members work together closely as a team, and their support for each other's personal and professional concerns is remarkable (Joffe, 1986). Many share social as well as professional ties.

This close working relationship allows the staff the opportunity to rely on one another when they encounter difficult counseling situations or find themselves in danger of burn out. It also allows them to share responsibilities for certain tasks. For example, certain members of the clerical staff have been called upon to do counseling, and counselors have been trained to do many medical tasks such as assisting the physician, taking vital signs, and assisting with potential emergencies. Many staff members have undergone special training as options counselors and provide problem pregnancy counseling on a limited basis.

Teamwork and shared responsibilities are especially important at the main clinic because it is the only department involved with providing direct abortion services, and those participating in abortion counseling can experience considerable personal and professional pressures and strain (Joffe, 1986). Each individual involved in the abortion service must examine her beliefs and value dilemmas. She helps clients with any physical, psychological and/or moral discomfort resulting from the procedure. The counselor must also confront the political issues surrounding abortion, including actions of anti-abortion groups and funding problems. Often, she has to defend her beliefs in discussions with family or friends.

One of the most difficult clients for family planning counselors is the poorly motivated contraceptor. When such a client becomes an abortion repeater, counselors can become especially frustrated. The special moral and philosophical issues surrounding abortion demand that the decision to terminate a pregnancy not be taken lightly. An important part of abortion counseling is to provide clients with the information and understanding they need to prevent future unplanned pregnancies. An abortion repeater is an indication of failure; for whatever reasons, the counselor was unable to communicate with that client effectively.

Case Description

Carol Downs is a thirty-three-year old, single, black woman who lives in a small city in suburban Philadelphia with her young daughter. Unable to maintain steady employment, Carol has been on welfare (Aid to Families with Dependent Children) for four or five years. She has an unsettled look about her which is reflected in her manner of dress and her actions. Her make-up is garish and makes her look older. In conversation, she jumps from one subject to another, often contradicts herself, and tends toward gross exaggeration.

Carol has been in contact with PPSEP on and off for about two years. She was a sporadic contraceptive patient at one of the county clinic sites near her home and had been at the main clinic for an abortion about six months before our first meeting. Because she has a reputation for being disruptive during clinic visits, only a few staff members will work with her.

Carol came to the clinic for her second abortion on a day when I was in charge. Because of her reputation for being difficult, I agreed to see her. We met in my office prior to the procedure to review her medical history and discuss her present situation. My goal for our meeting was to be certain Carol had carefully considered the decision to terminate her pregnancy and had sufficient information about the procedure to give informed consent. I was also to review information which might help Carol prevent future unplanned pregnancies.

Carol made it quite clear that she did not want to bother with these formalities and just wanted to get the abortion over with as quickly as possible. She preferred no other involvement with the agency, insinuating that we had provided her with questionable care in the past. Much of this animosity toward us appeared to be caused by a Class IV Pap smear report which Carol had received at the time of her last abortion indicating a possible precancerous condition. Although urged to obtain further evaluation on numerous occasions, Carol refused to do anything about the abnormal Pap smear.

Carol's rationale for the abortion was much the same as it had been six months before, and she appeared firm in her decision. She felt that her partner was not supportive of continuing the pregnancy, that having a baby would make it impossible for her to get a job, and that she could not manage on her welfare payments alone.

Both pregnancies involved the same partner. Although it was difficult to assess their relationship, it appeared that Carol wanted more commitment from this man than she was receiving. She had not informed him about her decision to have an abortion, and it seemed that she had arrived at the decision mainly to punish him for his lack of concern about the pregnancy.

Since Carol was unwilling to get involved in any discussion of her present situation, my role was a supportive one. I felt it important to accept her decision and to make her as comfortable as possible during the procedure. We also explored her contraceptive plans in some detail. Our relationship was a friendly one, and I did not confront Carol or delve into new areas. She came for an abortion, and that was all she wanted.

Carol's mother, a very flamboyant, well-dressed woman, joined her at the clinic while she was waiting for the doctor. Their conversation was loud, friendly, frank and amusing. Mrs. Downs told Carol repeatedly that it was high time she got a man and settled down. It was difficult to assess their relationship and the mother's influence, although Carol had mentioned that her mother lived in another town and that they rarely saw each other.

Carol's procedure went quite smoothly, but she encountered various problems during the post-abortion recovery period. Some of the trouble was related to the abortion itself; she experienced heavier than normal bleeding and had to return for reevacuation. Other problems were related to her unwillingness to follow post-abortion instructions and, possibly, her conflicting feelings about her decision. Carol expressed anger with the agency and a lack of confidence in the doctors whom she held responsible for her problems.

Ordinarily, Carol and I would have contact only on the day of the procedure. Because of her continuing problems and history, I continued to work with her. I also asked a nurse to visit Carol at home, as she called with various complaints but refused to return for evaluation. The nurse reported that Carol's complaints were highly exaggerated.

Carol's contraceptive plans were of special concern. She had already had intercourse without protection, even though advised to abstain for at least two weeks. Carol had informed her partner about the abortion, and apparently he had told her that she should have had the baby. Therefore her plans for future pregnancy were quite uncertain. She realized that she was not in the best physical, emotional or financial condition to have a baby. She expressed many concerns about her partner and their relationship. Her mother, however, was urging her to settle down, and her partner was now telling her that he would like a baby. In addition, Carol's contraceptive choices were limited. An IUD was not possible. Her age and several episodes of elevated blood pressure meant that the pill was not a good choice. She did not favor foam because she had experienced a previous failure with it, and she thought it very unlikely that her partner would use a condom. She did, however, decide on foam until she could return for a diaphragm fitting.

Carol and I discussed follow-up care. She was not interested in returning to the main clinic, which was about forty minutes from her home. Instead, she decided to return to her own physician for medical checks, and to consider the Planned Parenthood office near her home for contraceptive care. I contacted her physician who also thought he was not relating to Carol effectively.

It appears that Carol is using pregnancy to try to force her partner to make a permanent commitment to their relationship, or at least to pay more attention to her. Twice she has gotten pregnant only to discover that he was unwilling to make a further commitment; yet she wants to believe him when he mentions a desire for a child. Carol understands that emotionally and financially she is not prepared for another child. The need to establish a more permanent relationship with her partner, however, causes her to risk further pregnancy. Until Carol can understand this pattern, she will continue to be an unsuccessful contraceptor.

At the time of this writing, Carol is pregnant again. At first her partner seemed pleased. He gave her money for maternity clothes and took her out to buy things. But a month ago he disappeared and has not contacted her. At this point, Carol is desperate about what to do about the pregnancy. She hopes he will return but thinks that is unlikely. She is thinking seriously about having another abortion.

DECISIONS ABOUT PRACTICE

Definition of the Client

In this case, the client is Carol Downs. Although her mother was briefly involved and her boyfriend had great influence on Carol's abortion decision, neither of them were involved in the counseling process. One wonders, though, what the result would have been had someone been able to counsel the couple (O'Connell, 1984).

Goals

My goal was that Carol be a successful contraceptor. While I was working with her, I was not convinced that Carol could attain that goal; in fact, when I began to write this chapter, I hesitated calling because I thought Carol might be pregnant again.

Carol's goal changed from one occasion to the next, depending on what she saw as her boyfriend's goal. He was very ambivalent about Carol's pregnancy, reacting negatively to whatever solution she found. When she aborted, he was angry; when she became pregnant again, he was at first supportive, then abandoned her.

Carol rejected all offers of counseling. On the day of the procedure she did not want to discuss her decision in any detail, nor did she want to involve her partner or her mother. Her stated objective was to have the abortion as quickly as possible; so, the function of agency and counselor was to provide her with this service. She rejected my concern about the results of her abnormal Pap smear and refused recommendations for further evaluation. A suggestion to undertake ongoing counseling to help her explore and understand her goals, especially in regard to her partner, was also rejected.

Contract

Carol and I were unable to arrive at a clear contract. Carol wanted the agency and staff to respond to her needs as she saw them and as they changed. This angered many staff people who felt she was manipulating them. If I had insisted on outlining a firm contract, she would not have allowed me to help at all.

Meeting Place

We met in my office as is the tradition of the agency. Once, despite this tradition, a nurse was dispatched to Carol's home because she had many medical complaints but refused to come to the agency.

Use of Time

Timing is primarily dictated by trimester of pregnancy, possibilities for intervention, and the woman's goals. Within that time frame, need rather than agency structure determines the amount of time that social worker and client spend together.

Treatment Modality and Stance of the Social Worker

My treatment approach combines education and support. I educate clients about contraception and pregnancy and provide supportive counseling. In a situation like Carol's, where the client relates so poorly to professionals and seems destined to be a failed contraceptor, it is extremely important that I maintain enough detached concern to avoid getting angry with the client. I must also work quickly and directly because one cannot stop the clock of the pregnancy. While defense mechanisms work to protect the client or she expresses ambivalence about pregnancy, termination and contraception, while I develop the best interventions with which to help her, the pregnancy proceeds, waiting for neither of us.

Outside Resources

Counseling is a prerequisite for contraceptive devices and abortion which might be considered concrete services or outside resources in other agencies. In addition, as was mentioned before, Carol receives Aid to Families with Dependent Children.

Reassessment

While I wait for Carol to decide whether she wishes to terminate this pregnancy, I again assess our relationship and my ability to help. When Carol makes her decision, she and I will renegotiate our relationship and the kind of help which Planned Parenthood can offer.

Differential Discussion

If I were to begin again with Carol or someone like her, I would proceed differently. First, I would try to involve her boyfriend who played such an important role in Carol's life and in her decisions about family planning. Perhaps if I had tried to do this, neither of them would have come for help, but that decision might have been better than the extraordinarily ambivalent behavior I encountered.

Also, I would maintain my relationship with Carol longer, to allow her to use the relationship as a forum for decision making. That way, we could assess alternatives together rather than her expecting the agency to expedite her solution. I would also evaluate her relationship with her AFDC social worker. If they had an ongoing relationship, I would enlist the help of the AFDC worker to explore Carol's relationship with her boyfriend as well as her contraceptive use. perhaps, since her mother did accompany Carol to Planned Parenthood once, there may be a way to enlist her mother's help as well. Finally, I would refer Carol for psychotherapy to improve her self-image and ability to take control of her life. Franklin, I do not think that Carol is ready for a long term counseling commitment at this time, but perhaps she will be ready in the future.

PRACTICE IN CONTEXT

Both the legalization of abortion and the technology which provides for medically safe abortions at reasonable cost have revolutionized the family planning movement. The struggle to keep abortion legal and available to all, regardless of ability to pay, requires a strong commitment from the agency on both formal and informal levels. This seems to be possible for Planned Parenthood and its supporters because of their unique history of supporting controversial issues. On the formal level, the agency has united to take a strong stand against the constant threats to eliminate the right to choose when and if to have children. There is also special concern for those who are unable to pay for their own health care. Certainly discontinuation of Medicaid funding would have profound effects on those clients without financial means. Informally the staff must continue to support each other and the clients. Although statistically abortion is an important method for fertility control, it is considered a poor choice as a primary method of birth control by most family planning professionals. Yet Planned Parenthood cannot abandon clients such as Carol who make this choice. They require such services until they are able to use other means of contraception.

Planned parenthood is the common theme of the agency. An unplanned or unwanted pregnancy is seen as a failure. Other dimensions of the work exist in the shadow of this looming disappointment. Proper use of effective contraception decreases the incidence of unwanted pregnancy and most women find contraceptives safe and effective.

REFERENCES

Alan Guttmacher Institute. *Issues in Brief* 5:2 (Jan. 1985): 1-3.

Boston Women's Health Book Collective. *The New Our Bodies Ourselves: A Book By and For Women*. New York: Simon and Schuster, 1984.

Faria, Geraldine, Elwin Barrett, and Linnea M. Goodman. "Women and Abortion: Attitudes, Social Networks, Decision-Making." *Social Work in Health Care*, XI, No. 1 (Fall 1985), 85-99.

Forrest, Jacqueline D. "The End of IUD Marketing in the U.S.: What Does it Mean for American Women?" *Family Planning Perspectives*, XVIII, No. 2 (March/April, 1986), 52-57.

Forrest, Jacqueline D. "American Women—A Sexual Profile." *Contemporary OB/GYN* (April, 1987), 75-82.

Freeman, Edith M. "Interaction of Pregnancy, Loss and Developmental Issues in Adolescents." *Social Casework* 68, No. 1 (Jan. 1987), 38-46.

Gold, Rachel B. and Jennifer Macias. "Public Funding of Contraceptive, Sterilization and Abortion Services, 1985." *Family Planning Perspectives*, XVIII, No. 6 (Nov./Dec. 1986), 259-264.

Henshaw, Stanley K. "Characteristics of U.S. Women Having Abortions, 1982-83." *Family Planning Perspectives*, XVIX, No. 1 (Jan./Feb. 1987), 5-8.

Hutchings, Jane E. et al. "The IUD AFter 20 Years: A Review." *Family Planning Perspectives*, XVII No. 6 (Nov./Dec. 1985), 244-255.

Joffe, C. *The Regulation of Sexuality: Experiences of Family Planning Workers*. Philadelphia: Temple University Press, 1986.

Lincoln, Richard, ed. "Americans Exaggerate Health Risks of the Pill, Underestimate Effectiveness of All Contraceptives." *Family Planning Perspectives* XVII, No. 3 (May/June 1985), 128-129.

Luther, K. *Abortion and The Politics of Motherhood*. Berkeley, CA: University of California Press, 1984.

O'Connell, M. and C.C. Rogers. "Out-Of-Wedlock Births, Premarital Pregnancies, and Their Effect on Family Formation and Dissolution." *Family Planning Perspectives*, XVI, No. 1 (July/Aug. 1984) 157-162.

Ory, H.W., J.D. Forrest, and R. Lincoln. *Making Choices: Evaluating the Health Risks and Benefits of Birth Control Methods*. NY: The Alan Guttmacher Institute, 1983.

Petchesky, Rosalind P. *Abortion and Woman's Choice*. NY: Longman Inc., 1984.

Rodman, H., Lewis, S. and Griffith, J. *The sexual rights of adolescents*. NY: Columbia University Press, 1984.

Schwartz, D.B. and Darubi, K.F. "Motivation for adolescents' first visit to a family planning clinic." *Adolescence*, 21(83), Fall 1986, pp. 535-545.

Tanfer, K. and Rosenbaum, E. "Contraceptive perceptions & method choice among young single women in the United States." *Studies in Family Planning*, 17 Nov./Dec. 1986, pp. 269-277.

Responding Effectively
to the Crisis of a Gay Man
with AIDS

George S. Getzel

DESCRIPTION OF THE SETTING

The Gay Men's Health Crisis is a non-profit organization established in the summer of 1982 by a group of New York City gay professionals who recognized the desperate crisis engendered by the AIDS related deaths of friends and lovers. They felt fearful of contracting AIDS and at the same time overwhelmed by the increasing needs of persons with AIDS who did receive compassionate care from health and social welfare organizations.

They developed mutual aid groups to provide emotional support for themselves and much needed activities for persons with AIDS. Subsequently, social workers and other professionals were enlisted as the number and complexity of the caseload increased. From the beginning, social workers have strongly influenced GMHC's program directions and values stances. Social work's simultaneous concern with both private troubles and public issues corresponds to the range of activities of GMHC. The theoretical underpinning for the crisis services and community volunteer programs come in large measure from social work's biopsychosocial assessment and treatment orientations. The preponderance of GMHC's assistance still comes from volunteers for both direct and indirect services to persons with AIDS and their significant others.

Currently, there are over one thousand volunteers and approximately twenty-five hundred persons with AIDS registered as clients. By 1987, the full-time staff of GMHC had grown to more than sixty persons. The number of clients has grown steadily by the month, and so has the number of volunteers acting as buddies, caregivers and crisis intervention workers with individual persons with AIDS. A variety of groups for lovers, family members and friends of clients have been established. Long-term therapy and other specialized groups are offered, as are a variety of recreational activities including evening movies, cultural events, parties hosted by concerned community leaders, restaurant lunches and excursions. These experiences provide respite for caring loved ones and serve as a partial antidote to the loneliness and isolation experienced by persons with AIDS.

A growing area of activity at GMHC has been financial advocacy services. Ongoing training sessions are offered to keep financial advocacy volunteers abreast of the everchanging governmental income, health, nutrition and housing benefits for which clients may be eligible. Financial counselors see clients in the office and also make home visits. GMHC serves as a link and as a legitimizing instrument for persons with AIDS as they approach health and social welfare bureaucracies for vital material supports. GMHC also gives emergency relief to clients who are in desperate straits after not receiving services and income from traditional sources. Undocumented aliens with AIDS have been a special concern.

As this epidemic grows, an increasingly important service is community education, designed to reach every level of society in New York City. GMHC publishes recommendations for reducing the risk of infection. Information and education programs designed in concert with community groups are deployed to educate those at risk for AIDS—not only gay men (who still account for three out of four cases), but other risk groups as well. Especially important has been the GMHC effort to dispel superstition and fear concerning how the disease is contracted or transmitted. More than 25,000 calls have been received by the GMHC hotlines, and the demand for seminars and public education about AIDS to the public and professional groups is enormous. GMHC medical advisory statements are revised to reflect new developments, such as warning about the federally approved blood screening test for an antibody of the virus that most probably causes AIDS. GMHC publications are translated into Spanish and Haitian Creole (Kosterlitz, 1986).

Another area of increasing importance is legal services. A pro bono panel of volunteer gay and lesbian lawyers provides a bi-weekly clinic to help clients in writing legal instruments often required by those who have AIDS, such as wills and powers-of-attorney. Increasingly, persons with AIDS or even suspected of having AIDS need help defending themselves against discrimination in matters of employment, public accommodation, housing, and transportation (U.S. News and World Report, 1986). Discrimination by health care organizations and insurance companies is a frequent target for legal action.

Technology

AIDS is characterized by the presence of life-threatening opportunistic infections and rare forms of cancer such as Kaposi's sarcoma and lymphomas, caused by the progressive collapse of cellular immunity associated with HIV infection of T4 helper lymphocytes, a type of white blood cell.

The proportion of HIV-infected persons who go on to become full blown cases of AIDS is unknown, because the virus, once hosted in the body, may be activated by unknown co-factors. HIV infection is also related to AIDS related condition or ARC, a decline of immune capacity featuring a loss of T4 helper lymphocytes and very distressing symptoms: intermittent or continuous fevers over several months, weight loss, night sweats, malaise, diarrhea, rashes and generalized lymphadenopathy (swollen glands), but not cancers such as Kaposi's sarcoma, or major opportunistic infections such as pneumocystis carini pneumonia (occurring in approximately 60 percent of AIDS cases), Taxoplasmosis, disseminated tuberculosis, rare lymphomas or other diseases designated by the Centers of Disease Control (Joffe et al., 1985).

During the course of his or her disease process, a person with AIDS may develop one or more opportunistic infections that will not be responsive to medical technology. Treatments typically involve the use of powerful chemicals and radiation which are themselves clinically iatrogenic, causing physically distressing and stigmatizing side effects. To date, there has been slow progress in finding substances that either slow HIV's destructive activities or enhance the overall immune system. It appears that a vaccine to protect uninfected persons may take several years to develop and to test for broad applications. Therefore, medical technology must be largely directed at relieving symptoms of opportunistic infections and being palliative for patients whose illnesses do not respond to treatments and are dying in severe pain and discomfort (Cole and Lundberg, 1986).

Over a period of months or years, all patients die from complications arising from AIDS. Therefore the diagnosis of AIDS is a traumatic event for the patient's loved ones and health care professionals. As the number of new AIDS cases increases, doubling approximately each year since 1981, the capability of medical technology and health resources will be sorely tested. The social, economic and psychological crises of AIDS patients severely taxes health care professionals who try to respond empathically to this catastrophic epidemic (Oppenheimer and Padgug, 1986).

Doctors, nurses and other health professionals see AIDS patients, typically in their 20s and 30s, recover from one opportunistic infection (through the application of sophisticated, expensive procedures in hospitals, out-patient clinics and in the community), only to undergo additional health crises and painful deaths. The cost of caring for an AIDS patient routinely runs into tens of thousands of dollars and beyond. In large cities with high concentrations of PWAs, the cost of health care, public assistance and related services places enormous strains on extant resources. Unfounded fears of contagion through casual contact contribute to the unwillingness of some health professionals to work with PWAs in different health care contexts (U.S. Congress, 1986).

Family, friends and neighbors play as vital a role in providing PWAs support and assistance during hospitalizations and while PWAs are in the community as complex medical technology does in treating the opportunistic infections. The underlying fragility of PWAs' immune systems necessitate constant monitoring to detect the onset of episodic health crises. The ongoing experience of AIDS is analogous to a rollercoaster ride. Sudden changes in physical, instrumental and mental functioning are not unexpected.

AIDS is a progressively disabling condition. It can involve diseases that affect the central nervous system and cause dementia. Friends, kin and neighbors provide essential episodic and continuous assistance that maximizes PWA's autonomy and self-worth, especially when they remain in familiar situations at home. Clearly PWAs benefit when the gains of medical technology can be joined with their wishes to maintain previous levels of functioning. Much of GMHC's services are directed toward this end (Baumgartner, 1985).

Policy

As the twentieth century closes, AIDS has been identified as the most serious public health issue in the United States and the world (Nichols, 1986). Although AIDS occurs in central and eastern Africa in both heterosexual men and women, indicating bilateral transmission, the AIDS epidemic in the United States has taken its largest toll to date on gay and bisexual men, who account for 65 percent of all diagnosed cases since 1981. The second largest risk group for AIDS are drug abusers, 17 percent of all cases. The third largest risk category, with 4 percent of cases and the largest potential population at risk, are heterosexual men and women who are sexually active and not in long-standing monogamous relationships with uninfected partners. Of all persons diagnosed with AIDS since 1981, more than half have died (Curran et al., 1985).

The biological and medical ramifications of AIDS tend to become overshadowed in popular thinking by the social and cultural implications of the disease. AIDS brings together two areas of extreme societal dissensus: sexuality and death. It has long been noted that illness and disease are as much objects of moral valuation as of biological interest (Sontag, 1978).

GMHC volunteers and staff discovered early in their work that persons with AIDS did not always receive compassionate and just treatment from health care providers, social agencies, public agencies and communities (Bayer, Fox and Willis, 1986). Because of the stigmatization of the disease and its initial appearance within segments of the population that have traditionally suffered discrimination, there has occurred a potential erosion of services and human rights of persons with AIDS, AIDS related complex, and even those presumed to be carrying the virus thought to cause the disease (Casseus, 1985; Merrit et al., 1986).

The widespread use of a test for the HIV antibody to indicate the presence of the virus in the body poses a special problem for people who believe themselves to be at risk for the disease both before they take the test and if they find they have positive results. Consequently, GMHC has advocated that the antibody testing be voluntary and findings confidential. In cases of discrimination against PWAs and their loved ones, GMHC pursues legal recourses in the New York City and New York State Human Commissions as well as the courts. Am ombudsman program exists at GMHC to negotiate fair treatment from health and social service providers. Through GMHC's long active engagement with hospitals, the Social Security Administration, the New York City Human Resources Administration and other organizations, agreements have been created on how PWAs should be treated.

Over its first five years of existence, GMHC has supported a dual policy focus of advocating for humane and compassionate treatment from service providers, and developing a freestanding city-wide network of volunteers providing crisis service and groups support to PWAs and their loved ones. Clients served are gay and non-gay. Most importantly, the services include the available designated "lover" or life companion of a gay man as part of the agency's concept of family.

Organization

Gay Men's Health Crisis is governed by a volunteer board of fourteen who work very closely with one another and with the approximately 60 person staff. Board members typically have had direct experience with PWAs or with other aspects of the agency's social policy and educational activities. At least one member is a PWA, and thus represents that interest.

In 1985 over 80 percent of the agency income came from individual contributions, the remaining support cash from governmental sources. With an operating budget of nearly $1,000,000, approximately forty-one percent of the budget went for clinical service and thirty eight percent for AIDS education activities.

The agency is administered by an executive director and two deputy executive directors for program administration and social policy. The largest agency unit is clinical services, which provides crisis intervention, agency intake, recreation, group services ombudsman services and financial advocacy. AIDS education and research is the second largest unit providing public education and AIDS prevention programs. Other departments are volunteer services, legal services, public relations and development.

The growth of the organization has been rapid as has been its funding base. Office space is tight. The growth of full-time staff has required that the agency establish more formal ways of relating to the army of volunteers which has reached nearly 1,500 persons.

Recently a volunteer council has been developed to maintain lines of communication between the volunteers who provide the bulk of agency services and full-time staff. Periodic events are held to enhance socialization and education for volunteers about emerging developments at GMHC and to reward their activities.

Many social workers and health care workers have volunteered at GMHC. The staff of GMHC has provided technical assistance to health and social service agencies throughout the region and the country. Staff of GMHC has taken leadership in the establishment of public assistance for people with AIDS, Medicaid provision, and funded AIDS research in New York State and on the federal level.

The agency has formal linkages with a national network of AIDS organizations as well as local and national gay and lesbian organizations. GMHC from its beginning saw itself serving all people regardless of sexual orientation, gender, race, religion or nationality. Currently volunteer crisis teams exist in all boroughs of New York City serving people of varying backgrounds.

Case Description

Peter Phillips, thirty-nine, worked as a writer for a large corporation in New York city until he was hospitalized with *Pneumancystis carinii* pneumonia (PCP). When it became known he was diagnosed with AIDS, Peter was unceremoniously fired by his boss who said although it was not his decision to let Peter go, "higher-ups" felt his presence would jeopardize the well-being of other workers. Peter felt depressed, and embittered at his employer's treatment of him. Although AIDS is viewed as a disability in New York State,

Peter felt too ill and emotionally overwhelmed to pursue extensive legal action. He agreed to accept a modest financial settlement from his employer equaling two months salary. As Peter's health deteriorated after successive health crises, he ruminated about whether the acceptance of the settlement was a correct decision.

Peter came to New York ten years ago from Texas where his parents, sister and three brothers lived with their families. He lived alone in a small apartment. With a little smile, Peter noted that he was briefly married in his early twenties, but that was not meant to be. By the age of seven or eight he knew that he was gay because he felt strong attraction to his older brothers and cousins. Peter formally told his parents that he was gay when he left for New York City.

Greatly pained by Peter's sexual orientation, his father, a Baptist minister, addressed him with a great reserve on those occasional visits back to Texas. His mother remained a confidant and a link to his family of origin. Mrs. Phillips told Peter not to tell anyone outside the family he had AIDS, because she feared that his diagnosis would jeopardize her husband's job. Peter was enraged at his parents, who he felt were more concerned with themselves than with his deteriorating health; they did not visit him during five hospitalizations — two for PCP, two for chemotherapy of lymphomas, and one for an eye infection that partially blinded him.

Peter expressed a wish to visit his parents, if they would openly accept him as a gay man with AIDS. His younger brother and sister-in-law visited him during Christmas, which gave him a degree of psychological lift.

Peter's weight dropped from 150 to 110 pounds after undergoing chemotherapy. He experienced numbness in his legs and periodic bouts of pain which severely limited his ability to clean, cook and shop for himself. Several friends remained steadfast companions and assisted with chores when he was able to ask for help. Very prideful and stubbornly willful, Peter found asking for help excruciatingly embarrassing. Were it not for his considerable intellect and sense of humor, Peter's exacting and controlling manner would drive his friends to exasperation (Nichols and Ostrow, 1984).

As a result of illness and hospitalization, Peter used up all his small savings and received public assistance and Medicaid. He obtained high quality medical attention from his doctors in a large municipal hospital, but nursing care was very uneven. When he was in a designated unit for people with AIDS, care was excellent; but when he was placed in other areas due to the mounting number of AIDS cases in the hospital, his care was wanting.

Peter came to GMHC a week after his first hospitalization (for PCP) in February 1985. He was interviewed by an intake clinician, and two service needs were noted: first, assistance with his dire financial situation; second, group therapy for people with AIDS offered by GMHC professionally trained volunteers. I did an intake interview for group therapy in which Peter expressed interest in hearing how other people with AIDS dealt with their lives, so "I can understand my destiny," as he put it somewhat philosophically.

For Peter, the group therapy became the core experience to integrate the various twists and turns in his situation (Lopez and Getzel, in press). Peter could accept help from other group members, because he felt that he could contribute to others as well. He quickly assumed a "senior statesman" role, because he somehow survived five hospitalizations, each time returning to tell his survival story. He would emphasize how important it was to ask questions of doctors and nurses and not accept impersonal treatment. The group members were appreciative of Paul's courage, yet were quick to confront him when his need to control every part of his world got the better of him in or outside of the group.

Peter was the first group member to openly acknowledge his "prospective death," which allowed him and other members to make plans for what they had to do in their remaining time. Practical planning included the completion of wills, granting powers of attorney, funeral instructions, and the development of "living wills" stating what if any extraordinary means should be used if they could no longer give competent instructions to their doctors (Vinogradov and Thornton, 1984).

As Peter required help with household chores, he used the group to discuss having a GMHC "buddy" come to his apartment to help shop and clean. He developed a close, affectionate relationship with the buddy, a former pro hockey player. He spoke about having "funny" feelings because his buddy was a jock and he considered himself an intellectual. Group members joked that they would take the buddy's phone number and invite him to be *their* buddy.

An ongoing theme in the group was members' reconciliations with their families in the face of being gay and having AIDS. Peter's situation became a centerpiece for discussions of this kind. I engaged Peter and group members in discussing the hurt and loneliness they felt in not being able to discuss being gay with certain family members. Peter expressed powerful ambivalence at being dependent on his parents for money or that they might nurse him through his likely death. His angry feelings toward his parents were acknowledged and legitimated as very important by other group members. Peter was especially helpful to those members who gradually revealed their being gay to parents and siblings, in some cases after hiding the fact for more than thirty years.

The group helped Peter explore his powerful need for even a token expression of his parent's love for him, now that he was sick with AIDS. Members helped him prepare for telephone calls to his parents, and he was encouraged to tell his parents "how sick he really was." Consequently, his parents called more often, and intimated they might visit him.

Although Peter said he would not recommend AIDS to anyone, in some ways he felt his life had never been more meaningful and that he had never had such a sense of purpose. He had grown to appreciate small accomplishments, like making his bed himself or completing correspondence. The group members who had seen Paul rebound and deteriorate from successive opportunistic infections were realistically appreciative of Peter's comments at these moments, or when he would grieve the loss of his ability to bend over, or lament the disfiguring growths that appeared on his face and all over his body that he felt turned him into a "monster" (Hollan and Tross, 1985).

Toward the end of his life, Peter got a viral infection that caused partial blindness. He felt he was forced to have a Hickman catheter applied to his upper chest so he could receive an experimental antiviral medication. He was told after receiving the catheter that he needed it for life. He accepted it mournfully and resolved to discontinue chemotherapy now that his lymphoma in his jaw had disappeared. When I visited him in the hospital, he shared his resolve to remain in control of decisions, even if he could not remain in control of his body, now or in the future. I suggested he share his position with the group, which he did.

Three months later, Peter's jaw became cancerous. He told the group that he intended to ask his parents to come visit him for the last time. To his surprise, and the group's, they came to visit two weeks prior to his third and fatal PCP infection. I visited Peter at home after he was too weak to come to the group. He accepted my suggestion that he have a GMHC volunteer crisis worker come daily in addition to his buddy. The crisis worker focused on being there when Peter became anxious and helped him plan for his care, now that he rejected going back to the hospital to die (Lopez and Getzel, 1984). Peter organized his friends to be available to him. Until he became unconscious Peter held discussions with friends and gave them small possessions so that, as he said, "you might think about me from time to time."

The crisis worker, a close friend of Peter's, and I arranged a schedule so that Peter would not be alone. Funeral arrangements in New York City were made with Peter's participation just three days prior to his death. Peter died as his parents were coming back to New York. His father recited a brief biblical portion at his memorial service. Peter left his clothing and furniture to GMHC to distribute to needy people with AIDS and their families.

DECISIONS ABOUT PRACTICE

Definition of the Client

The client was primarily Peter Phillips, with a secondary emphasis on his friends and family who remain vital social supports. My participation with collaterals was dictated by Peter's wish for either direct or indirect assistance with informal or formal providers of emotional, social or instrumental support. Peter was seen as an autonomous person wanting and using GMHC services in or outside a hospital setting. The choice of services or modality remained wholly his throughout the helping process.

Goals

The goal of services rendered on behalf of Peter Phillips and other people with AIDS is to provide material and supportive service which allows for maximum individual autonomy and community participation. Peter was linked to his friends and family to support his sense of well-being and to counter the potential for isolation and loneliness. Also a group experience provided an antidote for isolation. Other goals with Peter were to maximize his choice of services and to help him advocate for sound treatment in the community and from health care providers. A major focus was helping to prepare for prospective illnesses, medical decisions, and his own death, through discussion and practical planning. I and other GMHC volunteers were flexibly available to Peter during those overwhelming periods of self-blame, anger, depression and fear as Peter faced life-threatening events that were evocative of past difficulties in his life (Weiner, 1986).

Contract

An explicit contract about commencing and terminating services between Peter and all GMHC service providers was made. At intake Peter explicitly picked or rejected services. Clients have the right to terminate for any reason at any time without recriminations. Clients' rights are detailed in a published client service directory given to Peter at intake. I endeavored to reiterate Peter's options, choices and rights throughout my work with him. Anytime Peter felt there was a lack of respect for him, or an unreasonable response, or a breach of confidentiality, or any other grievance, he could call a quality assurance committee. The development of a clear contract is especially important because this builds in rights and entitlement at GMHC which may be wanting elsewhere because of discrimination toward people with AIDS, gay men, drug abusers and other persons at risk.

Meeting Place

Peter and I met in agency buildings, his hospital room, his apartment and in the community. Flexibility and informality at times enhanced our work together.

Use of Time

I worked with Peter from May 1985 until his death in June 1986. The commitment I and GMHC have is "until death do we part" or until client terminates himself from service.

Treatment Modality and Stance of the Social Worker

The general service approach used can best be described as multimethod. In Peter's case, group therapy served as an integrating modality which cogwheeled into entitlement, advocacy and crisis intervention services provided by this worker and other members of the clinical volunteer team of GMHC. Case integration of service changed and shifted with Peter's biopsychosocial condition at different phases of the disease process. Different clients would receive different patterns of case integration (Christ, Weiner and Moynihan, 1980).

Stance of the Social Worker

In the early phase of intervention with Peter, the worker's stance tended to be supportive and non-confrontational to allow for Peter's controlled expression. Denial was supported as was maximum autonomy.

The worker explored the functional requirements of maintaining well-being after each successive health crisis. The worker monitored his responses particularly when he felt panicky that Peter would die suddenly and when he wanted to protect him or do too much. It was difficult experiencing Peter's anger and depression. As the relationship deepened, the worker used his own experience with PWAs to help Peter understand specific aspects of his emotional responses to disease. The worker at times did teaching about subjects like entitlements and AIDS transmission. He was direct and honest about his sadness and concern at Peter's health reverses. As Peter came to a closer recognition of his imminent death, the worker occasionally found himself the object of Peter's anger. The worker helped Peter explore his own grief and rage at becoming more disabled and ill. As Peter became more helpless, the worker found himself being there for him, neither offering over-optimistic nor morbid comments, but helping Peter make sense of what was happening to him. As Peter reached the end stage, the worker found himself more actively helping Peter reach out to others and advocating for his right to live and die as he wished (Nichols, 1985).

Outside Resources

Concrete services were an integral aspect of total service to Peter from the beginning of contact with GMHC to his death. The concrete services used by Peter included public assistance, disability insurance, Medicaid, will preparation, hospital advocacy and ombudsman services, funeral preparation, surplus food and food stamps as well as education on new medication and medical procedures (Arno, 1986). Access and referral services to the GMHC and external services eased a significant amount of stress for Peter from the point of diagnosis onward.

Reassessment

Peter's case necessitated constant reassessment at weekly group therapy meetings which provided opportunities to observe changes in his health and environmental conditions. If there were absences or instability in his health, follow up phone calls were made to him, his doctor, or designated friends. Peter understood and appreciated my concern. During the later phase of his illness, I reached him two or three times a week. I contacted his buddy, crisis worker, doctor, and a few close friends who took an active interest in his care. Toward the very end, I met with his mother.

Differential Discussion

Despite the complexity of the case, I would in retrospect not act differently given what I know. Peter's engagement in the helping process was constant and intense. However tragic the outcome, I found meaning and gratification in my work with him. The long-term nature of AIDS cases probably allows for midcourse corrections in approach. I constantly asked Peter for feedback and for explicit criticism directed toward me.

PRACTICE IN CONTEXT

The practice model described through the case illustration is a response to special needs. People with AIDS require complex medical intervention because of the uncertain course of their disease patterns culminating in likely death (Furstenberg and Olson, 1986). Their illnesses are expensive and greatly taxing on available health resources. The stigma of illness falls heavily on gay men and minority group members. GMHC's program and service model bear the considerable burden of meeting the epidemic's increasing toll by providing direct services, while simultaneously advocating for enlightened and humane social policies and education of the general public.

Emotional burdens of professionals working with dying young men are tremendous. Our belief systems are challenged when despite all our efforts, the people we have invested so much in die, only to be succeeded by new cohorts of ill people (Dunkel and Hatfield, 1986).

Of necessity, the GMHC approach weds armies of professionals, paid and volunteer, with lay helpers. The culture of GMHC organizations is delightfully — and at times exasperatingly — anarchistic and democratic. Its structure, operation and vision have been replicated and adapted to different parts of the United States and the world in an effort to provide humane care to people with AIDS.

REFERENCES

Anderson, G. R. "Children and AIDS: Implications for Child Welfare." *Child Welfare* 63, No. 1 (1984): 62-73.

Arno, P. S. "The Nonprofit Sector's Response to the AIDS Epidemic: Community-Based Services in San Francisco." *American Journal of Public Health* 76:11 (Nov. 1986): 1325-1330.

Baumgartner, G. H. *AIDS: Psychosocial Factors in the Acquired Immune Deficiency Syndrome*. Springfield, Ill.: Charles C Thomas, 1985.

Bayer, R., D. M. Fox and D. P. Willis (Guest Eds.). "AIDS: The Public Context of an Epidemic." *Milbank Quarterly* 64:1 (1986), entire issue.

Buckingham, S. L. and S. J. Rehm. "AIDS and Women at Risk." *Health and Social Work* 12:1 (Winter 1987): 5-11.

Caputo, Larry. "Dual Diagnosis: AIDS and Addiction." *Social Work* 30:4 (July/Aug. 1985): 301-364.

Casseus, B. J. "Social Consequences of the Acquired Immunodeficiency Syndrome." *Annals of Internal Medicine* 103:5 (Nov. 1985): 768-771.

Christ, Grace, Lori Wiener and Rosemary Moynihan. "Psychosocial Issues in AIDS." *Psychiatric Annals* (March 1986).

Cole, H. M. and G. D. Lundberg. *AIDS: From the Beginning*. Chicago: American Medical Association, 1986.

Coping with AIDS: Psychological and Social Considerations in Helping People with HTLV-III Infection, U.S. Department of Health and Human Services, Public Health Service, 1986, National Institute of Mental Health, Office of Scientific Information, Rockville, Maryland.

Curran, J. W. et al. "The Epidemiology of AIDS: Current Status and Future Prospects." *Science* 299 (1985): 1353-1357.

Dunkel, Joan and Shellie Hatfield. "Countertransference Issues Working with Persons with AIDS." *Social Work* 31:2 (March/April 1986): 114-117.

Furstenberg, A. L. and M. M. Olson. "Social Work and AIDS." *Social Work in Health Care* 9 (Summer 1984): 45-62.

Golan, Naomi. *Treatment in Crisis Situations*. New York: Free Press, 1978.

Hollan, J. C. and S. Tross. "The Psychosocial and Neuro-psychiatric Sequelae of the Acquired Immunodeficiency Syndrome and Related Disorders." *Annals of Internal Medicine* 103:5 (Nov. 1985): 760-764.

Joffe, H. W. et al. "The Acquired Immunodeficiency Syndrome in Gay Men." *Annals of Internal Medicine* 103:5 (Nov. 1985): 662-664.

Kosterlitz, J. "Educating About AIDS." *National Journal* 35 (Aug. 30, 1986): 2044-2049.

Lopez, Diego and George S. Getzel. "Helping Gay AIDS Patients in Crisis." *Social Casework* (Sept. 1984): 387-394.

Lopez, Diego and George S. Getzel. "Strategies for Volunteers Coping for Persons with AIDS." *Social Casework* (Jan. 1987): 47-53.

Lopez, Diego and George S. Getzel. "Groupwork with Teams of Volunteers Serving People with AIDS." *Social Work with Groups* 10:4) (Winter 1987): 33-48.

Merrit, D. J. et al. "AIDS: Public Health and Civil Liberties." *Hastings Center Report* 16:6 (Dec. 1986): 1-36.

Morin, Stephen, Kenneth Charles and Alan Malon. "The Psychological Impact of AIDS on Gay Men." *American Psychologist* (Nov. 1984): 1303-1307.

Nichols, Elizabeth K. *Mobilizing Against AIDS: The Unfinished Story of a Virus*, Cambridge, Mass.: Harvard University Press, 1986.

Nichols, S. E. "Psychosocial Reactions of Persons with the Acquired Immunodeficiency Syndrome." *Annals of Internal Medicine* 103:5 (Nov. 1985): 765-767.

Nichols, Stuart and David Ostrow. *Psychiatric Implications of Acquired Immune Deficiency Syndrome*, American Psychiatric Press, 1984.

Oppenheimer, G. M. and R. A. Padgug. "AIDS: The Risk to Insurers, the Threat to Equity." *Hastings Center Report* 16:5 (Oct. 1986): 18-22.

Peabody, Barbara. *The Screaming Rooms: A Mother's Journal of Her Son's Struggle with AIDS*, Oak Tree Publications, 1986.

Pearson, Carol Lynn. *Goodbye, I Love You: The True Story of a Wife, Her Homosexual Husband and a Love Honored for Time and All Eternity*, Random House: 1986.

Rubenstein, A. and L. Bernstein. "The Epidemiology of Pediatric Acquired Immunodeficiency Syndrome." *Clinical Immunology and Immunopathology* 40 (1986): 115-121.

Sontag, Susan. *Illness As Metaphor*, New York: Vintage Books, 1978.

U.S. Congress, Office of Technology Assessment. *Review of the Public Health Service's Response to AIDS*. Pub. No. OTA-TM-H-24, Washington, D.C.: Government Printing Office, 1985.

U.S. Congress, Subcommittee of the Committee on Government Operations. "Federal and Local Governments' Response to the AIDS Epidemic." *Hearing*, 99th Congress, 1st Session, Washington, D.C.: U.S. Government Printing Office, 1986.

U.S. House Committee on Energy and Commerce, Subcommittee on Health and the Environment. "Nonhospital Care for AIDS Victims." *Hearing*, March 5, 1986, 99th Congress, 2nd Session.

U.S. News and World Report. "AIDS Triggers Painful Legal Battles," March 24, 1986.

Vinogradov, S. and J. F. Thornton. "If I Have AIDS, Then Let Me Die Now." *Hastings Center Report* 14 (1984): 24-26.

Walker, L. A. "What Comforts AIDS Families," *The New York Times Magazine*, June 21, 1987, 16-22, 63, 78.

Weiner, L. S. "Helping Clients with AIDS: The role of the Worker." *Public Welfare* 44:4 (1986): 38-41.

Part 4

Mental Health Services

Acute Psychiatric Unit:
Two Hospitalizations in One Year

Toba Schwaber Kerson
Susan Steigner
Sally A. Neustadt
Tom Marshall

DESCRIPTION OF THE SETTING

The acute psychiatric unit (APU) at Francis Scott Key Medical Center is a 20-bed facility in a 600-bed general hospital owned since 1984 by Johns Hopkins Hospital. Until very recently, the institution was known as the Baltimore City Hospitals and was operated by the city. For many years, the hospital was one department of the Baltimore City Department of Public Welfare. In 1965, a city referendum mandated that the hospital become an independent department within the municipality. In 1980, another referendum determined that the hospital separate from the municipal bureaucracy and become a public benefit corporation. Although Baltimore City Hospitals is not the largest hospital in Baltimore, it has the second largest number of patients visiting the emergency room department annually and several large federally funded research programs in alcoholism and gerontology.

The APU was established in 1966 as a twelve-bed multidisciplinary unit and was the hospital's first step toward becoming a comprehensive community mental health center. Its purpose was to provide psychotherapy and chemotherapy for acutely disturbed people who might otherwise have had to leave the community and be hospitalized in a state facility. For the last ten years, the expanded and remodelled unit has had twenty beds and two seclusion rooms.

A five year demographic view of the APU population shows

male and female, black and white patients from age 13 to 81, with 20- to 40-year-old white, female patients as the majority. Most patients are from working class families employed by heavy industry in the area. Most women admitted are unemployed homemakers. Manic-depressive illness, including unipolar depression, has replaced schizophrenia as the most frequent functional psychosis diagnosis (Sands, 1985). For the past several years, severe psychoneuroses, character or personality disorders, acute situational reactions, as well as alcoholism and drug addiction, have also been treated. The usual length of hospitalization is about one month, although some patients are discharged within two weeks and others stay for a few months.

Policy

Several explicit policies affect the work of the APU. Acceptance of only voluntary patients, brief hospitalization, and intensive group and family work reflect the unit's philosophy of rehabilitation (Leibenluft and Goldberg, 1987). Both stabilized mental status and hospitalization coverage determine the length of stay. Flexible attitudes of the APU medical director and hospital administrators generally permit progressing patients to remain hospitalized past their coverage limit.

The admissions policy of the APU has shifted from patients with neuroses, situational reactions, personality disorders and acute schizophrenic episodes to those with chronic affective, schizophrenic and organic disorders. In order for treatment to reflect this change, the total therapeutic-community approach was replaced with individualized treatment plans. However, the policy of voluntary admission was continued because of staff preference for an open ward in which therapeutic contracting is possible. The Annotated Code of Maryland (Article 59, Section 11) provides that a person who signs a voluntary agreement may leave a hospital with three days written notice. As of 1980, the Medical Assistance Administration no longer specifies the number of inpatient days allowed for various psychiatric diagnoses (Uyeda et al., 1986).

Technology

The APU treats patients with a variety of medications (phenothiazines, Haldol, Lithium, tricyclics, monamine oxidase inhibitors, etc.) and psychotherapy (group, family and individual). Medications are given to stabilize patients and usually are continued after discharge. Manic depressive illness is viewed by the psychiatrists as a biochemical problem, and this orientation is taught in the psychiatric residency training program at Hopkins' Phipps Clinic (Johnson, 1984). Lithium and antidepressants are frequently used in the treatment of MDI (Matorin and DeChillo, 1984).

Group therapy is conducted by the social work, nursing and occupational therapy staffs. Social workers conduct discussion groups and request meetings on a twice-a-week basis. Social workers also provide psychosocial assessment and family therapy for nearly all patients and their families, using strategic and eclectic models, as well as disposition planning and coordination of services and resources outside the institution (Harris and Bergman, 1987). Individual therapy is routinely provided by residents and primary nurses using varied approaches. Two therapeutic community tools, patient government and the privilege system, complete the treatment approach of the APU. Patient government is an organized effort to help patients assume more responsibility for the therapeutic milieu. The privilege system allows patients to work for increasingly independent levels of activity, including leaves from the unit.

Organization

As a part of the Johns Hopkins Hospital system, Key is a training institution for many health professions including medicine, nursing and social work. Staff consists of rotating attending psychiatrists, rotating first-year psychiatric residents, nurses, aides, two social workers and two occupational therapists. Staff is divided into two teams, each with one resident who examines and admits the patient. Patients are assigned to whichever team has an empty bed, with no attention paid to previous relationship. Value seems to be placed on the expedient training of the rotating resident rather than on previously established staff-client relationships.

The APU social workers are part of the centralized hospital department of social work which has a staff of 25 MSWs and 4 BSWs. The department of psychiatry in which the APU is located and the department of social work are far apart; however, workers in both departments make an effort to close that gap through joint participation in professional and social activities. Camaraderie is nurtured by both. Social workers are well integrated into the hospital and the APU where they, along with nurses and occupational therapists, function very much as the backbone of unity in the face of rotating physicians. Ties between the APU social workers and those in community psychiatry are also strengthened through supervisory ties and frequent transfer of patients (Lecca and McNeal, 1985).

Case Description and Decisions About Practice

Fanny Zell was chosen for discussion because she is typical of people admitted to the APU in terms of age, race, sex, diagnosis and recidivism. Twice in one year, Mrs. Zell was admitted to the APU in a state of crisis. Since the APU team which cared for her in her first admission had no bed available for her second admission, she was assigned to the other team. Thus, three social workers were involved in Mrs. Zell's treatment; the social workers of the first and second teams as well as their supervisor.

Mrs. Zell was a twenty-five-year old divorced white female who was diagnosed as manic-depressive (Goldberg, 1987) and had had two previous psychiatric hospitalizations elsewhere. Referred to a community mental health center for Lithium maintenance and psychotherapy, Mrs. Zell had refused to take Lithium and had seen her therapist only intermittently.

Mrs. Zell is an only child who married at age eighteen, moved away from Baltimore with her husband and returned to her parents' house after her divorce five years ago. Her two sons, Lou and Bill, live with her and her parents and have had no contact with their father since the divorce. Mrs. Zell had a well-paying civil service clerical job on her return to Baltimore but resigned after her first manic attack three years ago. She now receives Social Security Disability payments and a small amount of support from her ex-husband. Her family is stable, and both of her parents work.

Mrs. Zell had been a competent mother before her first acute episode of manic-depression. However, prior to her first hospitalization on the APU, she had been very depressed, lying around in her bed and relinquishing most of her parental responsibilities to her parents. When her parents took the children to a carnival to which she was feeling too depressed to go, she overdosed on Stelazine, which had been prescribed for her depression. As a result of that overdose, Mrs. Zell was admitted to the Medical Intensive Care Unit and later transferred to the APU where she remained for two months on Team 1. Mrs. Zell's second admission to the APU ten months later was precipitated by a phone call from her mother to the social worker on Team 1 indicating that her daughter was acting manic and had stopped taking her Lithium. Mrs. Zell was staying up all night listening to the radio, writing poetry in a manner she did only when manic, feeling that she had special powers to predict and heal, and generally acting very strange. Mrs. Zell came to the APU with her mother and was seen by the attending physician there who assessed her mental state, suggested hospitalization and readmitted her, this time, to Team 2.

DECISIONS ABOUT PRACTICE

Definition of the Client

Generally, the APU staff defines the client as the individual patient. The social worker expands that unit to include the family system.

In accordance with APU policy, a psychosocial assessment was completed by the Team 1 social worker shortly after Mrs. Zell's admission. She was first interviewed alone and then was seen with her parents and her children. The initial assessment revealed that Mrs. Zell had not only MDI but also severe personality problems which persisted even after the acute MDI symptoms were alleviated. It became evident from the assessment that her psychiatric symptoms and personality problems profoundly affected her family. Mrs. Zell's sons had found her following the overdose, and neither they nor her parents were able to verbalize how frightened they were by her attempted suicide. Her parents were virtually raising her children, and Mrs. Zell expressed many ambivalent feelings about her roles as parent and daughter. Based on this information, the social worker defined the client system as the family and recommended family therapy as the modality of choice.

When Mrs. Zell was admitted for the second time, the Team 2 social worker also defined the family as the client; however, the family's great attachment to the Team 1 social worker made the transition very difficult.

Goals

If the patient is mentally capable, the social worker's initial goal is to promote a trusting, open relationship, to establish him or herself as a family therapist. Two types of factors determine a family's willingness to engage in therapy. Situational factors such as job inflexibility, transportation problems or financial limitations may limit the family's ability to participate. Internal determinants such as the family's physical and/or emotional state, motivation to change, and resistance to therapeutic intervention may also limit capability or willingness to establish goals and address family problems. None of these factors were present in Mrs. Zell's family.

Despite her deep depression, Mrs. Zell quickly established a positive identification with the social worker. She openly discussed problems which indicated the need for family intervention, and elicited help from the worker in setting goals. Initially, Mrs. Zell's parents were reluctant to participate in family therapy because of previous unsatisfactory experiences. However, both parents participated because they were frightened by their daughter's suicide attempt and were worried about her oldest son who was misbehaving in school and with peers.

The manic state which precipitated Mrs. Zell's second hospitalization prevented her from involvement in goal setting. After being stabilized on Lithium, she was able to participate in family meetings, but her personality problems interfered with setting goals (Wise, 1986). Mrs. Zell's family welcomed family therapy during the second hospitalization because of the positive experience they had had with the previous social worker.

Contract

During hospitalization 1, the psychosocial assessment from both Mrs. Zell and her family generated a problem list which became the basis for an oral contract which was documented in medical and social work records and renegotiated as new goals were articulated. The major problems defined by the client system were Mrs. Zell's living situation and physical condition, the children's behavior problems, and family communication. Mrs. Zell and her children lived, cooked and ate in her parents' basement and hated it. She felt she would be less depressed if she could move out of the basement and, perhaps, out of her parents' home. She felt she did not have enough money to move into a suitable place and could not support her children away from her parents' house. Her somatic complaints left her feeling too ill to do anything. In addition, both the boys, especially the eldest, were fighting with teachers and classmates, and Lou was doing poor work in science. The family was unable to communicate about deep feelings, especially anger. Mrs. Zell resented her father's reticence and was unable to talk to her parents about what bothered her.

Responding to Mrs. Zell's attributing her depression to the problem list, the social worker established the following objectives as part of the contract: (1) to improve the physical situation at home by examining alternatives; (2) to assess Mrs. Zell's work abilities and opportunities; (3) to encourage Mrs. Zell to contact school officials about the boys' behavior problems and Lou's academic problems; (4) to practice communication skills. It was agreed that Mrs. Zell's somatic complaints would be referred to her physicians and that the social worker would act as a liaison between the physician and family, if necessary. The social worker and family agreed to meet at least once a week during Mrs. Zell's hospitalization. In addition, Mrs. Zell and the social worker would meet for support and reinforcement of the work of family sessions.

Similarly, a contract was negotiated in the second admission, but the problem list changed. Mrs. Zell was no longer living in the basement, and she had given up the idea of working. However, Lou's problems had escalated to violence and verbal abuse. He was hurting his grandmother and brother and having increased difficulty with peers. Thus, the objective of the new contract became assessing and managing Lou's behavior.

Meeting Place

Both social workers have private offices on the APU, providing patients easy daily access to their workers, as well as easy retreat to their bedrooms when they feel upset or angry. The offices are large, with a desk, phone, one-way mirror, and a combination of chairs and a love seat that comfortably seats six. This seating arrangement allows families to be close together without feeling cramped. Office privacy permits them to express themselves freely without being overheard by others. However, since the offices are located on the unit, interruptions of family sessions by other patients and staff do occur.

Most family sessions are held in these offices because home visits take so much time. However, social workers have lately made home visits when patients live alone, families will not or cannot come to the hospital, disposition is in question, and when assessment of family dynamics in the home situation is important for treatment and disposition decisions. During Mrs. Zell's second hospitalization, no home visits were made.

Use of Time

In most cases, the length of time during which the client meets with the social worker on the APU is determined by the length of hospitalization rather than by the time frame necessary to achieve the goals established in the oral contract. In a few instances, the social worker will continue to see members of the client system as outpatients, but the policy and organization of the unit dictate that intervention begin shortly after the patient is admitted and end upon discharge. The length of hospitalization is generally based on two factors: financial resources and medical management. In Mrs. Zell's case, a high-option Blue Cross insurance policy could cover psychiatric hospitalization 365 days a year, if necessary; thus, there were no financial restrictions on length of treatment.

Mrs. Zell was first hospitalized for sixty days. Although the maximum stay of most patients with MDI is thirty days, Mrs. Zell's physicians decided to have her remain in the hospital until her acute symptoms had cleared and she was able to function reasonably at home. She had been released from a previous hospitalization while still symptomatic and had never regained a stable level of functioning.

Mrs. Zell's persistent somatic complaints during her second hospitalization resulted in a stay of forty-seven days. By extending the length of stay, the physicians were able to obtain adequate blood levels of Lithium for her. When she left the hospital, she was no longer experiencing psychotic symptoms but still exhibited many somatic complaints and personality problems.

Family sessions lasted one hour, as the contract specified and as is customary for the unit. The APU social workers maintain evening hours two nights a week to see those families who cannot come during the day. Mrs. Zell and her family were usually seen in the evening. The length of individual sessions varied from fifteen minutes to an hour depending on the patient's needs and the social worker's schedule. At the beginning of each session, the patient is usually told how much time the social worker would spend with her.

During the first hospitalization, the social worker met with Mrs. Zell at least once and often twice a week, and with Mrs. Zell and various members of her family once a week. Once, in family rounds, the family was interviewed by a consultant psychiatrist specializing in family treatment. During the second hospitalization, the new social worker had sporadic individual meetings of short duration with Mrs. Zell and five hour long meetings with the family.

TREATMENT MODALITIES
AND THE STANCE OF THE SOCIAL WORKER

Strategic family therapy (SFT) is the treatment used by both social workers on the APU (Braverman, 1986). It is used in modified form because of the policy, technology and organization of the inpatient unit. This model of family treatment is a problem-solving approach. It differs from other symptom-oriented therapies in that it emphasizes the social context of human problems.

> This therapy approach focuses on solving a client's presenting problems within the framework of the family. The emphasis is not on a method but on approaching each problem with special techniques for the specific situation. The therapist's task is to formulate a presenting symptom clearly and to design an intervention in the client's social situation to change that presenting symptom. (Haley, 1976)

Strategic family therapy makes four assumptions related to the following concepts: protection, units of three, sequences, and hierarchy. It assumes that family members want and act to protect each other from hurt and that children are most willing to sacrifice themselves to protect their parents and to keep the family together. Family structure and symptoms are viewed in terms of a unit of three to shift attention to sequences of behavior rather than causality. In general, the larger the unit worked with, the more possibilities there are for change and intervention.

The therapist is seen as part of the interactions. Underlying this approach is the belief that sequences of behavior seen in troubled families usually consist of confused hierarchies, stable coalitions, and rigid patterns. Hierarchy refers to the assumption that families, like all social groups with a past and a future, are organized according to different levels of power and ways of acting. These levels form boundaries of authority. In troubled families, the therapist attempts to change sequences of interaction and to reorder the hierarchy in order to make desired changes regarding the problem (Stanton, 1981).

Strategic family therapy was used because (1) the identified client was the family, (2) the short-term, goal-oriented, present-focused SFT approach was well-suited to the APU, (3) the social workers were trained in this treatment mode, and the orientation of their supervision enabled them to receive ongoing additional training, (4) the family was able to use this approach.

The APU's emphasis on the biochemical treatment of mental illness is an important factor which dilutes the pure practice of SFT.

Decision making by the physicians about medication and discharge adulterates the relationship between the therapist and the family, preventing the social worker from being at the top of the hierarchy, as pure SFT requires. Additionally, the primary nurse and the psychiatric resident have major responsibility for individual psychotherapy, and this detracts from the family therapist's ability to be truly in charge. Although ideally the work of all therapists involved with the patient is coordinated, in reality this often breaks down. Nurses do sometimes ask to sit in on family therapy sessions in order to learn about this therapy mode, and do participate when appropriate. Occasionally, medical students and residents also ask to observe.

The social workers deviate from the strategic family therapy model by taking the history and conducting the psychosocial assessment which are required by the hospital social work department and the APU when the patient is admitted to the unit. Once the history and assessment have been carried out, the social workers practice according to the tenets of strategic family therapy.

During Mrs. Zell's first hospitalization, family work began with a problem list made by the family and the social worker. Primarily, the list focused on Mrs. Zell's overdose and the family reactions to it, the boys' problems, communication difficulties and Mrs. Zell's somatic complaints (Shachnow, 1987). Family and social worker agreed to meet once a week to discuss reactions to the overdose and to aid communication. Since the boys were having emotional and academic problems in school, Mrs. Zell was told to contact the school counselor for clarification and help (Beardslee et al., 1983). Mrs. Zell's somatic complaints were referred to the physicians and to Mrs. Zell's primary nurse.

Within the family sessions, work on the child-centered problems consisted of helping the family correct the disturbance in the hierarchy. By the time Mrs. Zell was hospitalized, her parents, especially her mother, had assumed parenting responsibilities. Mrs. Zell had abrogated most of the responsibility but resented her parents' filling the void.

When the problem of Lou's poor performance in science was raised, the family was given the task of deciding who would help him with his homework. The grandmother suggested the grandfather had the best skills in this area; Mrs. Zell agreed, and the worker directed her to ask her father to help her son. It was agreed that grandfather would work with Lou during the week, his efforts reinforced by Mrs. Zell when home on a weekend pass. The social worker also authorized the grandparents to coach Mrs. Zell to be in charge of her children and of certain household decisions and activities.

In addition, the grandparents made up a schedule for the children which was approved by Mrs. Zell. Taking the problem-solving style used during sessions, Mrs. Zell and her family instituted round-table discussion at home to engage in decision making. During one session, the worker asked each boy to pick a recreational activity which he wanted his mom to share with him when she came home on a pass. Although she agreed to do this, Mrs. Zell did not follow through.

As therapy continued, Mrs. Zell's mother became increasingly dependent on the worker and called several times to ask how she should handle some aspect of her daughter's behavior when she came home. She was encouraged to raise these questions at family sessions.

Mrs. Zell's living, sleeping and preparing meals for her children in the basement of the house was a major family issue. Change in sleeping quarters was left to be worked out during outpatient treatment. After much discussion, the family agreed that Mrs. Zell was to go home daily during the last two weeks of her hospitalization and prepare dinner in the kitchen for the family when her mother was at work. Every possible detail was discussed during the sessions: who decided the menu, what each person's expectations were, and how the boys could help. The goal was to reintegrate Mrs. Zell into family life on a responsible and agreed-upon level. Issues relating to Mrs. Zell's ability to work were to be considered after she left the hospital.

Stance of the Social Worker — 1st Hospitalization

The social worker's stance during the initial session was one of reassurance and hope. The family was frightened and demoralized by the attempted suicide; therefore, the worker supplied an attitude of confidence, posing the possibility of positive change against Mrs. Zell's pronounced pessimism and her family's grief. During family sessions, the worker's stance became more authoritative and directive. Rapport was maintained with Mrs. Zell and her family partly because the worker was close to Mrs. Zell in age, had been divorced herself and had small children, and conveyed her empathy to the family.

Use of Family Therapy Consultation

One family each week was to be seen by a psychiatric consultant who helps to further explore family dynamics and educate the staff. The social workers find that this consultation provides a unique opportunity to gather information, raise anxiety levels and to push families to work harder and to feel aligned with the social worker. Mrs. Zell's family was seen by the family therapy specialist but her father failed to come because of parking problems. The session evolved into a highly emotional scene between Mrs. Zell and her mother. Although this confrontation increased professional insight into the mother-daughter relationship, the worker reassessed the situation and decided to set this issue aside in order to continue to work on the problems originally identified by the family.

Transfer

The staff supported the worker's decision to continue to see the family after Mrs. Zell's discharge from the unit. Mrs. Zell's psychiatric medication would be provided by the Johns Hopkins Hospital which was directed by the APU medical director. For organizational reasons, it was necessary to close Mrs. Zell's case and reopen it as an outpatient one. A family appointment was arranged for the week after discharge; however, Mrs. Zell requested and was granted individual therapy. She kept her first two, cancelled her third because she felt physically ill, missed the fourth, and called prior to the fifth saying that she felt too bad to come. Despite the worker's urging, offer to come to the house, and periodic telephone calls during the next few weeks, Mrs. Zell insisted that she felt too ill and too depressed to work on anything. She dropped out of treatment, and the case was closed.

Treatment Modality and Stance of the Social Worker—
2nd Hospitalization

During Mrs. Zell's second hospitalization, the patient and her parents were seen ten days after her admission because a manic psychosis precluded Mrs. Zell's participating in family meetings any earlier. She had numerous somatic complaints which continued throughout her hospitalization. Mrs. Zell left the office in the beginning of the first session and would not return. Her parents identified the primary problem as the oldest boy, Lou who had become increasingly aggressive toward his mother, his grandparents, and his peers. They wanted outside help to control his behavior, and agreed to include both boys in future sessions. The worker retained an objective, impartial stance in order to elicit information and to convey support and hope for change through family sessions.

When Mrs. Zell was home on a pass the following weekend, Lou became aggressive and angry about her hospitalization. She returned to the hospital extremely upset, feeling guilty and helpless.

Next, an agreement was made with the nurse-clinician on the APU that she could sit in on a family session to better understand the family dynamics. She understood that a contract had not yet been established. Mrs. Zell, her mother and the boys attended. Grandfather was working. The grandmother focused on Lou's misbehavior and her increasing frustration over failing to control him. Efforts to get Mrs. Zell to take charge in the session failed. She was passive, deferring to her mother and complaining about her physical problems. The boys were quiet. At this point, the nurse unilaterally suggested her own treatment plan of seeing the boys separately for a few sessions. Both Mrs. Zell and grandmother quickly agreed to turn the boys over to someone else. This intervention was inconsistent with the worker's assessment of the family problems and with the strategy needed to work toward the goal of putting Mrs. Zell in charge under her parents' supervision.

Subsequent family sessions included the entire family, and the worker used his authority to help the family define other problems and set goals. Mrs. Zell was confused about her role in the family, and in an attempt to increase and improve her mothering, a list was made of the tasks to do while she was at home on weekend pass. Mrs. Zell agreed to cook meals and spend recreational time with each boy several times that week. During the following week, Mrs. Zell went home infrequently and complained about physical ailments. Continuing the pattern that began in the first hospitalization, Mrs. Zell continued to use her home passes to remain in bed and allow her parents to assume all responsibility for her children.

An incident in the following family session again demonstrated a lack of coordination around family therapy on the APU. The worker told the parents to bring a crying Mrs. Zell back into the family meeting, but a unit nurse took over and sent them back without her. Mrs. Zell soon rejoined the family under the worker's prompting and was given support for this.

Mrs. Zell persisted in feeling guilty and inadequate as a mother. Support and direction were given for her to manage her jobs at home again that week. The worker later encouraged the nurse-clinician to terminate her work with the boys because it enhanced Mrs. Zell's feelings of incompetence, but the nurse continued until just before discharge.

Case Conclusion

Although Mrs. Zell continued to be extremely insecure about her mothering, she and the physicians agreed on a discharge date. During termination, Mrs. Zell was given support and encouragement by the family and the social worker for her accomplishments. An outpatient family therapy contract was set to continue to work on this problem. The family is currently in therapy working to improve Mrs. Zell's maternal functioning. The contract is open ended (Solomon, Gordon and Davis, 1984).

Differential Discussion

In considering whether alternate practice decisions could have affected outcome, the following ideas were agreed upon.

1. Mrs. Zell's somatic complaints should have been dealt with in family therapy, using SFT techniques. For example, Mrs. Zell could have been instructed to express all of her physical complaints in a session with all family members ministering to her. Then the family could have been assigned to minister to her twice a day at home for a week or two at specified times. This paradoxical tech-

nique aims at extinguishing her somatic complaints by providing Mrs. Zell with family attention without her having to feel sick (Lazarus, 1985-86).

2. Family therapy rather than individual therapy should have been the mode of treatment provided following the first APU hospitalization. Mrs. Zell's family hierarchy and sequences of behavior are too disturbed to solve identified problems through individual therapy (Johnson, 1986).

3. Both workers could have assumed a firmer stance in holding the patient and family accountable for task performance.

4. The social workers could have insisted that APU policy be relaxed to allow Mrs. Zell readmission to Team 1 or family therapy with the Team 1 social worker. Continuation with the same family therapist could have averted another beginning for Mrs. Zell and her family and increased the chances of making progress with the goals established in the first hospitalization.

5. Interference with family treatment by two nursing staff members should have been dealt with more effectively during the second hospitalization. In the first instance in which a nurse-clinician contracted with the family to see the boys separately, two interventions should have occurred: (a) the social worker and nurse should have talked beforehand and agreed upon goals for the session, and (b) the worker should have been more active in the session to prevent the nurse from forming any therapeutic subgroups. In the second instance, in which a nurse on the floor sent the parents back into the family session without Mrs. Zell, the worker should have instructed the nurse to allow the parents to take charge themselves and bring her back.

6. The APU lacks the necessary staff cooperation, knowledge and support to allow proper practice of SFT. In order to enhance this practice, education of the entire staff would be needed. If this were to occur, joint decision making about discharge dates would be possible, and social workers would be better able to reorder family hierarchies. Because this is a goal only for the social workers, and the social workers do not control critical decisions such as date of discharge, it is very difficult to obtain. Basically, this is an example of a way in which policy and organization can constrain practice.

PRACTICE IN CONTEXT

Policy influences patient care in numerous ways. High-option insurance coverage allows an unlimited period of time for treatment. The open ward policy and the use of privileges are useful to patients who must go home to practice new behaviors and generally to rejoin their families. On the other hand, the policy which allows the admitting resident to decide to which team a patient is assigned is sometimes detrimental because it may mark a new beginning with the social worker/family therapist. In this unit, a new beginning with a physician is not as detrimental because the physician's work with patients is based more on assessment techniques and technology than on relationship.

APU aftercare policies and practices also influence outcomes. Follow-up plans are sometimes arranged to be split with medical care provided at the Johns Hopkins Hospital Affective Disorders Clinic which is located several miles away from the Francis Scott Key Medical Center where psychotherapy is provided.

Technology has had a profound effect on psychiatry since the development of phenothiazines and Lithium in the 1950s. Use of these medications have allowed the APU to be an open unit since its inception. The use of Lithium and antidepressants usually helps to control severe depressions within two to three weeks of admission, and Lithium and a major tranquilizer promote an even quicker stabilization of manic episodes. Control of such disturbing symptoms as hallucinations, delusions, and extreme mood swings allows patients to behave in socially acceptable ways and thus to become integrated into the unit's milieu. Monitoring the correct level of medication in the patient's blood helps maintain stability (Berg and Wallace, 1987).

Some effects of technology are less desirable. The use of the medical model in hospital-based care emphasizes the sick role of the patients, and, in psychiatry, the physical, mental and affective components of patients' problems are emphasized because they are most likely to be controlled through medication and electroconvulsive therapy.

Organizational aspects of the APU have other specific effects of treatment. The multidisciplinary staffing of the unit has the advantage of providing comprehensive care and the disadvantage of creating communication coordination problems by virtue of staff size, difference in theoretical approaches and goals, and staff changes. The therapeutic milieu on the unit and its medically dominant hierarchy impinge on care by encouraging patients to assume and maintain a sick role. As is commonly observed, patients who gain attention for their medical problems or complaints often have their ineffective solutions reinforced. The medical staff frequently discourage patients' and their families' initiative in solving their own problems. Social work, by profession, works to enhance individual strengths and self-determination.

REFERENCES

Beardslee, W. et al. "Children of Parents with a Major Affective Disorder: A Review." *American Journal of Psychiatry* 57,1 (January 1987), 66-77.

Berg, William E. and Michael Wallace. "Effect of Treatment Setting of Social Workers' Knowledge of Psychotropic Drugs." *Health and Social Work* 12, 2 (Spring 1987), 144-152.

Braverman, Lois. "Social Casework and Strategic Therapy." *Social Casework* 67, 4 (April 1986), 234-239.

Christ, Winifred. "Factors Delaying Discharge of Psychiatric Patients." *Health and Social Work*, 9, 3 (Summer 1984), 178-187.

Davenport, Y. et al. "Early Child-Rearing Practice in Families with a Manic-Depressive Parent." *American Journal of Psychiatry* 141: (1984), 230-235.

Ferris, Patricia A. and Catherine A. Marshall. "A Model Project for Families of the Chronically Mentally Ill." *Social Work*, 32, 2 (March/April, 1987), 110-114.

Goldberg, Harold. "Affective Disorders" in *Conn's Current Therapy*, Ed., Robert E. Rakel. Philadelphia: W.B. Saunders Company, 1987, 941-943.

Haley, J. *Problem Solving Therapy*. San Francisco: Jossey-Bass, 1976.

Harris, Maxine and Helen C. Bergman. "Case Management with the Chronically Mentally Ill: A Clinical Perspective." *American Journal of Orthopsychiatry*, 57, 2 (April 1987), 296-302.

Johnson, H.C. "The Biological Bases of Psychopathology" in *Adult Psychopathology: A Social Work Perspective*, F.J. Turner, Ed. NY: The Free Press, 1984, 6-72.

Johnson, Harriette C. "Emerging Concerns in Family Therapy." *Social Work*, 31, 4 (July/August 1986), 299-306.

Kurtz, Linda F., Dennis, A. Bagarozzi, and Leonard P. Pollane. "Case Management in Mental Health." *Health and Social Work* 9, 3 (Summer 1984), 201-211.

Lazzarus, Arthur. "Factions Disorder in a Manic Patient: Case Report and Treatment Considerations." *International Journal of Psychiatry in Medicine* 15, 4 (1985-86), 15.4, 365-369.

Lecca, P.J. and J.S. McNeil. *Interdisciplinary Team Practice, Issues and Trends.* NY: Praeger Pub., 1985.

Leibenluft, Ellen and Richard L. Goldberg. "Guidelines for Short-Term Inpatient Psychotherapy." *Hospital and Community Psychiatry*, 38, 1 (January 1987), 38-43.

Levant, R. *Family Therapy: A Comprehensive Overview.* Englewood Cliffs, NJ: Prentice-Hall, 1984.

Madanes, Cloe. "Advances in Strategic Family Therapy" in *The Evolution of Psychotherapy*, Jeffrey K. Zeig, Ed. NY: Brunner Mazel, 1985.

Matorin, Susan and Neal DeChillo. "Psychopharmacology: Guidelines for Social Workers." *Social Casework* 65, 10 (December 1984), 579-84.

Nichols, M. *Family Therapy: Concepts and Methods.* NY: Gardner Press, 1984.

Sands, Roberta G. "Bipolar Disorder and Social Work Practice." *Social Work in Health Care* 10, 3 (Spring 1985), 91-105.

Shachnow, Jody. "Preventive Intervention with Children of Hospitalized Psychiatric Patients." *American Journal of Orthopsychiatry* 57, 1 (January 1987), 66-77.

Solomon, Phyllis, Barry Gordon, and Joseph Davis. "Assessing the Service Needs of the Discharged Psychiatric Patient." *Social Work in Health Care* 10, 1 (Fall 1984), 61-70.

Stanton, M.D. "Strategic Approaches to Family Therapy" in *Handbook of Family Therapy*, A.S. Gurman and D.P. Kniskerin, Eds. NY: Brunner/Mazel, 1981.

Uyeda, Mary K. et al. "Financing Mental Health Services." *American Behavioral Scientist* 30, 2 (Nov./Dec. 1986), 90-110.

Wetzel, J.W. *Clinical Handbook of Depression.* NY: Gardner Press, 1984.

Wise, Marilyn G. "Working with Medicated Clients: A Primer for Social Workers," *Health and Social Work* 11, 1 (Winter 1986), 36-41.

Psychiatric Halfway House:
To Achieve Independent Living

Carey Donovan

DESCRIPTION OF THE SETTING

Shalom House is a psychiatric halfway house in Portland, Maine. Founded in 1972 by local churches and synagogues concerned about deinstitutionalization, it was the first independent facility for psychiatric patients in our state.

Today, Shalom House is part of a larger organization, Shalom, Inc., which also runs a HUD 202 Demonstration Project for the Chronically Mentally Ill and a rooming house for mentally ill adults, and is developing a HUD 202 Section 8 housing project for the mentally ill. Shalom, Inc., is a private non-profit corporation which receives most of its funding from the Maine Department of Mental Health and Mental Retardation. Other funds come from United Way, Cumberland County, The Bureau of Rehabilitation, resident fees and private donations.

Shalom, Inc., has an executive director whose visibility is enhanced by his political involvement as a state senator, an administrative director, a clinical director (MSW) and a secretary. These staff members are shared by all the programs of the agency. Shalom House has two live-in house managers, a full-time BSW social worker, and a social work student.

Shalom House is a large, comfortable old house located in the heart of Portland. It is within walking distance of the hospital, mental health and social service agencies, the downtown area, a campus of the University of Maine, the city library, a major art museum, and many potential places of employment. It has room for 15 residents and operates at 95% capacity. Residents are adults with serious mental health problems who are felt to need a transitional program that will prepare them for independent living, which is the purpose of Shalom House. All residents who are accepted to the program are presumed to be capable of leaving Shalom House and living independently in the community within a year's time.

Policy

Social policy toward the mentally ill is very complex, for a variety of reasons. One is that mental illness is very complex: it can be short-term or long-term, mild or severe, chronic or episodic. Those afflicted can be very ill at times and very well at other times. In addition, mental illness is very scary and threatening; it is as stigmatizing as any illness can be and is the brunt of countless jokes and put-downs. To make matters worse, its prevalence is such that almost everyone will experience some form of mental ill-health in their lifetime, in themselves, a family member, or friend. Finally, the realities of severe mental illness run counter to some basic values and assumptions of our society; for example that every able-bodied person should be able to work.

Shalom House was created from the concern of private citizens toward a policy of deinstitutionalization that was discharging patients into communities unprepared to deal with them. Deinstitutionalization swept the country in the late 1960s due to a coincidence of changes in policy, law and technology. Up until that time, the states had cared for the mentally ill and had done so by running large state institutions for the insane (Goffman, 1961). The states had assumed this responsibility in the mid-1800s in response to the activism and fact-finding of Dorothea Dix.

Let me briefly describe the circumstances which made deinstitutionalization an irresistible option for state government in the late 1960s. First there was the discovery of psychotropic medications which had the potential to make mental illness much more manageable. Second were major changes in the law that restricted the states' power to hold and treat mentally ill persons. No longer could mentally ill people be confined against their will without severe cause (dangerousness) and due process. When they were held, it would be only for short periods of time unless the criteria (dangerousness) could be proved over and over. No longer could patients be confined for "treatment" without meaningful treatment being provided. A principle was established that persons should be treated in the least restrictive setting possible. Finally, patients could no longer contribute to the work of an institution (kitchen, laundry, housekeeping) without pay, as had been customary in the past.

In addition, some federal funding sources became available to the mentally ill. These included Social Security Disability payments, Supplemental Security Income, Medicaid and Medicare. These benefits allowed states to discharge patients to nursing homes, boarding homes or the community, with the federal government picking up the tab.

Finally, in 1962, the federal government established a funding mechanism for start-up costs for regional mental health centers. The idea behind these centers was to provide care for patients closer to home and in a less restrictive setting than the state hospital.

In the 1960s, deinstitutionalization was an idea whose time had come. In the 1980s it is a policy of failure and neglect. The homeless mentally ill are a national concern. Every city has actively disturbed people wandering the streets. State hospitals cost as much as ever, and employ as many staff, but hold far fewer patients. In our state, two-thirds of the patients who are admitted to the state hospital are sent home within two weeks. There are more services available in the community, but there is no one place where the buck stops.

Parents of the mentally ill are shocked to learn that they cannot get treatment for their desperately ill offspring (Wasow, 1978). Police are reluctant to transport; hospitals are full or are reluctant to process an involuntary commitment. When families finally win the battle and get the person committed, they lose the war when he is discharged five days later. At heart is a conflict between an individual's right to refuse treatment and the ability of a psychotic person to make sound judgements on his own behalf.

The concept of "community care" which seemed so bright in the 1960s has now faded. There are many more mental health services available in communities, but people who are "at large" must be motivated and functional enough to come in on their own for appointments. Also, while mental illness can be a very long-term problem, no one agency is assigned continuous responsibility for the mentally ill. In practice, "community care" looks a lot like "let people fend for themselves."

One result of these changes has been the recent activism of the families of the mentally ill. Family groups have sprung up all over the country, and a national network, The National Alliance for the Mentally Ill, has grown by leaps and bounds. These groups provide education and support to families, lobby for services and changes in legislation, and at times organize and run their own service-providing agencies.

At the same time, patients have become active and formed their own groups. They have lobbied for changes in the way services are provided and for more dignity in their treatment. As activists they want more control over treatment and are adamantly opposed to any encroachments on their right to refuse care. With both groups professionals can be in the uncomfortable position of not knowing whether they are considered friend or enemy.

It is within this complex environment that Shalom House operates as a halfway house for the mentally ill.

Technology

The technology that is relevant to the mentally ill is the technology of diagnosis, medication and treatment. Comprehensive care of the mentally ill transcends technology and includes a variety of concrete, supportive and educative services in addition to medical treatment.

Although great strides have been made in the treatment of the mentally ill, problems remain in the three key areas of diagnosis, medication and treatment. To some extent the problem lies not with the technology but with the way it is used. Mental illness can be a long-term problem; treatment often suffers from a lack of continuity.

Most people who are referred to Shalom House have already been in several other hospitals or treatment facilities. They are likely to have a different diagnosis from each one. There are two reasons for this. One is that mental illness is truly difficult to diagnose. The other is that hospitals tend to have policies that require a diagnosis to be recorded on admission but not necessarily reevaluated at a later date. As a result, diagnosis tends to take place when the doctor knows the least about the patient.

Inaccurate diagnosis and lack of continuity contribute to problems in prescribing medication. There are many possible medications and dosage levels. Each facility may go through a trial and error process with the patient rather than build on the knowledge gained in the last (Sheehan, 1983). A greater emphasis on documentation would be one way to alleviate this problem.

The right medication can make an almost unbelievable difference in a patient's ability to function. However, even the right medication doesn't work unless the patient takes it. Here we can appreciate how important it is for the patient and family to be included and educated in the process of treatment.

Nowadays there are many theories and therapies that are available to clients. Most have something to offer, but it is very easy for a patient and family to become confused and turned off to a mental health "system" that has a new theory or therapy at every turn. Patients can be helped enormously when they receive accurate diagnosis, helpful medication, supportive therapy, continuity in care, education, and concrete services. Mental health care is often ineffective because one service is provided without the others to back it up.

Organization

Shalom House provides a comfortable, secure and informal environment for patients and staff. It would not necessarily be easy for an outsider to distinguish those who live there from those who run the program. Shalom House provides a lot of structure with many rules and consequences; the staff has a lot of authority—including the authority to tell someone to leave; but the atmosphere is relaxed and egalitarian. Each staff member has a specific job description, but roles are flexible and everyone is involved in a little bit of everything. Many informal conversations between staff and residents occur in the kitchen, dining room and hallways. The offices for Shalom House and Shalom, Inc. are located on the second floor of the house, interspersed with bedrooms, bathrooms, and the laundry area. Most of the business (other than confidential matters) is conducted within earshot of the residents.

Shalom House is known as a good place to work. Live-in positions turn over every 18 months or so, but other staff positions are held for periods of five to ten years. Some permanent staff have risen through the ranks as students, back-up house managers, and house managers, before assuming a case manager position.

Shalom House has a cooperative arrangement with Portland's major hospital which provides a full range of psychiatric services and has a residency training program for psychiatrists. This hospital has an inpatient psychiatric unit, emergency room with psychiatrists on-call 24 hours a day, a Day Treatment program, and an outpatient clinic providing medication and treatment. Residents of Shalom House are generally treated at this hospital, although they are free to engage the services of a private psychiatrist if they wish and are able. Staff at Shalom House have to know enough to know when a client needs to be evaluated for medication or treatment, and must take residents to the hospital when an emergency arises.

Shalom House has cooperative arrangements with other service-providing agencies in Portland, including The Bureau of Rehabilitation, the aftercare agency, a social club for the mentally ill and a crisis intervention unit. Shalom House takes clients from all over Maine and sometimes from out of state, so we are in communication with hospitals and treatment centers all over New England.

Case Description

Bill Jones is a thirty-one-year-old, divorced veteran, who carries a primary diagnosis of chronic undifferentiated schizophrenia and a secondary diagnosis of alcohol abuse. He has had six psychiatric hospitalizations; all occurred within the past three years, and none lasted more than two weeks. His personal difficulties date back further. He reports a suicide attempt at the age of eleven and feeling "different" in high school. He was in the armed services for five years before being given a dishonorable discharge for being absent without leave for three months. He apparently drank heavily while in the service and during this time was briefly married and then divorced.

For the seven years since leaving the service, Bill has been a transient. He had one job that lasted two years during this time, but none of his other jobs have lasted more than a few months. He has gone through periods of heavy drinking and of minor involvement with the law. He was charged once with disorderly conduct and once with forging identification. He has not been involved with AA and does not consider himself an alcoholic.

His first psychiatric admission occurred three years ago. He was traveling on a bus from Massachusetts to Maine and created a disturbance when he got into a fight with a man he thought was making advances. The bus driver put him off the bus, called the sheriff, and Bill was admitted to a hospital in New Hampshire with a diagnosis of acute schizophrenic episode. He was paranoid and delusional at the time. Bill remembers being paranoid and delusional a couple of years before that, but he received no treatment and the feelings went away.

During the last three years, Bill has been drifting around Maine, living with relatives, holding jobs for a week or a month at a time, and being admitted to local psychiatric units. He has overdosed twice when despondent about not working and not being able to support himself. He was referred to Shalom House from a community mental health center. At that time he had no means of support other than living off relatives, was having increasing difficulty holding a job, and had been hospitalized four times in the previous year.

Definition of the Client

At Shalom House our client is the individual resident, not the family or the community. Unlike many social agencies, we choose our clients. Once accepted, the prospective resident may have to wait for a room to become available.

Over the years, Shalom House has developed a specific profile of the kind of client it is seeking. Acceptable residents are those who are judged to be currently incapable of independent living but who are felt to have both the ability and motivation to achieve independent living in a year's time. Screened out are those under eighteen, those with serious drug or alcohol problems, those who may be violent, and those whose suicidal impulses are not under control. Potential residents must be able to assume responsibility for their own medication and must be able to adjust to group living, including having a roommate. They must be in reasonably good health.

Bill's history reminds us that while the guidelines for admission to Shalom House are sound, they leave open a lot of room for interpretation. At Shalom House it is the job of the clinical director, a social worker, to make this determination in consultation with the rest of the staff. Bill had a history of alcohol abuse and suicide attempts; should he be barred from the program? The referring agency felt he was not suicidal, at least at present. We decided to offer Bill a place at Shalom House in exchange for a signed agreement that he would do no drinking while in the program. Bill agreed to this plan. At Shalom House, the consequence for breaking a contract of this nature is immediate dismissal from the program. Making these agreements gives us the latitude to offer a place to someone who is considered risky, knowing that if they break the agreement we can get them out of the program.

Mental illness is very often intertwined with drug or alcohol problems and very often includes some episodes of harm or threat to self or others. If we screened out everyone who had ever experienced any difficulty in these areas, there would be no one left to come to Shalom House. Judgements constantly have to be made.

A complicating factor in making these judgements is the anecdotal nature of psychiatric records. I have often received records stating that a person was "violent" or "very violent." In order to understand what that means, I have had to call the person who wrote the record and say, "what exactly did this person do that was violent?"

Bill's records were a case in point. His application to Shalom House was at first denied, without an interview being granted, because his hospital records indicated both a severe drinking problem and past that included arrest for attempted murder. Upon receiving this letter, Bill called me and denied that he had ever been arrested. In the ensuing interview, he was open and cooperative and denied the charges without being defensive or showing any hostility. I sent away to other hospitals that had treated him previously to see whether their records would show any evidence of such charges. A hospital in New Hampshire responded and described the incident in which Bill was psychotic, created a disturbance on a bus, and was brought to the hospital by the sheriff. There was no arrest, and no injuries were reported. Apparently, this was the incident which, when told by Bill to a doctor two years later, sounded like an arrest for attempted murder.

Contract

The person who enters Shalom House enters into an elaborate set of agreements. Shalom House is probably the most demanding environment the resident could choose: more demanding than being in an institution and more demanding than living alone. The resident makes choices every day about whether the benefits of Shalom House are worth the effort required to stay.

No drugs, alcohol, violence, stealing, sexual relations, or suicide gestures are allowed at Shalom House. Violation of any of these cardinal rules leads to immediate dismissal; one week's notice is given to move out. However, unless specifically contracted against, individuals are free to drink outside of the house, as long as this is not disruptive to the house and does not interfere with the resident's progress.

There is no curfew at Shalom House. Residents can come and go anytime. Everyone has his own key to the front door. Residents are free to go away on weekends. They are, however, expected to be at Shalom House during the week. They are required to be at house meetings Monday evenings and to be at dinner every weekday night unless excused. Everyone must cook for the house and clean up one night a week together with another resident. Everyone has one assigned house duty a week (e.g., cleaning the second floor bathroom). These duties are checked twice a week. Failure to complete a house duty results in being assigned extra duty the following week.

Each resident must maintain a day program. This could be working, going to school, going to day treatment, doing volunteer work or sheltered work, or looking for work. In any case, residents are required to be doing something constructive during the day. We discourage people from using sickness as an excuse to stay home. If a resident's day program is looking for work, he is expected to make a minimum of two job contacts a day and to hand in a job contact sheet describing these activities at the end of the week. Residents are also expected to take their medication as prescribed.

The first six weeks are a trial period. At the end of that time, the staff makes a decision whether the person should be fully accepted into the program. If the person is found not ready to meet the demands of the program, he is asked to move out.

The contract between the resident and the agency is complex and remains very much a live issue during the course of his stay. All of these policies are discussed at the time the individual comes for an initial tour, again at the interview, and again at the time of admission. New residents are given a handbook.

The agreement between the resident and the social worker is that they will meet regularly during the resident's stay to set goals, review progress, and deal with whatever personal matters are at issue. In addition, the social worker will direct the resident toward needed community resources and, if necessary, advocate for the client. Residents are told when they come in that anything they say will be shared freely with other Shalom House staff.

Goals

The goal for each Shalom House resident is to achieve independent living within a year's time. The specific goals that fall under this general guide are different for each client. Each has an individual care plan. "Independent living" is a general phrase that means living in the community as opposed to living in an institution or in the parents' home. It begs the question of work, and does not mean that one is no longer mentally ill or no longer needs medication and treatment. It may even be defined broadly enough to include infrequent, brief, and self-initiated psychiatric hospitalizations.

In Bill's case, his initial goals in coming to Shalom House were to find work and to rely on the support of the house to overcome the nervousness that had already caused him to lose, or let go of, several jobs. His longer-range goals, looking toward independent living, were to develop a support system and to save money for an apartment. Following is the care plan that was developed after Bill moved into Shalom House.

Goal: To achieve independent living

Objectives:

I. Obtain Employment

   A. Make at least two job contacts every day.
   B. Register with both city CETA and Cumberland County CETA.
   C. Apply to the office of vocational rehabilitation.
   D. Attend occupational meetings on Monday afternoons.

II. Maintain Employment

   A. Attend work regularly despite feelings of nervousness
   B. Discuss work problems with Shalom House staff

III. Develop a Support System

   A. Continue to spend two hours every day in common areas of the house.
   B. Make an effort to stay up until at least 8:00 p.m. four nights a week.
   C. Once income is obtained, do at least one recreational activity every week.
   D. Work with the social worker on developing interests and hobbies.

IV. Save Money

   A. Develop a budget with the social worker.
   B. Open a savings account and save for an apartment.

Meeting Place

Usually when I meet with residents, I do so in my office. Interviews with prospective residents and more informal contacts with residents are held downstairs in the manager's apartment, which is more comfortable and more accessible to the common rooms. Even more informal conversations with residents are held in the common areas. This leaves my office as the most formal of available settings. I preserve the formality of my office to emphasize that it is a place to talk seriously about things. When residents want to see me, they generally ask whether I am free or make an appointment rather than use my office as a drop-in center.

The house managers are encouraged to do the opposite. We do not want a line outside the manager's door of residents waiting to talk in private; we do want managers and residents out in the common areas discussing common issues and concerns.

Use of Time

The maximum stay at Shalom House is twelve months. The structured expectations of the house and the constant turnover tend to assure that as residents get their lives stabilized, they will want to move out of Shalom House and be on their own. We discourage residents from making hasty, unplanned exits from the house. We hope residents will stay at Shalom House until they have a stable means of financial support, have established some sort of routine for daily living, have made some friends in the community, and have made significant progress on the goals with which they entered Shalom House. If they are working a new job, we like to see them maintain that job for three months before leaving. We also like to see them give some notice to the rest of the group rather than move out suddenly.

The other social worker or I meet with each resident every week or two during their stay and for a few weeks afterward. The length of these interviews varies from a few minutes to an hour. The limiting factor is the resident's own tolerance for extended conversation. There are only a handful of residents at Shalom House who can tolerate an hour's conversation. My first sessions with Bill lasted only five or ten minutes. While being completely direct and to the point, he would answer questions with as few words as possible and introduce no new topics of conversation. Then he would fidget and ask, "Anything else?" Recently, he has become more relaxed and spontaneous and it has been possible to converse with him for half an hour.

Reassessment

A major reassessment occurred with Bill a month after he arrived at Shalom House. After looking for a month, he finally found a job washing dishes in a restaurant. He only held the job for a day. When I sat down with Bill he had just missed several days of work, calling in sick. He opened the discussion by saying he thought he should go back to the hospital. It was hard to elicit from Bill how he was feeling and why, because at this point he was still very non-verbal. Gradually, however, the picture emerged that he had been feeling suicidal for two weeks without telling anyone and that if he were to do anything to harm himself, it would probably be by over-dosing. He said that his grandmother, with whom he had previously been living, had sold her home and he would not be able to go back there, that he had been turned down by both CETA programs and that he simply could not tolerate the dishwashing job. If he could not do that, he did not know what else there was for him.

Rehospitalization was seriously considered, but I proposed an alternate plan for Bill to stay at Shalom House and be in a full-time day hospital program. Bill was willing to consider it and to make a contract that he would not make any suicide attempts. He agreed to come to the staff if he became too depressed to control his suicidal impulses so that we could get him to a hospital. Bill's doctor supported this plan and facilitated a speedy referral; within a day, Bill was in a full-time day hospital program. While still depressed, he appeared to have found some relief almost immediately from having brought his feelings out into the open and through experiencing this change of plan.

The focus of the plan changed from vocation to treatment. It was suggested to Bill that he apply for social security disability and supplemental security income, and procedures for doing so were explained. This option seemed reasonable since he had not been able to maintain a job in five years. This remained the general plan for a couple of months. However, the process of getting on SSI and SSDI is a long one, and as Bill began to feel better, there began a gradual refocusing back in the vocational direction. He was encouraged to try vocational activities again and try to determine what his tolerance for working might be. A medication change was also made, with good results: Bill began to feel less uncomfortable and to be more relaxed and spontaneous. The day treatment program was able to place patients in volunteer jobs, and a job in the hospital kitchen was arranged. At the same time, Bill was appointed chairman of the Coke Fund at Shalom House, a position that pays $5 a week and carries some status within the house. He is responsible for the Coke machine and all the business that goes with it: ordering, stocking, collecting the money, setting prices, paying bills, keeping the books, going to the bank, and supervising an assistant.

Bolstered by his positive experience doing volunteer work, Bill applied for a paying job in the hospital kitchen, and after several interviews he was hired as a full-time dishwasher. He began this job while keeping his case active with SSI and SSDI in case it turned out that he could not successfully hold this job.

Another reassessment occurred on the issue of alcohol use. Bill confessed occasional limited use of alcohol to me but denied it was a problem, saying that before he would have kept drinking all night but now he was able to stop at two beers and come home. The staff decided to change his contract to allow very limited drinking.

The issue of interests and hobbies was also reassessed. Bill insisted that he had no interests and hobbies and no intention of developing any. He maintained that this simply was the way he was and that he could live with it. I agreed to drop any mention of hobbies from his care plan.

Treatment Modality

In trying to define the type of treatment Bill received at Shalom House, it is easy to overlook the obvious. Concrete services are possibly the largest part of what makes Shalom House therapeutic. Many adults recovering from mental illness simply need a place to start. A temporary, no-rent, safe place to live within walking distance of potential jobs may be all that is needed.

In addition, the milieu of Shalom House has been carefully crafted for therapeutic benefit. Everyone has to cook dinner one night a week. Everyone has to go to his day program every day. The natural desire to be like everyone else in the group tends to reinforce higher levels of functioning. Since everyone has psychiatric problems, it also circumvents the argument, "I'm a sick person; you can't really expect me to do all this."

Teaching of daily living skills is also an important part of the Shalom House program. Shalom House residents should leave the program with some proficiency at cooking, cleaning, shopping, budgeting, banking, making friends, and structuring their free time. If they do not have a car, they should be familiar with the bus system. They should also be familiar with the social service system, and know what services are available and how to obtain them.

Shalom House also serves an educational function: residents should leave with some understanding of their illness and how to manage it, both in terms of medication and of awareness of vulnerable areas.

The work that goes on between social worker and client consists largely of emotional support, but also includes goal-setting, referrals, education, limit-setting and contracting. Many mentally ill adults desperately need someone to recognize their abilities as well as their disabilities and to treat them with respect. In addition, it is up to the social worker to provide focus to the efforts of client and agency by developing, with the client, a comprehensive Care Plan. Social worker and client review progress and write a new plan every three months.

Drawing up a Care Plan requires the social worker to accurately assess the needs, abilities, and motivations of the client. It doesn't do much good to write "Find a job" on the Care Plan of a client who has no intention of so doing. The social worker must be skilled at matching the complex resources of the community to the complex needs of the client. This is not simply an intellectual exercise; it involves facilitation, preparing the client for the service and the service for the client.

It is often the job of the social worker to better educate the client about his mental illness. It is also up to the social worker to enforce the expectations of the program since clients must fulfill certain responsibilities in order to remain at Shalom House. Contracting can be a useful tool.

Thus, the treatment offered by the social worker at Shalom

House includes assessment, emotional support, appropriate referrals, written comprehensive care plans with periodic review and
revision, education, enforcement of program expectations, and contracting. It must be admitted, however, that clients tend to be more
impressed with the concrete services provided (food, shelter, small
loans of money, someone to talk to) than they are with the aspects
of the program that are prized by the staff.

Stance of the Social Worker

I have to be active with Bill and draw him out. I must also listen
very closely for clues, since he gives out so little that indicates how
he is feeling, or what he is thinking. Drawing him out and sustaining a conversation is a goal in itself. I also have to work hard with
Bill to get him to link feelings to events. He tends to experience
feelings as facts that have no connection to any reality. For example, when he was suicidal and considering hospitalization, he had
no idea why. He said, "I'm just depressed, that's all." It was only
through a lot of probing that I was able to put together the puzzle
and say, "Gee, Bill, no wonder you're depressed. Your grandmother sold your home, you were turned down by both CETAs, it
took you a month to find a job and now you're not able to do it."

Outside Resources

Overall, one makes more headway with Bill manipulating the
objective realities of his life than talking to him about his feelings.
Bill's timely referral to day treatment can be considered a concrete
service. Clearly SSI and SSDI are concrete services. Bill did the
footwork on his own, but we provided him with the information he
needed to pursue it. Unfortunately, the system is set up in a way
that just about guarantees that if you walk in there naive, you will
end up with nothing. Bill has sometimes been without spending
money, and Shalom House has provided him with funds to fill his
prescriptions.

Residence at Shalom House is itself a concrete service. We provide shelter in an urban setting and charge 30% of a person's income for room and board. A person with no income is charged
nothing. We also provide a subsidy to people who are just begin-

ning to work, since we are cheaper than alternative living arrangements. This allows a resident to leave Shalom House with a security deposit, first month's rent, and some savings.

Transfer or Termination

We knew the decision to allow Bill to do some drinking and remain in the program was risky. I began to get feedback from house managers that Bill was drinking too much. Then we found money missing from the Coke Fund that Bill managed. Bill was dismissed from Shalom House for stealing. We believe he stole money in order to drink.

Bill did leave Shalom House with a full-time job. He had no particular difficulty finding a new place to live. He eventually paid back the money stolen and earned the right to return to Shalom House as an ex-resident visitor. My information through the grapevine is that he held his job in the hospital kitchen for approximately two years, then was fired. During this time he reportedly became increasingly involved in drug and alcohol abuse. I have no further information.

Differential Discussion

I see five major decisions that affected Bill's stay at Shalom House. The first was the decision to admit him to the program. This was a judgment call, but our finding was that he met the program guidelines and could be admitted to the program under a contract for no alcohol abuse.

The second decision involved what course of action to take when he quit his first job and became suicidal. In retrospect, the plan of full-time Day Treatment, a medication review, a contract not to act on suicidal feelings, applications to SSI and SSDI, and continuing at Shalom House, worked very well. It is important to realize that this decision, like every other, was a gamble. Despite his contract, he could have impulsively taken an overdose, precipitating another hospitalization and dismissal from Shalom House. I believe the plan we implemented addressed his concerns directly, taking away his need to make a dramatic statement by overdosing.

The next two decisions were somewhat contradictory: urging applications to SSI and SSDI, and encouraging continued vocational involvement. The first move creates for Bill a possible way out of the destructive cycle he has been in for the past few years: attempting work, failing, become psychotic, suicidal, or alcoholic; being admitted to a hospital, recovering, and starting the cycle all over again. The second suggestion allows for some more testing in this area, for keeping options open, and for clarifying what his problem with work really is.

The fifth and most risky decision was to allow some alcohol use while in the program. If we had enforced our original no alcohol contract with him, he would have been asked to leave. This would have upheld the sanctity of contracts at Shalom House and saved us the future trauma of having to ask him to leave for stealing money. It also would have undercut his denial and minimalization of alcohol as a problem in his life. However, it also would have denied him the opportunity to try drinking in a responsible way. Since he was certain to try drinking when on his own, and since he was not at all interested in alcohol treatment, it seemed reasonable to have him do his experimenting with us. The fact that he came on his own and told me that he had done some drinking made it harder for me to respond to his honesty by asking him to leave. In social work there is not always a right answer.

PRACTICE IN CONTEXT

The case of Bill Jones at Shalom House was clearly affected by technology, policy and organization. Without the technology of medication, Bill would not have been a candidate for a house like ours. Furthermore, a change of medication during his stay allowed him to feel much more relaxed and has probably contributed to his being able to work again.

Bill's experience with us was shaped by the organization of Shalom House. Once there, Bill faced a series of non-negotiable expectations that included maintaining a full day program, participating in house responsibilities and continuing to take medication. I believe Shalom House creates a very therapeutic environment for persons recovering from mental illness.

Some questions should be raised regarding the overall care Bill has received as a mentally ill person. Although we were able to coordinate a variety of services for him while he was at Shalom House, these were only minimally integrated with anything that has happened before or since. One problem with Shalom House is that it is a short-term solution to a long-term problem. Clients are with us on the average for six months, but they are mentally ill for much longer. Within our whole national system of health care and mental health care, there is a bias toward short-term care. The mentally ill and their families are subjected to many short-term interventions (brief therapies, brief hospitalizations) each of which "re-invents the wheel." In some cases a client is served by the same agency for many years, but the workers turn over every year or two, creating a series of fresh starts.

Perhaps if we had had more of a history with Bill we would have known that it was a mistake to condone any drinking or to put him in a position of responsibility with money. Was he "set up for failure" due to our ignorance? Conversely, in the six years that have passed since Bill left Shalom House, no one has ever written to us for information, despite the fact that we now know quite a bit about him.

When Shalom House was founded it was hoped that our efforts at education and rehabilitation would be effective in interrupting the pattern of recurring hospitalizations for our clients. Unfortunately, the more serious forms of mental illness tend to be more chronic than we wanted to believe. Over the years, Shalom House has adapted to this reality by taking clients back two or three times and by developing other, more long-term, residential programs.

As illustrated by the case of Bill Jones, mental illness is very often compounded by drug or alcohol problems. This is extremely common and very difficult to treat. Mental health programs often miss the boat on this issue. On the other hand, traditional drug and alcohol programs are very structured and have almost no ability to accommodate adults who are mentally ill. In recent years in Maine there has been an effort to provide more training on drug and alcohol abuse for mental health personnel, to have alcohol counselors employed in mental health settings, and to develop new programs for the mentally ill abusing client.

As noted, the function of Shalom House is to prepare clients for "independent living." This concept has also been called into question as Shalom House has evolved. In the past twenty years, Portland has changed from being a semi-depressed area to being a very popular and expensive place to live. It has become increasingly difficult for our clients to find any housing they can afford, and the housing they do find is often pretty terrible. At the same time, mental health services are becoming less available. Hospitals get full and stop accepting voluntary patients. Aftercare workers have full case loads and can't accept new clients. When clients are left to struggle under unfavorable circumstances, the question arises, "What's so great about independent living?" It is often hard to convince the parents of a mentally ill young adult that this is a desirable goal. They prefer to see their family member taken care of somewhere.

There are several trends that I think will affect how mental health services are provided in the future. I see a greater role for involvement of families; not just isolated treatment of the individual. Similarly, there will be greater emphasis on education for the patient and family as part of treatment. The value and need for concrete services will become increasingly apparent (housing, income maintenance, skills training, social clubs offering activities and support). There will be more research on the genetic components of mental illness and greater emphasis on accurate diagnosis and medication review. As the biochemical basis of mental illness is explored, stigma will decrease. Patient and family groups will continue to be active. Legal options, such as guardianship, which may create opportunities for involuntary treatment while safeguarding the rights of the individual, will be explored. The long-term nature of severe mental illness will be faced and states will assume more responsibility for assuring overall continuity of care.

REFERENCES

Altman, A. Collaborative Discharge Planning for the Deinstitutionalized. *Social Work*, 27, 5 (1982), pp. 422-429.

Bernheim, K. and Lehman, A. *Working with Families of the Mentally Ill*. New York: Norton, Inc., 1985.

Bernheim, K., Lewine, R., and Beale, C. *The Caring Family*. New York: Random House, 1982.

Bernheim, K. and Lewine, R. *Schizophrenia: Symptoms, Causes and Treatments*. New York: Norton, Inc., 1979.

Budson, R. *The Psychiatric Halfway House: A Handbook of Theory and Practice*. Pittsburgh: University of Pittsburgh Press, 1978.

Chacko, R. *The Chronic Mental Patient in a Community Context*. Washington, D.C.: American Psychiatric Press, 1985.

Ennis, B. and Siegel, L. *The Rights of Mental Patients: The Basic ACLU Guide to a Mental Patient's Rights*. New York: Avon, 1973.

Fairweather, G., Sanders, D., and Maynard, J. *Community Life for the Mentally Ill: An Alternative to Institutional Care*. Chicago: Aldine, 1969.

Foley, H., and Sharfstein, S. *Madness and Government: Who Cares for the Mentally Ill?* Washington, D.C.: American Psychiatric Press, 1983.

Glasscote, R. et al. *Halfway Houses for the Mentally Ill*. Washington, D.C.: Joint Information Service of the American Psychiatric Association and the National Association for Mental Health, 1971.

Glasscote, R. et al. *Rehabilitating the Mentally Ill in the Community*. Washington, D.C.: Joint Information Service of the American Psychiatric Association and the National Association for Mental Health, 1971.

Goffman, E. *Asylums*. New York: Doubleday, 1961.

Hall, J. and Bradley, A. Treating Long-Term Mental Patients. *Social Work*, 383-86, Sept., 1975.

Lamb, H.R., ed., *The Homeless Mentally Ill: A Task Force Report of the American Psychiatric Association*. Washington, D.C.: American Psychiatric Press, 1984.

Lamb, H.R. et al. *Community Survival for Long-Term Patients*. San Francisco: Jossey Bass, 1976.

Lamb, H.R. *Treating the Long-Term Mentally Ill: Beyond Deinstitutionalization*. San Francisco: Jossey Bass, 1982.

Liberman, R., ed. *Psychiatric Rehabilitation of the Chronic Mental Patient*. Washington, D.C.: American Psychiatric Press. 1987.

Maines, D., and Markowitz, M. Elements of the Perpetuation of Dependency in a Psychiatric Halfway House. *Journal of Sociology and Social Welfare*, 6:52-69, 1979.

Markowitz, M.A. and Nitzberg, M.L. Communication in the Psychiatric Halfway House and the Double Bind. *Clinical Social Work Journal*, 10, 3 (1982), pp. 176-189.

McCreath, J. The New Generation for Psychiatric Patients. *Social Work*, 29 (1984) pp. 436-441.

Menninger, W. and Hannah, G. *The Chronic Mental Patient/II*. Washington, D.C.: American Psychiatric Press, 1987.

Raush, H. and Raush, C. *The Halfway House Movement: A Search for Sanity*. New York: Appleton Century Crofts, 1968.

Sheehan, S. *Is There No Place on Earth for Me?* New York: Random House, 1983.

Talbott, J., ed. *Our Patients' Future in a Changing World*. Washington, D.C.: American Psychiatric Press, 1986.

Talbott, J., ed. *The Chronic Mental Patient: Problems, Solutions, and Recommendations for a Public Policy*. Washington, D.C.: American Psychiatric Press, 1979.

Wasow, M. For My Beloved Son David Jonathan: A Professional Plea. *Health and Social Work*, 3:127-45, 1978.

Wilson, D.C. *Stranger and Traveler: The Story of Dorothea Dix, an American Reformer*. Boston: Little, Brown and Company, 1975.

Long Term Family Therapy: Community Mental Health Center

Toba Schwaber Kerson
Lyne Iris Harmon

DESCRIPTION OF THE SETTING

One of four divisions of the Northwest Center for Mental Health/ Mental Retardation, the Children and Family Division consists of outpatient services, a partial hospitalization unit and a base service unit. The center employs over 350 people and serves all parts of the city. Clientele is low to middle income. In the children's division, school-aged patients are generally referred by schools, courts and other agencies. A referral of a child is not accepted unless a parent or legal guardian calls to request evaluation.

Policy

In October, 1963, Congress enacted the Community Mental Health Centers Act (Public Law 88-164) which authorized federal funds for a new kind of organization, the community mental health center. This would help ill people to remain a part of their communities. Centers were to be partly defined according to "catchment area," a geographical area in which they would be responsible for a range of mental health services. Although services for children were not specified, the Northwest Center established a children's outpatient department in 1970. Not until 1975, in an amendment to the Community Mental Health Act, did Congress mandate services to children to begin by 1977 (Larsen, 1986). The centers were established with the premise that the federal government would provide "seed money"; declining subsidies meant that in order to survive, local centers had to develop increasing amounts of nonfederal funding. After eight years centers were expected to be self-sufficient (Goplerud, Walfish and Apsey, 1983).

Presently clients are limited to seven psychotherapy hours plus three chemotherapy visits a month. Because the patient population often presents with very serious problems, intensive outpatient contact is used to prevent hospitalization. Contact beyond the number of visits set by policy is noncompensable and therefore increases the center deficit. Recently, the center decided to provide free evaluation and six psychotherapy visits for children whose family liability is $100 or less. This policy also contributes to the deficit.

It is not always possible to offer effective service while adhering to governmental guidelines. Once I returned from vacation to find that a partial hospitalization reimbursement rate increase (the first additional state funding in eleven years) had been tied to what was then an eight hour psychotherapy limit a month. The state secretary said that because of limited funds, the partial hospitalization rates would not be increased as originally proposed. In fact, there would be no further action on the rate increase until the judge ruled on the eight-hour limit. If the ruling was in the state's favor, the rates were almost certain to be raised as originally proposed. If the ruling was against the state and there was no specific limit to outpatient services, the future of the rate increase was unknown.

This change in external policy severely affected the organization of the children's division. Because there was great need and a rate increase was anticipated, the Center had allowed the program to operate at a deficit throughout the year. Since the rates were not increased and no one knew how and when the court case would be settled, the director of the Center closed the program.

The children who had been in partial hospitalization were transferred to the outpatient unit. Staff members increased caseloads, assumed additional responsibilities, and worked with parents to determine which outpatient services would best meet their needs, recognizing that such services were second best to the closed programs. Staff and clients were left in limbo, waiting to see what happened.

Organization

As a result of budget cuts, staffing of the children and family division depends increasingly on graduate students completing their field assignments during the academic year, and on social workers who are paid a fee for service during the summer months. The center provides excellent student supervision.

In addition to social workers, the children and family division is staffed by psychologists, mental health workers, child-care workers and one half-time psychiatrist. The other five divisions of North West Center are responsible for services to adults, the developmentally disabled, the addicted, those requiring after care and short-term care. The last two divisions have been added recently to work with the chronically ill, many of whom would have remained in state hospitals before the courts mandated deinstitutionalization (Lerman, 1982; Keisler, 1985). All divisions plus units for consultation, education, research and evaluation are responsible to the center administrator, clinical and executive directors. A Community Advocacy Board (CAB) organized in 1974 and consisting of ten elected representatives and eight appointed organizational delegates, all of whom live and/or work in the catchment area, advises the Center.

Case Description

The Richardsons are a lower-middle-class, black family: Mrs. Richardson, aged thirty-seven, Jossie, fifteen, and Stephen, seventeen. Mrs. Richardson requested an emergency appointment after Jossie threatened to run away following an argument with her mother. In the first session Mrs. Richardson was also concerned about Jossie's drinking, smoking pot and underachieving scholastically. At that point, Jossie's Catholic school was threatening expulsion. Jossie minimized the drinking and smoking while admitting the academic difficulties. She and her mother both acknowledged that the tension within the family was the primary problem and noted that Stephen had suggested family therapy. Once family sessions began, it became clear that Stephen felt entrapped in his role as peacemaker and surrogate husband-father. Although he wanted to join the Navy after high school graduation, he felt that the family needed him.

One major problem was the lack of separation and individualization among family members; each felt responsible for the others' happiness, especially the children for their mother's. Divorced for nine years, Mrs. Richardson remained embittered toward her ex-husband. She felt that Mr. Richardson had been lazy, immature, and incapable of responding to the needs of the family. She had worked as a laboratory technician during the children's preschool years because Mr. Richardson was usually unemployed. He had remarried and had two additional children, but he remained close to Jossie and Stephen, seeing them at least every other week. Because Mrs. Richardson had never forgiven her husband, the children felt disloyal and unable to admit their warm feelings for their father. Also, though Mrs. Richardson was lonely, her embitterment allowed her little dating.

DECISIONS ABOUT PRACTICE

Definition of the Client

Funding sources, the county and the medical assistance program, require that the client be an individual. Thus, Mrs. Richardson, Jossie and Stephen are each clients. In treatment terms, during the two years of work, the client changed from the family to mother and daughter, each seen individually.

Goals

The initial family goal was to listen to one another without the need to attack and defend. Recording the interviews, we measured progress by playing back interviews at appropriate times within the sessions. When there was disagreement about what had been said, we listened to that portion of the interview. In this way, family members became acutely aware of problems and were able to reinforce their progress in hearing one another.

Another family goal, which was more difficult to measure, related to each member's wish to separate and individuate within the family system (Rhodes, 1977). As the relationships evolved, the ability to assert one's feelings and ideas was an indication of the willingness to claim individual feelings and not feel responsible for the feelings of other family members (Reid, 1986).

In addition to family goals, each member had individual goals. Stephen's primary goal was to alter his role in the family (White, Brinkerhoff and Booth, 1985; Wallerstein, 1985). He wanted to be the son, to be able to love both parents without feeling guilty and not to be responsible for his mother's happiness. Stephen's joining the Navy while maintaining positive family relationships was a specific goal.

Jossie's goals included learning to differentiate herself so that her self-image did not depend on her mother's image of her, improving her academic performance, and convincing her school not to expel her. Continued enrollment in school, improved grades, and the elimination of smoking and drinking problems were all objective indicators of progress. Another goal Jossie noted was to become more mature, that is, to develop age-appropriate behavior in relation to her peers (Youniss, 1985). In family sessions, Jossie made minimal progress toward this goal. At the end of eleven months of family therapy, Jossie contracted with me individually to continue to work in this area. She is musically talented, and we decided to use her competencies in music and dance to help her find new friends who would reward age-appropriate behavior. In the past, Jossie had avoided these activities because she thought they were babyish.

Mrs. Richardson's goal within the family system was to allow her children the freedom to separate. She wanted to stop displacing her anger and pain onto them. Once the family sessions were over, Mrs. Richardson wanted to continue working on this goal as well as others. A personal goal was to decide whether she would remain in a state of depression now that she was truly experiencing her "single" status or whether she would use her emotional strength to make a life for herself (Berman, 1985). Choosing the latter, she joined a women's support group, began taking college courses, and began dating.

Contract

Northwest Center's policy is to work in six-month blocks with contracts to be drawn at the beginning of each time period. As long as goals are agreed upon by clients and social worker, additional treatment can be planned and the contract extended.

Everyone who was involved in the sessions signed contracts. Since two of the various phases lasted for almost a year, it was imperative that everyone be clear about the reasons for his or her participation and the viability of the contract. In addition to the written contracts, there were many oral ones as the need for reassessment occurred.

The means used to attain the goals were at times clearly defined and at other times illustrated on a metacommunication level. For example, when Jossie's goal was appropriately assertive behavior with peers, the means and the helpfulness of role play were clearly explained. In family sessions, means were often more implied than stated.

Meeting Place

The sessions were held in a comfortable room with furniture that could be moved around and allowed people to move in and out of the family circle.

Use of Time

Agency policy indicated that each family session last one and one half hours and each individual session, one hour. Sometimes as a family and sometimes individually, the Richardson's were in treatment for two years. Family treatment continued for eleven months, and Jossie's, until we had fulfilled the goals of the short-term contract. Mrs. Richardson's individual work lasted for one year; eight months of weekly sessions and four months of biweekly visits. The decision to work biweekly was Mrs. Richardson's means of practicing what she had learned in therapy while weaning herself from the relationship. Extra sessions were held when requested.

Treatment Modalities

Treatment modalities included analytical methods, a cognitive-behavioral approach and crisis intervention within family and individual models of intervention (Werner, 1982; Berlin, 1982; Golan, 1986). Depending on the needs of the family, approaches were used alone or in combination. Although the family approach was eclectic, structural family therapy and family-of-origin work were emphasized (Minuchin, 1981). Techniques teaching communication skills, separating generational boundaries, joining with family members, and helping them to retrace their family tree were all used in relation to specific goals (Hartman, 1978; McGoldrick, 1982).

At one point early in family therapy a tremendous power struggle occurred between Stephen and Mrs. Richardson. We subsequently did a "sculpturing" of the family, a rigid, immobile positioning of the way in which each family member saw himself or herself in relation to the others. In order to depict every view of the family system, each person took a turn positioning everyone. Then, everyone discussed whether he or she wished to stay in that position.

At the end of eleven months of family therapy, we felt that the Richardson's family goals had been attained and that the remaining goals could be best achieved through individual therapy. Jossie's problems involving an examination of thought processes and immature behavior indicated a cognitive-behavioral approach (Berlin, 1983). Jossie and I used role playing and behavioral rehearsal to try out new behaviors before she went out either with her friends or on dates. In the last few weeks of therapy, Jossie brought in a trusted friend who did some role playing with us (Haber, 1987). A minimal amount of analytical work helped her to understand her projections and the projections displaced on her by her mother.

Mrs. Richardson benefitted from an analytical approach that allowed her to explore her relationships with her father and husband and partially dealt with her deep-seated anger toward men. Later in the process, she was able to use a cognitive approach that examined the self-defeating assumptions she had carried into her adult life. Finally, a behavioral approach involving role playing helped her to approach male companions more confidently (Nelson, 1983). As she was fearful about going places alone, we used deep relaxation and self-hypnosis to overcome the anxiety (Long, Machiran and Bertell, 1986).

Stance of the Social Worker

My long-term relationship with the Richardsons deepened as they weathered many crises and experienced many levels of growth. At different points in the process, I directed, confronted, supported, taught and listened. In family sessions, I was direct and active. Since mood and tone could change rapidly and unexpectedly, it was essential that I be on top of the situation. This was especially necessary in the initial sessions, where a failure to intervene might have allowed an explosive situation with the family consequently dropping out of treatment.

I was direct and active in individual work with Jossie based on previous experience with teenagers, the short-term contract, and her tendency to withdraw and avoid problems whenever she was allowed to do so. Sessions with Mrs. Richardson were varied. Sometimes, I confronted her with using her strength for self-destructive purposes. At other times, I sat back and allowed her to consider how she was using her energy (Hepworth and Larsen, 1982). When Mrs. Richardson discussed her past, I tended to be more passive, helping her to think about the material as she became aware of it.

At times, it was beneficial to the family that I share personal experiences. The decision to do so depended on the process preceding the disclosure. If the sharing was ill-timed, the family heard the words differently than they were meant (Dowd and Boroto, 1982; Reynolds and Fischer, 1983). For example, although I wanted to share a personal experience with Mrs. Richardson when she was extremely depressed and angry, it would have been counterproductive because she was furious with me and needed to keep me at a distance.

Outside Resources

The Richardsons were helped to negotiate with Jossie's school, to budget money and to apply for scholarship aid. With Jossie's permission, I asked her teachers to give her a chance to improve her grades and behavior. Jossie also spoke up in her own behalf.

Mrs. Richardson also asked for help with budgeting as increased activities were straining her budget. Together, we reviewed her income and expenses, method of paying bills (charge accounts with high interest), sources for food and clothing, and home-heating costs. As a result, Mrs. Richardson found some new places to shop, joined a food co-op (which also added friends), and borrowed money to convert to gas heat and insulate her house.

Jossie was willing to take a part-time job, which helped financially and enhanced her relationship with her mother. When she was helped to apply for scholarships, I suggested that she obtain a Pennsylvania Higher Education Assistance Agency application from her school counselor through which she could apply for a grant or loan, check the scholarship catalogue held on reserve in the public library and apply to a bank for a low-interest loan.

Reassessment

Reassessment was linked to goals and contracts. Monthly, we informally assessed our progress toward established goals, and when family members seemed uninvolved, I used the process of reassessment to help everyone get back to work. Often, members used the process of reassessment to decide whether therapy should continue; whether the ordeal of family work was worth the potential benefit.

At one point, Mrs. Richardson threatened not to come to sessions because she was deeply hurt by the children's stating that they loved their father. She grew sullen and would not talk to her children in sessions or at home for two weeks. For her, reassessment meant examining the bind in which she placed her children and accepting individual therapy in order to complete an emotional divorce from her ex-husband.

Transfer or Termination

Termination differed with each phase of treatment. Family therapy was terminated because everyone concerned felt that family goals had been met. Jossie's work terminated when the terms of the short-term contract were met; she had learned more appropriate behavior and knew she could call me if she encountered a problem she could not handle. On two occasions, she did call for an appointment. Mrs. Richardson decided to terminate when we concluded that she had integrated new feelings and behaviors.

Case Conclusion

At the end of the family work, Stephen no longer carried the role of husband/father or mediated between his mother and sister and had told his mother that he loved his father and refused to be responsible for her unhappiness about her divorced state. Although Mrs. Richardson was still unhappy about Stephen's relationship with his father, she tried to understand his feelings. Once Stephen had joined the Navy, he remained supportive but individuated.

Jossie's presenting problems of drinking and smoking pot were symptomatic of the family disturbance and therefore decreased significantly after the first few months of treatment. Improved grades and college board scores helped her gain admission to college. By the end of the family sessions Jossie was still afraid of her mother's anger but had gained strength in separating her feelings from her mother's. She also learned that her rebellious attitude was a cover for her dependency (Applegate, 1984). Slow work in individual sessions on Jossie's independence-dependence issues gained momentum once she found positive peer support in college.

In family sessions, recognizing that this could leave her feeling alone and depressed, Mrs. Richardson still allowed her children to separate from her emotionally (Argles, 1984). As Jossie responded well to her mother's limits, Mrs. Richardson began to accept herself as a good parent. Her self-image improved along with her relationship with her children. Rather than trying to induce guilt, she learned to speak directly and assertively. When her individual sessions were terminated, she had come to terms with the children's love for their father. Most importantly, she had learned to think about her present and future needs. Facing the fear and anxiety which she had previously denied, she became involved in a women's group, singles activities and career aspirations. Although relationships were not yet what she wished for, her dating increased. She felt less lonely and could take vacations by herself and enjoy them.

Differential Discussion

At the end of therapy I felt a sense of incompleteness which may have reflected Mrs. Richardson's wish for a permanent male relationship. Although it is not the social worker's responsibility to meet that need, I was left feeling that Mrs. Richardson never really resolved her feelings about her ex-husband and her father, except on an intellectual level. Because of his relationship with the children and his place in Mrs. Richardson's emotional life, he remained part of the family. In retrospect, Mr. Richardson's participating in some of the family sessions might have allowed Mrs. Richardson to divorce him emotionally (Wylder, 1982). Rather than attacking a ghost, she would have been confronting reality. Perhaps then she could find a resolution that recognized their inability to live together but did not detract from their value as parents. Although Stephen and Jossie told their mother that their father viewed her as the giving, responsible parent, hearing it directly would have been helpful.

In addition, I would have been more insistent on seeing Mrs. Richardson along with her parents and sisters. She was strongly encouraged to do so but felt it was too difficult. In doing family-of-origin work, Mrs. Richardson became blocked in confronting her father who had always delivered double messages: she was to achieve because she was smarter than her sisters, but she was not to be given the attention and warmth they received because she could do without it.

The message to be independent and achieve even though you may suffer is what Mrs. Richardson understood as her script. If family-of-origin sessions could have taken place concomitantly with nuclear family sessions, she could have entered into brief therapy with her ex-husband from a different perspective. I wonder, however, if Mrs. Richardson would have been willing to do this after nine years of separation. Although ideally I wished more resolution for Mrs. Richardson, she may well achieve this for herself in time.

PRACTICE IN CONTEXT

Because of Northwest's Center's fiscal dependence on state and county funding, the types of services offered are the result of fiscal and clinical decisions, with the former taking precedence when budget cuts are imminent. Jossie and her family were patients at a time when the agency was partially financed by a federal grant; today, fiscal demand for an increased caseload might have ruled out using the same timeframe and subsystem treatment modalities. Dependence on government funding underscores the notion of practice in context. The therapeutic relationship cannot be isolated from agency structure. The Richardsons were fortunate in that the practice relationship, policies and organizational structure matched their needs.

REFERENCES

Adelson, J. (ed.). *Handbook of Adolescent Psychology*. N.Y.: John Wiley & Sons, 1980.

Argles, Paul. "The Threat of Separation in Family Conflict." *Social Casework* 65:10 (Dec. 1984): 610-614.

Berlin, S. "Cognitive-Behavioral Approaches." In *Handbook of Clinical Social Work*, pp. 1095-1119. Edited by A. Rosenblatt and D. Waldfogel. San Francisco: Jossey-Bass, 1983.

_____. "Cognitive-Behavioral Interventions for Social Work Practice." *Social Work* 27:3 (May/June): 218-226.

Berman, W. H. "Continued Attachment After Legal Divorce." *Journal of Family Issues* 6:3 (Sept. 1985); 375-392.

Billings, R. S. et al. "A Model of Crisis Perception." *Administrative Science Quarterly* 25 (June 1980): 300-316.

Dowd, E. T. and D. R. Boroto. "Differential Effects of Counselor Self-Disclosure, Self-Involving Statements, and Interpretation." *Journal of Counseling Psychology* 29:1 (1982): 8-13.

Faust, R. G. "A Model of Divorce Adjustment for Use in Family Service Agencies." *Social Work* 32:1 (Jan./Feb. 1987): 78-80.

Golan, N. "Crisis Theory." In *Social Work Treatment: Interlocking Theoretical Approaches*, pp. 296-340. Edited by F. J. Turner. N.Y.: The Free Press, 1986.

Goplerud, E. N., S. Walfish and M. O. Apsey. "Surviving Cutbacks in Community Mental Health." *Community Mental Health Journal* 19:1 (1983): 62-76.

Haber, R. "Friends in Family Therapy: Use of a Neglected Resource." *Family Process* 26:2 (June 1987): 269-281.

Hartman, A. and J. Laird. "Family Practice." In *Encyclopedia of Social Work*, 18th ed., pp. 575-587. Edited by Anne Minahan et al. Silver Spring, MD: NASW, 1987.

Hartman, A. and J. Laird. *Family-Centered Social Work Practice*. N.Y.: Free Press, 1984.

Hepworth, D. H. and J. A. Larsen. *Direct Social Work Practice: Theory and Skills*. Homewood, IL: Dorsey Press, 1982.

Keeney, B. and J. Ross. *Mind in Therapy*. N.Y.: Basic Books, 1985.

Keisler, C. H. et al. "An Assessment of Deinstitutionalization." *American Journal of Psychiatry* 38 (1985): 1292-1297.

Kolevzon, M. S. and R. G. Green. *Family Therapy Models: Convergence and Divergence*. N.Y.: Springer Pub. Co., 1985.

Laird, J. "Sorcerers, Shamans, and Social Workers: The Use of Ritual in Family-Centered Practice." *Social Work* 29:2 (March/April 1984): 123-129.

Larsen, J. K. "Local Mental Health Agencies in Transition." *American Behavioral Scientist* 30 (Nov./Dec. 1986): 174-187.

Lerman, P. *Deinstitutionalization*. New Brunswick, N.J.: Rutgers University Press, 1982.

Long, J. M., N. M. Machiran and B. L. Bertell. "Biofeedback: An Adjunct to Social Work Practice." *Social Work* 31:6 (Nov./Dec. 1986): 476-478.

McGoldrick, M., J. Pearce and J. Giordano (eds.). *Ethnicity and Family Therapy*. N.Y.: Guilford Press, 1982.

Minuchin, S. and H. Fishman. *Family Therapy Techniques*. Cambridge, MA: Harvard University Press, 1981.

Nelson, J. C. *Family Treatment: An Integrated Approach*. Englewood Cliffs, N.J.: Prentice-Hall, 1983.

Pinderhughes, E. "Power, Powerlessness, and Practice." In *Empowering the Black Family*, pp. 29-39. Edited by S. Grey, A. Hartman and E. Saalberg. Ann Arbor: National Child Welfare Training Center, University of Michigan School of Social Work, 1985.

Prinz, R. J. (ed.). *Advances in Behavioral Assessment of Children and Families*, Vol. 2. Greenwich, CT: Jai Press, Inc., 1986.

Reid, W. J. and K. Helmer. "Session Tasks in Family Treatment." *Family Therapy* 13:2 (1986): 177-185.

Rich, R. F. (ed.). "Mental Health Policy: Patterns and Trends." *American Behavioral Scientist* 30 (Nov./Dec. 1986): 85-245.

Rubenstein, H. and M. H. Block. *Things That Matter: Influences on Helping Relationships*. N.Y.: McMillan, 1982.

Schinke, S. P. "Social Skills Training with Adolescents." In *Progress in Behavior Modification*, Vol. II, pp. 66-115. Edited by M. Hersen, R. M. Eisler and P. M. Miller. N.Y.: Academic Press, 1981.

Thomlison, R. J. "Behavior Therapy in Social Work Practice." In *Social Work Treatment*, Chapter 6. Edited by Francis J. Turner, N.Y.: The Free Press, 1986.

Wallerstein, J. S. "The Over-Burdened Child: Some Long-Term Consequences of Divorce." *Social Work* 30:2 (March/April 1985): 116-122.

Werner, H. D. *Cognitive Therapy: A Humanistic Approach*. N.Y.: The Free Press, 1982.

White, L. K., D. B. Brinkerhoff and A. Booth. "The Effect of Marital Disruption on Child's Attachment to Parents." *Journal of Family Issues* 6:1 (March 1985): 5-22.

Wylder, J. "Including the Divorced Father in Family Therapy." *Social Work* 27:6 (1982).

Youniss, J. and J. Smollar. *Adolescent Relations with Mothers, Fathers, and Friends*. Chicago: University of Chicago Press, 1985.

Placement of a Developmentally Disabled Man: A Delegate Agency of a Regional DD Center

Toba Schwaber Kerson
Susan Freeman

DESCRIPTION OF THE SETTING

The Regional Center of the East Bay (RCEB) is one of twenty-one regional centers throughout the state of California providing comprehensive assessment and specialized services for developmentally disabled individuals. Regional centers are central points for developmentally disabled people to obtain or be referred for necessary services.

To be considered developmentally disabled, a person must be substantially handicapped by mental retardation, autism, epilepsy, cerebral palsy, or a condition closely related to mental retardation or requiring similar treatment. Handicaps that are totally physical are excluded. The handicap must have occurred prior to the age of eighteen and continue or be expected to continue indefinitely (Grossman, 1984).

Clients may be referred at any age by various sources, including schools, hospitals, parents or community agencies. Their eligibility is determined by an assessment team usually consisting of a social worker and a physician but which may also include a psychologist, an occupational therapist, a nurse, and a nutritionist. Once a client is determined eligible, the case is transferred to a case manager.

Only a small percentage of case management services is provided "in-house" by the Regional Center of the East Bay staff. The majority of cases are delegated to one of seven agencies which are under contract to the Regional Center of the East Bay to provide case management services. Home, Health and Counseling is one of the delegate agencies.

A case manager working for Home, Health and Counseling is responsible for advocating, counseling, coordinating, and obtaining necessary services for the developmentally disabled client (Kurtz, Baggarozzi and Pollane, 1987). A case manager is additionally responsible for developing, implementing and reviewing an individual program plan for each client. This should pinpoint developmental objectives and plans to achieve these objectives.

An individualized program plan as defined by the Accreditation Council for Services for Mentally Retarded and Other Developmentally Disabled Persons must (NASW, 1982; Keenan, 1983):

1. Be a written plan of action for the ongoing development of the individual based on the developmental model.
2. Result from a comprehensive assessment of the clients' developmental status.
3. Be formulated through an interdisciplinary process with the participation of the client, client's family, relevant staff of agencies serving the client, and other persons who may be significantly involved with the client's development. Participants must share all information and recommendation and develop, as a team, a single, integrated plan to meet the individual's identified needs.
4. Specify separately stated developmental goals and objectives written in behavioral terms, be time-limited, and provide measurable indices so that effectiveness of services and programming may be evaluated.
5. Contain written plans and strategies for the achievement of objectives, including names of individuals and agencies and their specific responsibilities.
6. Identify an overall client services coordinator — a single locus of responsibility to ensure the plan's implementation and success.
7. Be distributed and held in common by those directly involved.
8. Ensure periodic assessment of client progress toward achieving the objectives.
9. Be evaluated at least annually with the participation of all concerned after reassessment of the client.

The manual says, "Counseling is an integral part of case management and is a problem-solving process in which alternatives are jointly explored with the DD person and his family to find resolutions to situational stresses at various developmental stages of life." The policies would be excellent guides to practice if each case manager did not carry 62 cases. Often case managers feel like case manag*ees*, since all of the people involved tell them what to do (Intagliata, 1982). A minimum of four client contacts annually is required. There is no fee for services.

Policy

California established the regional center system with the enactment of the Lanterman Developmental Services Act. The intent of this law was to provide service to developmentally disabled individuals in their local community in the least restrictive manner and the most normal environment possible. Prior to this act, services were provided only at the time of institutionalization (DeWeaver, 1983).

The law explicitly states who is to be considered developmentally disabled. In addition, once an individual is so diagnosed and accepted into the system, with rare exceptions as long as he remains in California, he is a regional center client. A seventeen-year-old accident victim with severe brain damage, for example, is eligible for regional center services for as long as he lives. Had the accident occurred a year later, he would be ineligible. Numerous accountability procedures, such as the individual program plan, are mandated by law, thereby placing an emphasis on paper work and limiting direct client contact. Each year the California Legislature determines the funds to be allocated to each regional center.

The policy of each local regional center determines how these funds will be used. Funding priorities for the Regional Center of the East Bay range from a high priority for residential placement and day programming to a lower priority for respite, speech therapy, and equipment purchases. Also, the Regional Center of the East Bay's policy has been to increase case loads in order to stay within funding limitations. Case loads have been raised from forty-five to sixty-two, and this drastically affects case managers' abilities to provide services.

Home, Health and Counseling's policies also affect our relationship with the client. Some delegate agencies have elected to hire case aides to handle some of the paperwork and less complex cases. Home, Health and Counseling has only master's degree social workers and no case aide support.

On occasion, the policies of the two agencies, Regional Health Center of the East Bay, and Home, Health and Counseling, are in conflict. For example, RCEB case managers are permitted to transport their clients in their cars, whereas Home, Health and Counseling's case managers are not. A board and care facility operator who has residents from several different delegate agencies may be confused and angry over differing rules.

Technology

Treatment includes providing services and intervention according to the principles of the "developmental model." A comprehensive assessment of the individual's developmental status and needs is the basis for designing and maintaining a program of services. In delivering these services, special emphasis is given to the social integration of the person and to the least restrictive, effective service alternative. Services are continuously coordinated, reflecting planned and active participation by the individual and/or the family, the provider of service and the case manager (Slater and Wekler, 1986).

Much of the treatment is purchased or provided by other community agencies that specialize in services to the developmentally disabled population. These services might include infant stimulation programs, behavior modification consultation, speech therapy, and, less often, individual psychotherapy. Genetic counseling services are sometimes provided by outside specialists, and this helps both to advance the knowledge about various genetic disorders and to enable families to understand the risks entailed in having more children (Mealey, 1984).

In some instances, recent technological advances have enabled the developmentally disabled client to make significant progress. This is clearly evident for the nonverbal cerebral palsy client whose world is changed by an electronic communication device. Another example is a typewriter that has been adapted for a young client of mine with above average intelligence who has muscular dystrophy. He is able to talk well, but his upper extremities are too weak for him to write or use a conventional typewriter. This special typewriter has been adjusted so that he can type by touching but not exerting pressure. Another youngster in my case load with severe cerebral palsy but superior intelligence is nonverbal and spastic. She is being evaluated for a computerized device which will produce words on tape, and there is a possibility that someday a voice-box will reproduce her thoughts. As a case manager, I might arrange for consultation with a speech therapist and evaluation by a rehabilitation engineer to determine the most useful device. The regional center can sometimes further help with purchases of the equipment.

Many of our clients carry a dual diagnosis of developmental disability and mental illness. They are often followed by psychiatrists and treated with a variety of drugs. Clients with epilepsy also receive a combination of drugs for seizure control from their general physician or their neurologist (Kerson, 1985).

Organization

The regional centers were organized by the California legislature as part of a network of private, nonprofit agencies under contract to the California Department of Health. The Regional Center of East Bay is governed by a board of trustees representing various categories of developmental disabilities and reflecting the geographic and ethnic characteristics of the regional center's population. At least one-third of the board must be composed of people with developmental disabilities or members of their families. The board appoints a director who sets policies with the help of his administrative staff. The current director is in the process of a reorganization that will give him more direct control over all aspects of the agency.

Home, Health and Counseling is also a private, nonprofit agency governed by a board of directors and an administrative director. It primarily provides home care services to the elderly. The developmental disabilities unit, as part of the contracts division, is directly accountable to a director of contracts. In the unit there are six case managers and a supervisor.

There are often conflicts between the Home, Health and Counseling (HHC) staff and the Regional Center of the East Bay staff. Home, Health and Counseling is located farthest from the regional center. Because all the RCEB consulting staff is housed in the central building, HHC staff members often have a feeling of isolation and powerlessness and experience difficulties in procuring consulting services for our clients. Salaries and benefits differ for RCEB case managers, who are unionized, and delegate agency case managers, who are not. While conflict mars the inter-agency relationship, intra-agency relations are excellent. The Home, Health and Counseling DD unit consists of a small staff well supported by administration. The supervisor respects different styles and allows for flexible interpretation of policy.

Case Description

Joseph Wolfe is a twenty-nine-year-old, mild to moderately retarded white man with a diagnosis of Williams syndrome. In addition to retardation, Joseph has many features consistent with Williams syndrome. He is short, microcephalic, coarse featured and has an open mouth with a prominent, thick lower lip and dental malalignment. Joseph is neat, clean and well dressed, and although he is unusual looking, he is not really unattractive. His personality is also typical of those with Williams syndrome in that after initial nervousness subsides, he exhibits what is sometimes described as a "cocktail party personality." Joseph is a warm, outgoing, "huggy-touchy" person. Despite his graying hair and "crow's feet," he gives the impression of a young, vulnerable boy. I tend to feel protective and maternal toward him and find him very likeable.

Joseph was referred to the regional center by his mother at the suggestion of a physician from a genetics clinic. Mrs. Wolfe explained that for the past six years, Joseph had been living at a convalescent hospital with geriatric patients. He had no day programming. She was requesting the regional center's services to help find a more appropriate living situation and a day program. In the convalescent hospital, the majority of patients are nonambulatory. There is a limited activity program, but it is geared to the elderly, including, for example, throwing a softball from one wheelchair to the next. This type of facility is structured for the chronically ill patient; it makes someone like Joseph appear chronically ill. He received a lot of attention, being the only young patient and was the "pet" of the nurses and many other patients.

Mrs. Wolfe is fifty-one years old with bleached blond highly teased hair. She dresses in tight-fitting, seductive clothing and is a hostess in a cocktail lounge. She treats Joseph like a child, always referring to him as a "boy" and reinforcing his medical needs, and his dependence on her (Falck, 1984). She triggers much of his vomiting. Her last words to him as she left the first placement in a family care home were, "Now darling, don't disappoint Mommy and vomit." She is not a particularly likeable person — domineering and pushy.

Mrs. Wolfe provided sketchy information about Joseph's early years. He was the product of a full-term pregnancy. Labor was induced after Mrs. Wolfe slipped and fell down the stairs. Joseph was born with the cord wrapped around his neck and required resuscitation. As a baby, he had severe feeding problems, including frequent vomiting, and he failed to gain weight. Developmental milestones included holding his head up early, walking without support at thirteen months, and speaking single words at thirty months.

Medically, Joseph had frequent serious respiratory illnesses requiring hospitalization as a child. At sixteen, he had a severe drug reaction with hypertension and a stroke which resulted in paralysis of the left side. He shows some neurological difficulties, particularly in fine motor coordination, visual perceptual abilities, and mild left-handed ataxia that may be related to Williams syndrome, birth trauma, or the residuals of the stroke. His only current health problem is diverticulitis. It is recommended, however, that Joseph have his blood pressure checked frequently, since individuals with Williams syndrome often have renal failure stenosis, closing of the arteries that lead to the kidneys.

Joseph's parents were divorced when he was young, and he has no contact with his father. He sees his mother frequently and maintains contact with his sister. As a child, Joseph was placed in various residential schools for mentally retarded youngsters. He carried the diagnosis of isolated mental retardation until the age of twenty-eight, when he was referred by a friend to a genetics clinic and diagnosed as having Williams syndrome.

Joseph has good self-care skills, is able to read and write simple words, print his name and order from a menu. He speaks clearly and has good receptive language skills. He is weakest in community-living skills such as using public transportation, crossing the street, cooking, and managing money.

Once Joseph was accepted as an RCEB client, the assessment worker arranged placement at a small family care home near Joseph's sister; a private, licensed residence with three other men run by a couple. There were shared bedrooms, home-cooked meals eaten in the kitchen, and a weekly "family" outing to a restaurant and to a shopping center. There were no planned activities in the home, although the residents were taken to the local handicapped recreation program one night a week. A joint visit by the assessment worker and the case manager was made at the time of the placement. To me, this was the most normal, homelike type of environment available. A disadvantage was that this particular couple tended to overprotect and control their residents.

Immediately after placement, Joseph began vomiting and crying. His vomiting was not polite or controlled. He sat at the dinner table and threw up all over the food (not only his) and then continued to throw up anywhere and everywhere so that everyone knew he was vomiting and in distress. The caretaker felt she could not keep him. He was sent to his sister's for a brief time and then returned to the convalescent hospital because his mother, stressing his medical needs, refused to accept any other options for his care.

A team conference was set up soon after and was attended by the case manager, the assessment worker, a regional center psychologist, and the regional center physician. It became clear during this meeting that Mrs. Wolfe had been brought up in foster homes and viewed Joseph's placement in a small care facility as a reenactment of her childhood and a threat to her own mothering abilities. It was decided to pursue day programming and consider placement only at a large residential facility.

Plans were made, working with Mrs. Wolfe and Joseph, to have Joseph attend a workshop and travel by a bus, with both activities funded by the regional center. The workshop coordinator visited Joseph at the convalescent hospital prior to placement. In addition, Mrs. Wolfe and Joseph went to visit a large residential facility for mentally retarded clients in the area and were placed on a two-year waiting list.

The facility is a self-contained residence and program for seventy-six developmentally disabled adults, who live in cottages in a country-like setting at a distance from the town. The residents all work in the workshops on the campus, which has a college-like quality. There are different personnel for different shifts, allowing staff the strength to deal with more difficult clients. Disadvantages of the facility are the isolation and the institutional atmosphere. For example, meals are taken in an impersonal central dining room with little homelike character. There is also significant staff turnover.

The workshop in which Joseph was placed is one of a number sponsored by a county association for the retarded. Generally, it is a place for people unable to function in competitive employment. The workshop program has educational and training components with classes in, for example sex education, food skills, and self-help skills as well as assembly line type jobs for which the employee is paid on the basis of what he produces (a percentage of the minimum wage based on what a nondisabled worker could produce). There is also a social component with dances, camping trips, lunches at restaurants, etc.

Once Joseph had begun at the workshop, the case manager contracted behavior modification services for him. The program that was set up stressed Joseph's "manliness" and "healthiness" and was monitored by Joseph and the workshop staff. It included a daily notebook that was scored morning and afternoon on "manliness" and "healthiness" at the day program. The scoring was done by Joseph and checked by his teacher with a goal of gradually decreasing any statements suggesting weakness, ill health, nervousness, or lack of ability. It was gradually extended to the convalescent hospital and withdrawn from the day program. An additional program was set up by the behavior modification specialist to improve Joseph's physical strength and included jogging with the behavior modification specialist and participation in the special olympics.

After several months at the workshop, placement needs were again explored. It was decided, with Joseph's and his mother's concurrence, to place him at a middle-sized board and care facility where other workshop clients lived. The new residential facility houses twenty people and consists of a series of cottages behind a larger home, in a residential area in the same city as the convalescent hospital. There is different supervision for different shifts, although the owner/manager is there during the day and sleeps close by. Each cottage has several shared bedrooms and an occasional single room, as well as a TV room. All residents eat together in a central dining room. During the day, the residents go to their programs, which include various workshops as well as a special adult education school. Some go by public transportation, some are transported in minibuses. There is active programming many evenings and weekends. It includes movies, scouts, dances, and adult education by teachers from the local school district, who provides classes in singing and crafts. It is somewhere between the small family home and the large residential facility. It certainly does not have the warmth or homelike atmosphere of a smaller facility; yet, it provides an active, stimulating environment.

After a series of preplacement visits, placement was recently successfully completed. I think Joseph was able to make the transition from the convalescent hospital to the residence not so much because he knew other people from the workshop but because he had developed social skills and a better self-image from his workshop and behavior modification program (Hall et al., 1983).

DECISIONS ABOUT PRACTICE

Definition of the Client

According to strict policy terms, the regional center client is defined only as the developmentally disabled individual. In practice, however, a family member or a board and care facility operator is often also a client. In Joseph's case, it would have been impossible to do successful planning without considering his mother as a client (Mueller and Leviton, 1986). This became clear after her needs were not taken into account in the first placement. If a relationship had not been established with Mrs. Wolfe, she would have sabotaged any future programming.

Goals

Goals or objectives for the regional center client are formally written into the individual program plan, which is developed with the client and significant community and family members, reviewed quarterly, and rewritten annually. It is based on a developmental model. Since the case manager is not only the direct provider of service but often the coordinator as well, Joseph's goals depend on the relationship between himself and the case manager, the behavior modification consultant, the workshop staff, and the convalescent hospital staff. Joseph's initial goals were less refined and broader-based, becoming more confined once he entered a workshop program.

Contract

The contracts, or plans for achieving the goals, are also explicitly stated in the individual program plans. These plans are exact, with clear reference as to who is responsible for implementing the goals and in what way. In Joseph's case, the behavior modification consultant developed an additional contract with Joseph to increase his feelings of healthiness and reinforce his being a responsible adult.

Meeting Place

Meetings often take place in the client's home, school or day program and, less rarely, in the agency. For Joseph, all visits took place at the convalescent hospital or the workshop. Because our meetings required a feeling of warmth, support and attention and one goal was to increase Joseph's sense of healthiness, we met on the patio outside the sterile atmosphere of the convalescent hospital.

Use of Time

Duration and frequency of visits varies depending on the client's need and the case manager's time restrictions. Joseph was anxious, often talkative, and required long visits, particularly in the initial phase of the relationship. As he became more comfortable and familiar with the case manager, visits were shorter. Joseph was seen for seven months.

Regional center policy dictates that once an individual is accepted as a developmentally disabled client, in most instances he remains a client as long as he remains in California. If the regional center is not funding any services and if there is no need for case manager intervention, the case can become inactive. At one point, when Mrs. Wolfe was rejecting all alternatives and seemed intent on sabotaging plans, the option to make Joseph inactive was considered, but never used.

Treatment Modality

For Joseph, the most effective treatment was a behavior modification approach to deal directly with his vomiting and to enable him to integrate successfully into a day program. Relaxation techniques were also utilized (Blumenthal, 1985; Peveler, 1986; Herson, 1985; Thyer, 1983; Harris and Bergman, 1987). It was recommended to Mrs. Wolfe that she and Joseph receive some family therapy to help them deal with their symbiotic relationship, but thus far this has not occurred (Boyer, 1986).

Stance of the Social Worker

It was important to take an active role with Joseph. Since he lived in a convalescent hospital, he had assumed the role of a weak, sick person. His resistance to giving up that role required active intervention to effect any change. Mrs. Wolfe had ambivalent feelings about making any change in Joseph's lifestyle, and needed direct confrontation, as well as recognition of her feelings. Joseph profited more from a warm, supportive approach, since any confrontation made him anxious and immobile. While an active stance remains necessary with Joseph, currently, the social worker's stance with Mrs. Wolfe can be more passive, taking her into consideration when important changes are to take place in Joseph's life. Neither Joseph nor Mrs. Wolfe would benefit from sharing the case manager's life experience, since each would view such sharing as an imposition on their needs.

Outside Resources

Joseph required the use of many resources from the onset of his relationship with the assessment worker. These included arranging for the placement, having the regional center fund it, and actually transporting Joseph to the home. Once the case manager became involved, concrete services were again needed (Miller, 1983). These included setting up the workshop program, arranging for transportation to the workshop, and arranging for behavior modification consultation. Because of Joseph's retardation and his child-like self-image, these services had to be carefully arranged by the social worker and to be explained clearly both to Joseph and his mother, and required much support and coordination. For example, prior to Joseph's entering the workshop, the workshop coordinator visited him at the convalescent hospital to reassure him and explain the program.

Reassessment

Reassessment of needs and goals takes place quarterly according to the individual program plan. In Joseph's case a reassessment and then a change of goals took place after the failure of the original placement. At that point, it was decided by the regional center team and the case manager to slow down and place the highest priorities on programming and therapeutic intervention in order to prepare Joseph for placement.

Transfer or Termination

Joseph was transferred to another case manager for geographic reasons. Joseph and his mother require frequent intervention. When there are large case loads, localizing clients can help provide more effective service. The decision to transfer Joseph was made once it was felt he had sufficient support in his life to be able to accept the change. Once he was in the workshop, adjusting well, and involved in a behavior modification program, the transfer took place. The actual transfer occurred in the workshop with a joint visit by both the old and new case managers.

Case Conclusion

Joseph has, so far, adjusted well to the new residential facility. Mrs. Wolfe does not view the new caretaker as a threat to her mothering ability. The behavior modification program terminated successfully.

Differential Discussion

Different practice decisions might have resulted in a different outcome. Mrs. Wolfe's involvement was critical. Additionally, had the goals and contract been drawn with placement as the first priority, Joseph would probably not have had the social skills to interact successfully with peers and would have returned to the convalescent hospital. The workshop setting allowed him to develop and incorporate these skills at his own pace. If the therapeutic approach had been to involve Mrs. Wolfe and Joseph in psychotherapy with the exclusion of a behavioral modification approach, progress would have been slower or limited; I do not think I would have made a difference. The key factors is not Joseph's level of retardation, but his emotional dependence on his mother and his consequent lack of sense of self as a competent adult. If he were not retarded, Joseph might have benefitted from other treatment techniques requiring more insight.

Were I to begin again, I would urge the family as a unit, and Mrs. Wolfe, to receive psychotherapy (Falck, 1984; Munro, 1985). Certainly, Mrs. Wolfe remains a needy woman with many unresolved conflicts. She has gained absolutely no understanding of her relationship with Joseph and could still sabotage treatment. When she dies, Joseph's sister will probably assume Mrs. Wolfe's role. His mother is preparing his sister for this eventuality and creating enough guilt so she will feel responsible for Joseph. I think Joseph's sister allies with his mother and could not have helped Mrs. Wolfe gain perspective. Our range of options is not as great as it seems, given both Joseph's and his mother's needs, program openings, transportation limitations, etc.

PRACTICE IN CONTEXT

Regional Center of the East Bay and Home, Health and Counseling are both influenced by technology, policy and organization. The basic policy goal is to create the most normal, least restrictive environment; it means many fewer state hospitalizations. Continually changing policy also seems to have a major effect, particularly in terms of priorities for service, case loads and accountability procedures. When a case load jumps from forty-five to sixty and continues to creep upward, it is impossible to provide clients the same quality of service. Technology has also had its effect. A developmental model, more refined behavior modification techniques, electronic communication devices, drugs for seizure control, and a more advanced body of genetic knowledge have profoundly influenced the progress of many of our clients. Both formal and informal factors of organization influence practice. Home, Health and Counseling has its own structure, yet we are accountable to RCEB. We often feel isolated and distant from the source of power, which can make it more difficult and certainly more time-consuming to receive services for our clients.

These, then, are some of the factors that have influenced my relationship with Joseph. Joseph probably would not have been a client of RCEB had he not been referred to a genetics clinic that recognized his Williams syndrome and referred him to us. The policies of striving for normalcy and of choosing the least restrictive alternatives most certainly led to an emphasis on a workshop and a move from the convalescent home. Both day programming and residential placement are high priorities within the regional center system, so Joseph was assured of funding for these programs. On the other hand, the size of case loads and paperwork requirements are both policy decisions which definitely limited the time Joseph and I spent together and also made a transfer based on geographic centralization imperative. It seems also that if I had maintained a strict definition of Joseph as the only client, not including his mother, no progress could have taken place. I also feel the relationship benefitted from having a flexible meeting place and variable durations and frequencies of meetings. We could meet outside the sterile atmosphere of the convalescent hospital and thereby not reinforce Joseph's illness, and we could meet as often and for as long as needed. Both an active stance in dealing with Joseph and a continuous provision of concrete services were necessary because of Joseph's retardation and his image of himself as a child. Although there are many ways in which any case manager will always have to act assertively on Joseph's behalf, it is hoped that as he gains more emotional distance from his mother, he can better advocate and provide for himself. For it is that emotional dependence which severely limits his abilities to act more independently and assertively on his own behalf—within the limits allowed by his retardation.

REFERENCES

Agosta, J.M. & V.J. Bradley. *Family Care for Persons with Developmental Disabilities: A Growing Commitment*. Boston: Human Services Research Institute, 1985.

Blumenthal, J.A. "Relaxation Theory, Biofeedback & Behavioral Medicine." *Psychotherapy* 22.3 (1985): 516-530.

Boggs, E. "Feds and Families: Some Observations on the Impact of Federal Economic Policies on Families with Children Who Have Disabilities," in M.A. Slater & P. Mitchell, Eds. *Family Support Services: A Parent-Professional Partnership*. Stillwater, Oklahoma: National Clearinghouse of Rehabilitation Training Materials, 1984.

Boyer, Patricia A. "The Role of the Family Therapist in Supportive Services to Families with Handicapped Children." *Clinical Social Work Journal* 14.3 (Fall, 1986), 250-261.

Budley, J. Living & Stigma: The Lives of People Who We Label Mentally Retarded, Springfield, Ill.: Charles C Thomas, 1983.

DeWeaver, K.L. "Deinstitutionalization of the Developmentally Disabled." *Social Work* (Nov./Dec. 1983), 435-439.

DeWeaver, K.L. "Producing Social Workers for Practice with the Developmentally Disabled." *Arete*, 7 (Spring, 1982), 59.

Dudley, J.R. "Speaking for Themselves: People Who Are Labelled as Mentally Retarded." *Social Work*, 32.1 (Jan./Feb. 1987), 80-82.

Falck, H. "Mental Retardation: A Family Crisis" in T.O. Carlton, Eds. *Clinical Social Work in Health Settings*. New York, Springer, 1984, pp. 198-207.

Grossman, H. *Manual on Terminology & Classification on Mental Retardation*. Washington, DC: American Association on Mental Deficiency, 1984.

Hall, J.A. et al. "Evaluation of Group Treatment for Improving the Social Skills of Mentally Retarded Adults." Paper presented at the Annual Convention of the Association for Behavioral Analysis. Milwaukee, WI: May 27, 1983.

Hams, Maxine and Helen C. Bergman. "Case Management with the Chronically

Mentally Ill: A Clinical Perspective." *American Journal of Orthopsychiatry*, 57.2 (April, 1987), 296-302.

Herson, M. & A.S. Bellack. *Dictionary of Behavioral Assessment Techniques & Methods*. NY: Pergamon Press, 1985.

Intagliata, J. "Improving the Quality of Community Care for the Chronically Mentally Disabled: The Role of Case Management." *Administration in Mental Health*, 8.4 (1982), 655-674.

Keenan, M.P. "Standards for Social Workers in Developmental Disabilities" in L. Wikler & M.P. Keenan (Eds.), *Developmental Disabilities: No Longer a Private Tragedy*. Silver Springs, MD: NASW, 1983.

Kruzich, Jean M. "The Chronically Mentally Ill in Nursing Homes: Issues in Policy & Practice." *Health & Social Work*, 11.1 (Winter 1986), 5-14.

Kurtz, L.F., D.A. Baganzzi and L.P. Pollane. "Case Management in Mental Health." *Health & Social Work*, 9.3 (Spring 1984), 201-211.

Kusserow, R.P. *A Program Inspection on Transition of Developmentally Disabled Young Adults from School to Adult Services*. Washington, DC: U.S. Department of Health & Human Services, 1984.

McDonald-Wikler, L. "Disabilities: Developmental" in *Encyclopedia of Social Work*, 18th ed. A. Minahan et al., Eds. Silver Springs, MD: NASW, 1987.

Mealey, L. "Decision Making & Adjustment in Genetic Counseling." *Health & Social Work*, 9 (Spring 1984), 124-133.

Miller, G. "Case Management: The Essential Services" in *Case Management in Mental Health Service*, C.J. Sanburn (Ed.), NY: The Haworth Press, 1983.

Mueller, M. and A. Leviton. "In-Home vs. Clinic-Based Services for the Developmentally Disabled Child: Who is the Primary Client-Parent or Child?" *Social Work in Health Care*, 11.3 (Spring 1986).

Munro, J. Dale. "Counseling Severely Dysfunctional Families of Mentally & Physically Disabled Persons." *Clinical Journal of Social Work*, 13.1 (Spring 1985), 13-31.

NASW. "Standards for Social Work in Developmental Disabilities" in *NASW Standards for Social Work Health Care Settings*. Silver Springs, MD: NASW, 1982, 15-21.

Peveler, R.C. and D.W. Johnston. "Subjective & Cognitive Effects of Relaxation." *Behavior Research & Therapy*, 24.4: 413-414, 1986.

Rothman, David J. & Shiela M. Rothman. *The Willowbrook Wars: A Decade of Struggle for Social Justice*. NY: Harper & Row, 1984.

Schilling, R.F., L.D. Gilchrist & S.P. Schinke. "Coping and Social Support in Families with a Developmentally Disabled Child." *Family Relations*, 33 (Jan. 1984), 47-55.

Slater, M.A. and L. Winkler. "Normalized Family Resources with a Developmentally Disabled Child." *SW*, 31.5 (Sept./Oct. 1986), 385-390.

Thyer, B.A. "Behavior Modification in Social Work Practice" in *Progress in Behavior Modification*, G. Herson, R.M. Eisler & P.M. Miller (Eds.). NY: Academic Press, 1983, 173-216.

Wikler, L., M. Wasow, and E. Hatfield. "Seeking Strengths in Families of Developmental Disabled Children." *SW*, 28 (July/August 1983), 313-315.

Wikler, L. and M.P. Keenan (Eds.). *Developmental Disabilities No Longer a Private Tragedy*. Silver Springs, MD: NASW, 1983.

Yule, W. and J. Carr (Eds.). *Behavior Modification for the Mentally Handicapped*. London: Croom-Helm, 1980.

Private Practice:
Policies and Their Effect on Practice

Carol Silbergeld
Toba Schwaber Kerson

Social workers are increasingly recognized as autonomous mental health professionals (Marquis, 1982). According to recent National Association of Social Work estimates, twenty-five percent of clinical social workers are engaged in some form of independent practice at least part of the time. The number has greatly increased over the past decade; it is thought that 10,000 to 30,000 practice privately part-time and 4,000 to 10,000, full-time. Growth has been aided by trends encouraging private practice of all kinds, increased professional endorsement, cutbacks in agency budgets, increased thirty party financing and the willingness of many social workers to view themselves as autonomous (Neale, 1983).

POLICY

The independent practice of social work is increasingly regulated by state governmental agencies. In 1945, California became the first state to register social workers. In the mid 1960s, Oklahoma, Virginia and California became the first states to license clinical social workers. Currently, forty-five states regulate social work and the others are developing some form of regulation (NASW, 1985).

Licensing raises may issues for social workers (Johnson, 1983; Lund, 1987). Professional licensure, certification and registration (referred to here as "licensing,") serve to protect the consumer, the practitioner and the profession. Proponents of licensing argue that it encourages the highest standards of professional performance (Barker, 1987; Golton, 1983), enhances social work status by subscribing to the more autonomous medical model, and ultimately increases possibilities for third party reimbursement. In addition, it increases the likelihood of a middle and upper middle class clientele. Focusing on the egalitarian roots of social work and its commitment to the eradication of racism and poverty, opponents within the social work community think that social workers should not be competing with other mental health professionals for middle class clientele. "Since 1964, the National Association of Social Workers has officially recognized private practice as a legitimate area for social workers but stated the position that practice within agencies should remain the primary avenue for the implementation of the goals of the profession" (Kelley, 1985).

Licensing, with its often concomitant requirements for continuing education, postgraduate training and supervision, also compels clinical social workers to acquire advanced skills (Goldmeier, 1986). Along with a small but growing number of graduate schools, a number of institutes and clinics have developed educational programs which enable the MSW to earn a clinical PhD or a postgraduate certificate. The evolution of such programs seems to parallel the spread of licensing across the country.

Vendorship

A goal for independent practitioners is to be included by law in health plans, disability plans, self-insured employee welfare benefit plans, and hospital service contracts offering mental health care (Barker, 1983; Barker, 1987). In 1977, California passed the Torres Bill, the first state vendorship bill requiring insurance policies which included mental health coverage to recognize licensed clinical social workers as reimbursable providers. Such laws vary. Some require a referral from a licensed physician, others may require documentation of supervision or specified periodic consultation with a licensed psychiatrist or psychologist. Coverage for out-of-state vendorship also varies. Most social workers strive for maximal autonomy.

Third party reimbursement is critical in order for most independent social work practitioners to compete with other professionals for clients. Liberal reimbursement policies expand the client pool to include such groups as students, union members, and civil servants. Fees paid by insurance companies can approach those paid to psychiatrists and psychologists. Receiving substantial payments for most cases also permits the private practitioner to reduce fees for needy patients (Barker, 1982).

Insurance companies typically limit their reimbursement for psychotherapeutic services by setting a maximum hourly fee, limiting the client's total dollar expenditure, defining the treatment modes, or restricting qualifying diagnoses (Lechnyr, 1984). Some patients may be unable to continue treatment when they are no longer eligible for reimbursement (Sharfstein, Maszynski and Myers, 1984; Jackson, 1987). Issues related to diagnosis create conflicts for the therapist, especially when diagnoses such as sexual perversion, psychosis and substance abuse are particularly stigmatizing. At the other end of the diagnosis quandary are the clients who may want to discuss a social or situational problem but who have to receive a psychiatric diagnosis in order to receive reimbursement. For example, some insurance companies will not reimburse for treatment of transient situational disturbances or adjustment reactions since the current *Diagnostic and Statistical Manual* (1980) does not consider these to be psychiatric diagnoses. People coping with life-circumstance problems such as divorce, death, problems with spouse, child or job may be experiencing prolonged emotional stress and be in need of psychotherapeutic help. If therapists solve this problem by assigning a psychiatric diagnosis, they must discuss the diagnosis and the release of the diagnosis to the insurance company with the patient. Issues relating to informed consent and release of information are complex (Reamer, 1987).

Vendorship sometimes allows for manipulation by patients and occasional collusion by their therapists. For example, when the insurance company has agreed to pay a specific percentage of the therapist's hourly fee, a patient may suggest that a therapist bill the insurance company at a higher rate to reduce the patient's percentage of the fee. Some companies reimburse for specific modes of treatment such as individual therapy but will not reimburse for family or couple therapy, and patients ask the therapist to alter the facts to meet insurance requirements. Such arrangements are fraudulent and clinically contraindicated. A therapist who colludes with a patient communicates poor ethical standards and confederacy in illegal, manipulative behavior. The integrity and credibility of the practitioner is seriously impaired (Schultz, 1982).

Third-party involvement also affects confidentiality. Generally, insurance companies require that patients sign forms consenting to the release of certain information regarding their treatment. In addition to diagnosis, some insurers request treatment summaries in order to justify continued reimbursement. This information may be on file and/or accessible to the patient's employer. Thus, reimbursement policies directly influence the relationship between social worker and client.

Organization

Clinical social workers in private practice are not guided or controlled by agency or supervisory mission or structure and consequently are free to make their own decisions about case selection, treatment, and fees. Basically, one must establish one's own organization with a sound structure, referral base, consultant network, physical environment, accounting system, contractual arrangements, malpractice insurance and means of accountability.

Because they function autonomously, private practitioners must find alternate routes for maintaining referrals and for professional consultation. Successful private practitioners establish a network of referral sources and market themselves as a small business (Borenzweig, 1981; Levin, 1982). One aspect of marketing means defining oneself clearly to possible sources of referral. Defining oneself more specifically is helpful. For example, one may hold oneself out to the public as a specialist in a particular treatment mode such as family or group treatment, a certain problem area such as divorce-adjustment, depression or substance abuse, or a particular type of client such as children or adolescents. In terms of professional consultation, clinical social workers utilize specialists in areas such as psychiatry, neurology, speech pathology, law, other social work specialties and psychiatry when other kinds of diagnostic information is needed.

To organize my practice, I have an accounting and billing system, a tax plan, rules about delinquent fees and malpractice insurance (Rosen, Procter, and Livne, 1985; Bernstein, 1981). The manner in which the patient handles fee payment is an important communication to the therapist. Close scrutiny of the meaning of unpaid bills, late payments, or the reluctance to take responsibility for processing claims to the insurance company illuminates the patient's feelings about the treatment, the therapist, or past significant relationships. If the issue of fee payment is clouded by complicated forms, bureaucratic procedures, or substantially delayed reimbursements, this aspect of treatment may no longer be a clear basis for insight. I clarify the issues by asking the patient to pay me directly and seek reimbursement from the insurance company. I do not do this when patients are financially unable to manage this arrangement.

In addition to other carriers, NASW sponsors malpractice insurance coverage for clinical social workers. It is said that the following circumstances heighten the possibility of malpractice suits: lack of informed consent regarding treatment method, misusing the relationship to exploit the client, inappropriate treatment, faulty diagnosis, providing treatment without qualification, abandonment or premature termination of clients who still need service, and failure to warn others when the client has indicated intent to harm (Barker, 1987).

Within these realities is the contractual arrangement between therapist and patient. The patient agrees to pay the practitioner for a service and the practitioner renders a service based in her clinical judgement and expertise. Thus, the primary differences between private practice and agency based practice is the independence of the social worker to determine the conditions of work and direct payment from client to worker. This also means that the social worker has no one with whom to share responsibility. Missing is the comfort and support which one receives in teamwork or being able to dash into the office of a supervisor or colleague, call on another worker with expertise in a particular area, or transfer or get direct and immediate help with a problem. Thus, the independent practitioner may spend more time pondering the client's problems away from the treatment situation than she might in an agency setting. This aspect of practice is a challenge. It sometimes indicates the need for a literature search and/or consultation. Issues of countertransference and transference may also emerge, providing another reason for private practice to be the bastion of the highly experienced and trained clinical social worker.

My office is located in a building with the offices of many other psychotherapists. Patients come to a comfortable waiting room and press a button which rings in my office to let me know they have arrived. With a desk chair, two other chairs, an ottoman and a couch, I have several seating possibilities.

Primarily, my referrals come from other professionals, former clients, or, very occasionally, colleagues at work. From my twenty-four hour a week, agency based work as Director of Social Work and the Divorce Project and a supervisor for a two year, post-master's training program in child psychiatry at the Reis Davis Child Study Center, I have developed a reputation as a divorce and custody specialist. Lately, one dimension of my private practice has been court custody evaluations. Aside from the divorce and custody work, I am interested in long term therapy with individuals who would like to resolve issues in their lives. Some of my clients continue weekly therapy for three or four years. I screen out highly disturbed clients by suggesting they should have a therapist who can provide hospitalization and medication. Cases referred to me are primarily young adults with problems including identity confusion, low self-esteem, anxiety, depression, relationship difficulties, and separation-individuation issues. According to Goldmeier, more than half of all patients seeking psychotherapy services are adults between the ages of eighteen and forty. The three categories of mental disorder that are most prominent are anxiety disorders, adjustment disorders, and affective disorders (Goldmeier, 1986).

Case Description

At the time of referral, Nancy was a thirty-one-year old single woman who sought help for recurrent depression (Kahn, 1986). One of many children in a farm family with alcohol and incest problems, Nancy felt isolated and unloved. Her mother was highly critical and her father favored the boys. After an older sister left to marry, no one was there for Nancy. A early marriage to a self-centered and emotionally unavailable man was brief and unsatisfying. Recently, she had ended a relationship with a man who resembled her ex-husband.

A large, nice looking woman, Nancy wept easily. She was intelligent, verbal, interesting and had a warm sense of humor. When we began, Nancy was an assistant administrator in a small hospital and postgraduate student in public health. Concerned about her unsatisfactory relationships with men and a chronic weight problem, Nancy sometimes considered suicide. Having had previous psychotherapy experiences, Nancy was sophisticated about the role of unconscious processes in her difficulties.

Definition of the Client

In this situation, it was clear that the client was Nancy. Even if she had been married, had children or other significant biological or social relationships, Nancy's need to be viewed and valued as an individual would have indicated that she receive individual psychotherapy. Although the decision regarding definition of the client was clear, definition of the therapist was not. Patients assessed to be suicidal may be more appropriately treated by a psychiatrist who can medicate and hospitalize if necessary. After working together for several sessions, Nancy and I determined that she was not suicidal and that we could work well together.

Goals

Some initial goals were unarticulated at the beginning of treatment and were elaborated as work progressed (Saari, 1986). Nancy wanted to "feel better," and we used the initial phases of treatment to identify and clarify the nature of her discomfort. Nancy recognized that feeling better was contingent upon gaining psychological insight and resolving conflicts especially regarding closeness and intimacy (Cohen, 1983). She hoped that treatment would improve her self-esteem, allowing her to become involved in healthier relationships, and would reduce her depression and overeating. Each goal is observable or can be evaluated through self-report.

Contract

Contract primarily involved the structure of treatment: visit schedule, fee, insurance and billing arrangements. Nancy was billed once a month. Some therapists also discuss their cancellation policies, but I prefer to wait until the issue presents itself (Rothary, 1980). Agreement between patient and therapist about goals and methods unfolds as the therapist learns more about the patient. Areas for work are elaborated upon and reworked in the treatment process. Once treatment begins, patients frequently "challenge" the structure by not paying, cancelling, requesting a change of time or criticizing some aspect of the therapist's behavior. These may be manifestations of the patient's problems and can be used to help the patient to gain insight.

Use of Time and Meeting Place

At the beginning of treatment, Nancy and I agreed to meet weekly at a set time for a prescribed period. There was no discussion about the expected duration of treatment. It was clear that Nancy understood, perhaps as the result of a lengthy previous therapy experience, that treatment would take as long as she needed and that its duration would depend on her progress. We worked together for three years, always meeting in my office and assuming the same seats each week.

Treatment Modality

The primary treatment modality was psychoanalytic psychotherapy (Leiberman, 1982; Strean, 1983; Fraiberg, 1982). Psychoanalytic psychotherapy alleges that unless a person becomes aware of certain wishes, admonitions and defenses and recognizes that she is distorting the present and perceiving it as if it were part of her childhood, she cannot be helped (Strean, 1979). Important in this modality are such concepts as the unconscious, resistance, defense mechanisms and transference (Fraiberg, 1982). Transferential reactions, for example, are unconscious attempts by the patient to recapitulate with the therapist types of interpersonal interaction similar to those he or she expressed with significant persons in the past. Transference suggests experiencing the therapist in terms of how one wishes the therapist to be and/or fears he might be (Strean, 1979). Here, a primary goal is insight about one's intrapsychic state and how situations affect one's responses (Cohen, 1983).

Through exploration of Nancy's feelings, particularly those in the transference, we were able to relate many of her current difficulties to her early object relations (Saari, 1986). For example, during the first year of treatment, Nancy did not pay her bill for several months. In reality, she had a tight budget and had difficulty paying other bills as well; however, close scrutiny of her reactions to my inquiries about unpaid bills revealed underlying psychodynamics. Nancy resented my concern and interpreted it as distrust. After some exploration, it became evident that Nancy felt she had to pay me in order for me to care about her. By not paying, she was testing to see how long it would take for me to abandon her. As we gained more understanding about the meaning of the fee to Nancy, she managed payment more appropriately (Strean, 1979).

Stance of the Social Worker

My stance follows that of psychoanalytically oriented psychotherapy. It is primarily reactive and interpretive. I do not offer suggestions, but rather help the patient to explore the meanings and ramifications of her feelings, thoughts and actions. Self-disclosure, advance giving and the use of outside resources or concrete services are not part of this stance.

Reassessment and Termination

Nancy recognized that her fears of rejection and criticism were feelings she frequently had as a child (Strean, 1977). She gained insight into her tendency to defend against hurt and anger with depression and overeating. As her fears were understood, Nancy improved her ability to separate fantasy from reality. She developed a more realistic view of herself and was less fearful of intimacy. As her self-esteem improved, in an effort to be more attractive, she began to change her eating habits and lose weight. She experienced fewer and less intense depressions and had no serious periods of depression during her third year of therapy. At termination, Nancy was seriously involved in a gratifying relationship with an emotionally available, caring man.

PRACTICE IN CONTEXT

Differentiating this kind of practice from others is the relative autonomy of the social worker to set the conditions of her own work. Unlike social workers in other contexts, in independent practice, I have the freedom and autonomy to select and screen cases and structure treatment as I wish. Therapy decisions are guided by my training and theoretical orientation and the particular needs of the individual case. Treatment is limited by the patient's ability to use this particular kind of therapy and to pay for services, and by the limitations imposed by insurers. Diminished organizational and policy constraints and the resultant heightened therapist-patient control of practice decisions is highly challenging and rewarding (Matorin, 1987).

REFERENCES

American Psychiatric Association. *Diagnostic and Statistical Manual for Mental Disorders*. Third Edition. Washington, D.C., 1980.

Barker, R.L. *The Business of Psychotherapy: Private Practice Administration for Therapists, Counselors, and Social Workers*. New York: Columbia University Press, 1982.

Barker, R.L. "Supply Side Economics in Private Psychotherapy Practice: Some Ominous and Encouraging Trends." *Psychotherapy in Private Practice*, 1, 1 (1983), pp. 71-81.

Barker, R.L. *Social Work in Private Practice: Principles, Issues, and Dilemmas*. Silver Spring, MD: NASW, 1984.

Barker, R.L. "Private and Proprietary Services," in *Encyclopedia of Social Work*, Volume 2, 18th ed., pp. 324-329. Edited by A. Minahan. Silver Spring, MD: NASW, 1987.

Bernstein, B.E. "Malpractice: Future Shock of the 1980's." *Social Casework*, 62 (March 1981), pp. 175-181.

Borenzweig, H. "Agency vs. Private Practice: Similarities and Differences." *Social Work*, 26, 3 (1981), pp. 239-244.

Briar, K. and S. Briar. "Clinical Social Work and Public Policies," in *Practical Politics: Social Work and Political Responsibility*, pp. 45-65. Edited by M. Mahaffey and Jim Hanks. Silver Spring, MD: NASW, 1982.

Bunston, T. "Mapping Practice: Problem Solving in Clinical Social Work." *Social Casework*, 66, 4 (1985), pp. 225-236.

Cohen, R.J. and W.E. Marano. *Legal Guidebook in Mental Health*. New York: Free Press, 1982.

Eagle, M.N. *Recent Developments in Psychoanalysis: A Critical Evaluation*. New York: McGraw-Hill Book Co., 1984.

Fausel, D.F. "Profiles of Independent Social Workers: Rudolph Calabrese." *Journal of Independent Social Work*, 1, 1 (Fall 1986), pp. 81-87.

Foreman, J. "More People Shifting to Psychologists and Social Workers for Psychotherapy." *Boston Sunday Globe*, February 17, 1985.

Furrow, B. *Malpractice in Psychotherapy*. Cambridge, MA: Lexington Books, 1980.

Gabriel, E. Private Practice in Social Work. *Encyclopedia of Social Work*, 2 (1977), pp. 1054-1060.

Gartner, A. "Four Professions: How Different, How Alike." *Social Work*, 20 (1975), pp. 353-358.

Goldmeier, J. "Private Practice and the Purchase of Services: Who Are the Practitioners?" *American Journal of Orthopsychiatry*, 56 (1986), pp. 89-102.

Grossner, R.C. et al. "Clinical Social Work Practice." *Clinical Social Work Journal*, 11 (Fall 1983), pp. 245-262.

Jackson, J.A. "Clinical Social Work and Peer Review: A Professional Leap Ahead." *Social Work*, 32, 3 (1987), pp. 213-220.

Johnson, D.A., and D. Huff. "Licensing Exams: How Valid Are They?" *Social Work*, 32, 2 (March/April 1987), pp. 159-161.

Kelley, P. and Alexander, P. Part-time Private Practice: Practical and Ethical Considerations. *Social Work*, 30 (1985), pp. 254-258.

Kutchins, H. and S.A. Kirk. "DSM-III and Social Work Malpractice." *Social Work*, 32, 3 (May/June, 1980), pp. 205-211.

Lechnyr, R. "Clinical Social Work Psychotherapy and Insurance Coverage: Information on Billing Procedures. *Clinical Social Work Journal*, 12 (Spring 1984), pp. 69-77.

Levin, A.M. *The Private Practice of Psychotherapy*. New York: Free Press, 1984.

Lund, H. "The Effects of Licensure on Student Motivation and Career Choice." *Social Work*, 32.1 (January/February 1982), pp. 75-77.

Marquis, W. "Private Practice: A Nationwide Survey" *Social Work*, 27 (1982), pp. 262-67.

Matorin, S. et al. "Psychopharmacology: Guidelines for Social Workers. *Social Casework*, 65 (December 1984), pp. 579-589.

Matorin, S. et al. "Private Practice in Social Work: Readiness and Opportunity." *Social Casework*, 68,1 (January 1987), pp. 31-37.

Middleman, R.R. *A Study Guide for ACSW Certification*, rev. ed. Washington, D.C.: NASW, 1982.

The National Association of Social Workers. *State Comparisons of Laws Regulating Social Work*. Silver Spring, MD, 1985.

Pressman, R.M. Private Practice: *A Handbook for the Independent Practitioner*. New York: Gardner Press, 1979.

Reamer, F.G. "Ethical Dilemmas in Social Work Practice," *Social Work*, 28, 1 (1983), pp. 31-35.

Reamer, F.G. "Ethics Committees in Social Work." *Social Work*, 32, 3 (1987), pp. 188-192.

Rosen, A., E.K. Proctor, and S. Livne. "Planning and Direct Practice." *Social Service Review*, 59, 2 (1985), pp. 166-177.

Rubin, A. and P.J. Johnson. "Direct Practice Interests of Entering MSW Students." *Journal of Education for Social Work*, 20, 2 (1984), pp. 5-16.

Rothary, G. "Contracts and Contracting." *Clinical Social Work Journal*, 8 (Fall 1980), pp. 179-187.

Schultz, B.M. *Legal Liability in Psychotherapy: A Practitioners Guide to Risk Management*. San Francisco, CA: Jossey-Bass, 1982.

Sharfstein, S.S., S. Maszynski, and E. Meyers. *Health Insurance and Psychiatric Care: Update and Appraisal.* Washington, D.C.: American Psychiatric Press, 1984.

Sharwell, G.R. "Legal Issues in Social Work Practice" in *1983-84 Supplement to Encyclopedia of Social Work*, Washington, D.C.: NASW, 1983, pp. 69-75.

"Social Workers Vault into Leading Roles, in Psychotherapy." *New York Times* April 30, 1985.

Wallace, M.E. Private Practice: A Nationwide Study. *Social Work*, 27 (1982), pp. 262-267.

Weil, M. et al. "Impact of the Tarasoff Decision on Clinical Social Work Practice." *Social Service Review*, 57 (March 1983), pp. 112-124.

Williams, J.B.W. "DSM III: A Comprehensive Approach to Diagnosis." *Social Work*, 26, 2 (1981), pp. 101-106.

Rehabilitation Center
for Multi-Faceted Treatment
of Alcoholism

Susan A. Balis

DESCRIPTION OF THE SETTING

The Strecker Program is an in-patient rehabilitation program for the treatment of alcoholism and other dependencies. Located in a private psychiatric hospital in a large city, it is ideally situated to treat dual diagnoses of alcoholism and other psychiatric illness. The decision to create a specialty unit for the treatment of alcoholism means that the institution defines alcoholism as a primary illness which must be treated along with any other physical or mental disorder (Freed, 1982).

Location in a private psychiatric hospital influences the patient population, and thus the nature of the treatment. The majority of patients have private health insurance because they are employed or have other financial resources. A small percentage of patients are publicly insured. That most have private health insurance is an indication that some of their resources are still intact. Their alcoholism has not progressed to the point where they have lost everything. Since, as social worker, I secure necessary concrete services, the fiscal situations of most of our patients means that I can concentrate more on treatment issues and less on securing resources.

Strecker is a short term treatment program with a required minimum length of stay of twenty-eight days, an average stay of five to six weeks, and occasionally as much as two or three months. Length of stay is determined on an individual basis and influenced by each patient's responsiveness to treatment as well as his or her economic resources. Responsiveness to treatment may be influenced by duration and severity of the alcoholism, severity of the psychiatric diagnosis, and complicating medical factors (Pattison and Kaufman, 1982). Responsiveness also includes the patient's receptivity to recommendations for aftercare plans and the availability of appropriate post-hospitalization services for the particular needs of the patient (Nadel et al., 1983). Influencing factors may include the severity or intransigence of family conflict, and the availability (if needed) of satisfactory living arrangements, support groups and out-patient therapy.

A multidisciplinary team consisting of a private attending psychiatrist, an addictions counsellor, a primary nurse, an activities therapist and a social worker provide individualized attention for each patient as well as group and milieu intervention. The goal is to provide a structured environment where patients can be safely detoxified if needed and then given education, individual addictions counselling, group therapy, psychotherapy, family or marital therapy if indicated, medical treatment, wellness therapy and leisure time counseling.

The goal is to reduce enough of the denial of illness so that patients can make a commitment to an aftercare plan that will help them maintain life-long sobriety. This will include recommendations from a multi-disciplinary staff based on their assessment of the patient and his or her family regarding use of AA, NA, out-patient individual and/or group therapy, marital or family therapy, the need for residential treatment or a half-way house, and the restructuring of free time.

Alcoholism is seen and treated in this setting not only as a disease but as a family illness (Balis and Zirpoli, 1982). The effects of the alcoholism are devastating not only to the alcoholic but to those living with the alcoholic (Kerson, 1985). These effects are so profound that the co-dependents (those living with and "adapting" to the alcoholism) develop symptoms as well, assume unhealthy roles within the family based on a life now organized not around the needs of the individual family members but around the alcoholism (Wegscheider, 1981; Peyser, 1980; Berenson, 1979).

Each patient is seen by a social worker for a psychosocial assessment shortly after admission. This is to determine which are the most pressing problems impinging on the patient's recovery. These include the strengths and problems in the family system and any living and financial problems that will affect either the current hospitalization or the discharge planning.

The majority of the social worker's time is spent working with families. This may mean individual work with the spouse, parents or children of a patient, or joint work with patient and spouse or with the entire family. The purpose is to bring the family back to the premorbid level of functioning, or to begin work on an always-poorly functioning system that must be addressed if it is to support the patient's recovery.

Policy

Public attitudes towards the use and abuse of alcohol and other drugs affect social policy. This in turn affects the nature of the laws governing alcohol use and abuse and the nature of treatment that society encourages or discourages. Pattison (1982) describes the shifts in public opinion from 1900 to 1970 and its implications for treatment. He describes the shift in public attitudes toward the substance abuser, from moral blame to a medical model with a concomitant shift from control of the substance to treatment of the abuser, and from a punitive position to a therapeutic one. However, he also points to an even more recent shift of this position, to less emphasis on the illness and more on the responsibility of the substance abusers for their own behavior. This has led public opinion away from a rigid medical model and toward a demand for more social control of the substances and the abuser.

Alcoholism treatment is affected by state laws, which determine who can get treatment, where, and for what. State laws regarding insurance coverage and policies of insurance agencies also affect treatment (Kerson, 1985). Laws differ from state to state, resulting in significant differences in the nature of treatment in different localities. These laws cover three different aspects that impinge on treatment.

The first are the commitment laws. The Mental Health Commitment Act of 1966 in Pennsylvania states that no one can be committed to a hospital for treatment of alcoholism or drug addiction. However, a recent Mental Health Bulletin (January 16, 1987), which updates the most recent guidelines for interpretation of that act, lists intoxication with drugs and/or alcohol as one factor to be considered in the assessment of one's danger to self or others. The strictness of the commitment laws and whether or not someone can be committed vary from state to state.

The second set of laws, the mandatory reporting laws, also vary from state to state and reflect each state's attitude toward addictions: whether they be regarded as an illness requiring treatment or a moral weakness deserving of punishment and containment, but not treatment. Methods of identifying impaired professionals fall into this category. In Pennsylvania, the Medical Practice Act of 1985, for example, provides that the Pennsylvania State Board of Medicine evaluate each physician brought to their attention and decide whether the physician is impaired or acting unethically. If the former is found to be the case, the physician is then given the opportunity for rehabilitation under the careful scrutiny and supervision of the medical board. If the latter is found to be the case, then punitive action is required (Moyer, 1987).

The recent federal regulations regarding drug testing of government personnel reflects these positions. If the emphasis is on detection and then punishment (such as dismissal from a job after a positive urine) then this reflects the moral position. If emphasis is placed on detection *and* intervention, such as how to get a person who has been identified as an alcoholic or substance abuser into treatment and use the pressures of the job or licensing bureau to get that person to accept adequate treatment, that is the disease concept model. Laws as such become either punitive or rehabilitative in nature; this is usually a local matter and reflective of local public attitudes.

The third area has to do with insurance policy and laws. In Pennsylvania a new act was passed that requires insurance companies to pay for treatment of alcoholics, but in non-medical settings (Pa. Senate Bill 935, 1986). This could adversely affect alcoholism treatment in general and psychiatric hospital settings unless the patient has another, more primary diagnosis than alcoholism. In some states there are no laws mandating insurance coverage. But both state and federal government and private insurance companies have policies regarding treatment of alcoholism, duration of stay and nature of the setting where treatment may occur.

Technology

There are several ways that technology impinges on the treatment of alcoholism in this setting. Given the devastating impact of alcohol on the various systems of the body, tests are sometimes used to determine the extent or existence of damage: psychological and neuropsychological testing and brain scans can be ordered when needed to determine the extent of brain damage caused by the substance of abuse (Kerson, 1985).

The use of drugs is one of the ways that treatment differs in medical and non-medical rehabilitation programs. Selected use of drugs in a hospital setting may occur for a variety of reasons. Drugs are sometimes used in the detoxification process. Anti-depressants, Lithium and major tranquilizers may be used for patients who are dually-diagnosed, to treat the psychiatric problems concomitantly with the substance abuse (Solomon, 1982). Two other drugs are used selectively with certain patients. One, Antabuse, is used for certain alcoholic patients. Antabuse is an inert drug until combined with alcohol, at which point it can make the user gravely ill. Knowledge of the potentially toxic effects of combining Antabuse and alcohol can be a deterrent for some patients to the impulsive taking of a drink (Ewing, 1982; Fuller et al., 1986). Naltrexon provides a similar dynamic for opiate abusers. Naltrexon blocks the body's ability to get high from opiates and so renders any use of opiates ineffective, and thus provides a deterrent effect for the user (Kleber and Kosten, 1984). Both of these drugs are prescribed on an individualized, case by case basis, and are seen only as useful adjuncts to other forms of treatment. They are also never prescribed for patients who are suicidal, psychotic or with very poor impulse control, for each can be potentially fatal if used injudiciously.

Drug-testing is also used judiciously and always in conjunction with other treatment modalities. In this setting it is used in two ways. Random weekly urine testing within the therapeutic community is used as an ego support and preventive device for patients more than as a meaningful means of detection of drug use. Knowing that they could be tested at any time often provides unstable or wavering patients with a useful structure that helps them control their impulses to use, particularly in the early stages of treatment. Testing is also used when there is/are clinical signs or suspicion that a patient has used drugs or alcohol. This too is never done by itself but in conjunction with clinical observation and intensive work with the patient. There is never sole reliance on the results of such tests. They are not infallible, and too much reliance on them tends to result in an abdication of clinical responsibility and judgment, which in the long run is the more effective and enduring treatment for the majority of cases.

Organization

The organization of this program is a reflection of the medical model of treatment. Strecker is directed by a psychiatrist who is responsible for clinical and medical administration. There is a nursing co-ordinator and assistant co-ordinator to whom the staff nurses and psychiatric technicians are responsible. The nursing co-ordinator, activities therapists and social workers are each responsible to directors within their own disciplines, rather than to the medical director of the unit. The addictions counsellors and the two (psychiatrist) assistant directors are directly responsible to the medical director. There is an all-hospital Medical Director to whom each of the directors is responsible. This organization enables the social workers to take advantage of the resources both of the specialty programs and the Social Service Department. Social workers in different parts of the hospital can use specialized resources for substance abuse, housing and treatment of the elderly, half-way houses for the psychiatrically impaired, treatment resources for eating disorders, etc.

The staff on Strecker is divided into two treatment teams, each composed of two mini-teams to provide individualized attention to each patient. Each mini-team is led by one of the assistant directors of the program and includes an addictions counsellor, an activities therapist, a primary nurse and a social worker. The team meets twice a week to coordinate work being done with each patient by each discipline and to make decisions about the patient's treatment, privilege levels, and aftercare planning.

Case Description

Kevin is a twenty-six-year old married dentist who came to Strecker for treatment of his long-standing alcoholism. He reported a history of conflict with his intrusive, controlling and demanding father from early childhood. Endowed with native intelligence and pushed by his father's needs, he did well in school academically but always had trouble socially. He started drinking in early adolescence. Because of the on-going family conflicts he was "sent to therapy" in mid-adolescence and was in and out of therapy from then until the present. One of the psychiatrists he saw prescribed Valium for his on-going and unrelenting anxiety and Kevin had been using it ever since. When he entered treatment for his alcoholism he did not realize that his Valium use had also turned into abuse, and he required detoxification and treatment for both substances.

Kevin married Maggie three years prior to his hospitalization. With no history of chemical dependency in her family of origin, Maggie knew that Kevin's drinking was problematic, but she never identified it as alcoholism, Very quickly, it began to take a toll on the marriage. Maggie found herself trying to control Kevin's drinking, arguing with him about it, emptying out liquor bottles, making sure she drove him from parties when he was obviously drunk. As his drinking increased, their arguments increased and the frequency and satisfaction in their sexual relationship decreased. Kevin spent more and more time alone, the alcohol and pills becoming increasingly his only companions. Maggie felt that somehow this was all her fault. Ever since they married his drinking seemed to get worse and worse. Was this because she was an unsatisfactory wife? She seemed unable to please him anymore. And when she complained about this or about his drinking it always ended in an argument that sent Kevin running for the bottle. She felt unloved and undesirable, helpless and inadequate to save a rapidly failing marriage. She also felt isolated and alone, ashamed to tell anyone what was happening and unable to talk to Kevin. She began sleeping poorly and eating poorly.

Kevin also saw his marriage deteriorating. His "solution" was to drink more, to take more Valium, to cope, to block out the pain he was also feeling. It was only when his dental practice was on the verge of collapse because of his addiction that he finally went for help.

My first contact with Kevin occurred when I met with him shortly after his hospital admission to do a "Social Service Assessment" for the purpose of determining his psychosocial status. This initial interview is also used to determine who should be invited to attend the Family Program and who should be the major focus of the social work intervention. At that time I discovered that Kevin's father, a retired physician, had suffered a severe stroke several years ago and was paralyzed and often bed-ridden, and that Kevin's mother spent most of her time tending to her husband. Kevin also had a married sister who lived far from the hospital and was kept busy with her two young children. From this information it was decided that none of Kevin's family of origin would be expected to participate in the family program, though they could all be informed about it and invited to attend. Kevin did not want his parents informed of his addiction or his admission to the hospital, insisting that they had too many problems of their own and that nothing would be gained from informing them.

This is a common initial response and was not challenged at this time. However, Kevin's position was seen as a reflection of some of his attitudes toward his own alcoholism, and was examined with his counsellor. Secrets are a frequent phenomenon in the alcoholic family system and often support the alcoholism. Sometimes it is appropriate and self-protective to withhold such information; at other times, it is more protective of the alcoholism than of the recovery. Kevin eventually decided to tell his parents about his treatment, though they were never able to participate in our family program. He also eventually told his sister, and found her to be a good support within the family.

Kevin's twenty-five-year old wife, Maggie, worked full-time as an office manager for a center-city accounting firm. They had no children. Kevin said that his wife supported his being in treatment and wanted to get involved in our family program.

The philosophy supporting the family program is that alcoholism is such a devastating, far-reaching illness that anyone who lives with it is touched by it. Family members may also develop symptoms that often parallel the symptoms of the alcoholic. In addition, they may contribute to the perpetuation of the problem by their attempts to control or cope with the alcoholism. With this in mind we fashioned a program for family members that parallels, though with less intensity, the program for the patients. This includes group therapy, education through lectures, workshops and films, encouragement to attend self-help groups such as Al Anon, Nar Anon and Families Anonymous. Individual assessment for the primary people in the patient's life is followed by whatever treatment is indicated: individual sessions, couple or family therapy during the patient's stay and a recommended aftercare program for the family member.

As a result of talking with Kevin it was determined that Maggie be involved in the family program. According to Kevin, their marriage was under great stress and he felt it needed immediate attention. While Maggie was pleased that he was in treatment and intended to participate fully in the family program, Kevin felt that she was very angry at him, that their conflicts seemed unresolvable and that their communication was almost entirely unproductive. What Kevin described are fairly typical presenting problems of a family struggling with an addiction. Kevin gave his permission for Maggie to be contacted, and an initial interview was set up. Maggie's perceptions of the marriage paralleled Kevin's. She too cited anger on both sides, poor communication, seemingly unresolvable conflicts and a diminished capacity to problem-solve as a couple, and added dissatisfaction with their sexual relationship to the already-long list of problems.

After the initial meeting with Maggie we decided that the following sessions should be with the couple to work on some of the most acute problems in the relationship (Berenson, 1979). In the couple's first session they were both initially reluctant to speak, both keenly aware of how talk in recent months had so quickly degenerated into bitter, non-productive arguing. They had lost their faith in their ability to speak to each other and were afraid, at this point, of upsetting each other by talking about how they felt. Maggie was afraid that if she let Kevin know how angry and frightened and hopeless she felt, it might precipitate another round of drinking and perhaps even make him leave treatment. He had blamed his drinking on her many times in the past. Kevin, on the other hand, was afraid that if he told Maggie how angry, unsupported and alone he felt, she might leave him. She had threatened to do so many times recently.

They were afraid to speak honestly and, expecting blame and criticism from one another, had lost the ability to listen. In the first marital session, the theme was manipulation. Both realized they had been trying to manipulate each other; she to control his drinking, he to continue to drink. Both were surprised at what the other had to say. As the very tense session ended, both felt some relief from talking.

The theme of the second session, held the third week of Kevin's hospitalization, was their anxiety about his coming home. Less afraid to talk, they had spent the week discussing how they would manage the Christmas parties to which they had been invited. Kevin wanted to avoid drinking situations but was reluctant to tell people, especially Maggie's parents, that he was alcoholic. It was easy to agree on which friends to tell and what excuses to make but much harder to decide what to tell Maggie's family and whether to visit them, since there was always drinking there on holidays.

In the third session, we talked about the problems they would face soon after discharge, what they would do if Kevin had a relapse or if Maggie sensed he was heading for one. To discuss the possibility of relapse recalls painful memories of previous, unsuccessful attempts to abstain and often raises anxiety for both the alcoholic and the family member. It enables them to come to an agreement, at a calm time when there is no crisis pressing at them, to make a reasoned, sober decision about the best way to proceed should there be a relapse. Kevin and Maggie were able to come to some reasonable decisions about what they could do for each other in such a situation, and despite their initial resistance to discussing this, found that it actually lowered their anxiety to be able to devise a mutually agreed upon plan.

The last part of this final session revolved around the formulation of an aftercare plan for them as a couple. Kevin had already worked on his plans for individual and group therapy and attendance at AA. Maggie had decided to forego therapy for herself, group or individual, feeling that their financial resources were stretched and that Kevin's needs for therapy were more pressing than her own at that point. However, they both wanted to continue with marital therapy, since they were finding it so helpful. But again, because of their limited resources, it would mean that Kevin would have to give up some of his own therapy. The highest priority is always given to maintaining sobriety. It was decided that it would be better for each to work separately at this time, Kevin through therapy and AA and Maggie through Al Anon and four post-discharge Family Group sessions. Maggie and Kevin knew they could call if they felt that their marriage was in trouble, and they did so approximately one year after discharge.

Definition of the Client

In this psychiatric hospital, the client is always the hospitalized patient; yet on Strecker, the family is my client. Although the treatment plan was written for Kevin, it also served his family by stating that I would assess Maggie's role in their relationship and help her to understand alcoholism and the part she might play in Kevin's recovery.

Goals

Maintaining sobriety is always the first priority. Unless drinking is in remission, there can be no effective work. Again, with the hospitalized patient defined as client, my goal was help Maggie to support Kevin's recovery, specifically to educate her about alcoholism, offer her a place to ventilate and solve problems, and help her to address her marriage through brief marital therapy. Goals for our work together were formulated first with Kevin and then with Maggie. The formulation of goals is part of the process of treatment.

Contract

Goals are written only for the treatment plan which Kevin signs but to which Maggie has no access. In this situation, the contract is mutually determined, informal and general. The means for attaining the goals are dimensions of the general treatment plan of the organization.

Meeting Place

Kevin, Maggie and I always met in the hospital, primarily within the Strecker program. Making Strecker the meeting place helps family members be part of the hospital experience, emphasizes the fact that the illness profoundly affects family members as well as the patient, helps reduce isolation and serves as a model for the use of self-help and other support systems after discharge.

Use of Time

That Kevin, Maggie and all staff knew that he would be in the hospital for a minimum of twenty-eight days helped prioritize treatment objectives, and set reasonable goals and an appropriate aftercare plan.

Treatment Modality

Treatment modalities such as psychoeducational groups, lectures, self-help groups, individual, group and marital therapy are typical in the treatment of addictions and were used to help Kevin and Maggie (Kirn, 1986; Peyser, 1980). Given the time constraints, work is oriented to short-term intervention, always with an emphasis on the addiction and the work needed to arrest it and maintain abstinence. In addition to the weekly marital sessions, Maggie attended the Family Education Hour held weekly on topics related to addiction. She also attended Family Group, a weekly social work led therapy group for family members which offers support, education, and a safe place for significant others to examine their contribution to addiction and to begin to devise strategies for change for themselves (Balis and Zirpoli, 1982).

Discharge planning begins on the day of admission. Transition

Group is held weekly and led by members of the nursing staff and trained volunteers who are successful "graduates" of the program. This group presents family members with ideas such as a "dry house" (we recommend that no alcohol or drugs be kept in the home to which the patient will return), the importance of AA and NA and the use of AA or NA sponsors.

Stance of the Social Worker

Treatment of alcoholism, where denial in both alcoholic and family member is always present to some extent, requires an active, direct, sometimes confrontational approach. Social, emotional, physical and financial problems overwhelm the family. By understanding the nature of alcoholism, and its effects on family dynamics and values, I help clients to order priorities. I am the facilitator, not the doer. The choice of content belongs to the family.

I never assume that I understand the person just because I understand the illness. Even when the decision-making abilities of the family have been compromised by alcoholism, they must make their own decisions. Maggie, for example, saw that I was not criticizing or blaming her for Kevin's alcoholism. Education, support and gentle confrontation of her denial, expressed as curiosity rather than accusation, furthered our work.

I also combined structuring and careful listening in the marital sessions. If Kevin or Maggie started to accuse, I would interrupt, taking an educational approach, so that I did not parallel their tendency to blame. As discomfort rose, I allowed them to struggle to express difficult issues. Otherwise, I interrupted only if the process was denigrating or they were avoiding critical issues.

Outside Resources

Patients take as much responsibility as possible. I provide information about community services for higher functioning families. A more frail and disabled person might require help in changing living arrangements, or in negotiating the Medical Assistance, Public Assistance and Social Security systems. Referrals to drug and alcohol long-term residential treatment programs or half-way houses are managed by addictions counselors, and the social worker provides support to the family.

Reassessment

Reassessment is on-going and fluid. Certain structures, however, ensure periodic reassessment. A preliminary treatment plan must be completed within seventy-two hours after a patient's admission. Within ten days, a comprehensive plan designed by the treatment team designates aspects of the patient's treatment such as specialized groups, privilege levels, family involvement, restrictions and medications or detoxification regimen. In a "Review and Planning Conference" held during the third week, staff, private attending psychiatrist and the patient formally review the patient's progress and aftercare plans.

Transfer or Termination

Termination begins with admission. Since there is no cure for alcoholism, maintaining lifetime sobriety can only begin in a twenty-eight day program. Here, termination means the end of the in-patient phase of treatment. Success is measured by the adequacy of aftercare and the patient's willingness and ability to implement it.

Case Conclusion

Kevin and Maggie maintained their aftercare program. Kevin remained in an outpatient therapy group and individual therapy and attended AA daily (Kurtz, 1985). Maggie attended the follow-up sessions in Family Group and became active in Al Anon. Marital therapy which they began one year after discharge continued for two years. At that time, Maggie began individual treatment which she continued for about ten months until the birth of their first child. Having lost his dental practice, Kevin did not immediately resume work but spent the time immediately after discharge maintaining his sobriety through great involvement in AA and therapy. Three years post discharge, Kevin's new dental practice was thriving, and he and Maggie had bought their first house. Kevin has maintained sobriety since his discharge.

Differential Discussion

Since Kevin had very serious conflicts with his father, I could have involved his father in the treatment. Maggie's family offered support but their prejudice about alcoholism prevented Maggie and Kevin from telling them about his disease for many months. Although work in these situations could have helped ease tensions and increase family support, it seemed my time was best utilized in working with Maggie.

Also, I might have continued to work with Maggie alone. I often work with a spouse individually until I hold a discharge session in the last week of hospitalization. I thought, however, that Maggie primarily needed the educational and support groups, reading materials, and help with her marriage during this chaotic period. Not an introspective person, Maggie tended to withdraw from her own affect.

Marital sessions were more productive than individual work at that time. Seeing Kevin with Maggie helped him become more aware of her and of her needs, and helped them both to recognize their dominance and control issues. While these sessions could not resolve years of marital conflict, they (in conjunction with other help) enabled the marriage to function while Kevin secured an alcohol-free lifestyle supported by Maggie.

PRACTICE IN CONTEXT

Public attitudes about alcoholism influence insurance and government policies. Defining alcoholism as a moral weakness or an illness determines whether an alcoholic is sent to a prison or a rehabilitation program (Kirn, 1986; Pattison, 1982). Within the field, the treatment someone receives depends on the philosophy of the particular program he enters. Also, the structure of the program will largely determine the role of the social worker. In terms of technology, sophisticated tests measure the effects of alcohol abuse on physical and mental functioning. Although they do not have great impact on my program, detoxification and psychotropic medications and drug testing apparatus have become increasingly sophisticated.

At Strecker, I specialize in one aspect of the treatment, the family illness (Humphreys, 1983), and share responsibility for treatment as part of an inter-disciplinary team. The short term nature of the program requires that I take an active, focused role and emphasize aftercare for this chronic condition. Since the effects of alcoholism are far reaching, our multidimensional treatment approach parallels the course of alcoholism in its active phase.

REFERENCES

Balis, S., & Zirpoli, E. Four Plus Four: A Short-Term Group for Relatives of Alcoholics. *Social Work with Groups*, V, No.1:49-55, 1982.

Berenson, D. The Therapist's Relationship with Couples with an Alcoholic Member, in *Family Therapy of Drug and Alcohol Abuse*. Edited by Kaufman, E. and Kaufman, P. New York: Gardner Press, Inc., 1979.

Ewing, J.A. Disulfiram and Other Deterrent Drugs, in *Encyclopedic Handbook of Alcoholism*. Edited by Pattison, E.M. and Kauffman, E. New York: Gardner Press, 1982.

Freed, E.X. Mental Hospitals: Hospitalization and Treatment of the Alcoholic, in *Encyclopedic Handbook of Alcoholism*. Edited by Pattison, E.M. and Kauffman, E. New York: Gardner Press, 1982.

Fuller, R., L. Branchey, D. Brightwell, R. Derman, C. Emrick, F., Iber, K. James, R. Lacoursiere, K. Lee, I. Lowenstam, I. Maany, D. Neiderhiser, J. Nocks, S. Shaw. Disulfiram Treatment of Alcoholism, *Journal of the American Medical Association*, 256, No. 11:1449-1455, 1986.

Humphreys, N.A. Social Workers: Roles in Alcohol and Drug Abuse Services. *Alcohol Health & Research World*, Vol. 8, No. 1:28-29, 1983.

Kerson, T.S. "Substance Abuse," *Understanding Chronic Illness*, New York: The Free Press, 1985.

Kirn, T. Advances in Understanding of Alcoholism Initiate Evolution in Treatment Programs, *Journal of the American Medical Association*, 256, No. 11:1405, 1411-1412, 1986.

Kurtz, L.F. "Linking Treatment Centers with Alcoholics Anonymous," *Social Work in Health Care*, 9,3 (1984), pp. 85-92.

Kleber, H.D. and Kosten, T.R. Naltrexone Induction: Psychologic and Pharmacologic Strategies. *Journal of Clinical Psychiatry*, Vol. 45, No. 9, Section 2:29-38, 1984.

The Medical Practice Act of 1985. The General Assembly of Pennsylvania Senate Bill No. 1158, Session of 1985.

Mental Health Bulletin, No. 99-87-07. Commonwealth of Pennsylvania, Department of Public Welfare, p. 4. January 16, 1987.

Moyer, J.H. The Medical Practice Act of 1985, *Pennsylvania Medicine*, 69-76, March 1987.

Nadel, M., Petropoulos, A.W. & Feroe, N. Alcoholism Treatment Resources; Which One When? in *Social Work Treatment of Alcohol Problems*. Edited by Cook, D., Ferwell, C. & Riolo, J. New Brunswick, N.J.: Rutgers Center of Alcohol Studies, 1983.

Pattison, E.M. Alcohol Use: Social Policy, in *Encyclopedic Handbook of Alcoholism*, Edited by Pattison, E.M. and Kauffman, E., New York: Gardner Press, 1982.

――― & Edward Kauffman. The Alcoholism Syndrome: Definitions & Models, op cit.

Pennsylvania Code Title 55. Department of Public Welfare, Chapter 5100. Mental Health Procedures. 1984.

Pennsylvania Senate Bill 935, Session of 1986.

Peyser, H.S. The Roles of the Psychiatrist, Psychologist, Social Worker, and Alcoholism Counselor, in *Alcoholism: A Practical Treatment Guide*. Edited by Gitlow, S. & Peyser, H. New York: Grune & Stratton, 1980.

Solomon, J. The Role of Drug Therapies in the Context of Alcoholism, in *Encyclopedic Handbook of Alcoholism*.

Wegscheider, S. *Another Chance: Hope and Health for the Alcoholic Family*. Palo Alto, Calif.: Science and Behavior Books, 1981.

Part 5

Long Term Care

Reestablishing
a Coordinated Care Program:
Home Health Services

Nancy V. Lotz
Denise DuChainey

DESCRIPTION OF THE SETTING

Community Home Health Services of Philadelphia (CHHSP) is a voluntary non-profit, Medicare certified home health agency, which provides multidisciplinary health services to any resident of Philadelphia. Services provided are skilled nursing, physical, occupational and speech therapies, medical social work and home health aid. Two hundred employees, of whom 3/4 are field staff, work from three area offices. The central office is responsible for administration, billing and intake.

CHHSP provides home visiting services to patients from 8AM until 9PM. A telephone reassurance program operates from 5PM until 8AM. CHHSP is the oldest and largest home health agency in the state. In April 1986, The Visiting Nurse Association of Philadelphia, an affiliate of CHHSP, celebrated its centennial. In fiscal 1986, 181,901 home care visits were made to 9,926 patients. The primary health problems treated were heart disease and circulatory ailments (26%), diabetes (15%) and cancer (14%). The majority of patients are at least 65 years old and female, and they are approximately half white and half black (Garner, 1984).

Policy

The agency adheres to a medical model, and services are provided only by order of a physician. Medical orders are certified every sixty days. Most referrals are made by area hospitals, other

373

health organizations such as HMOs or outpatient clinics, and private physicians. Private individuals can also initiate contact, but medical orders are required before services are rendered.

Most common requests are for skilled nursing and rehabilitation services. Most fees are paid by insurance. When consumers are billed directly, the fee is determined by an income based sliding scale.

Each social worker is assigned to one area office and provides consultation and direct service when a need is determined by intake or field staff. Appropriate problems must be clearly related to the care of a patient's medical condition. For example, social workers secure financial entitlement, coordinate long term care plans, mobilize support networks, and expedite protective service referrals. On receiving a referral, the social worker schedules a home visit for psychosocial assessment and the establishment of goals and a treatment plan (Kirschner and Rosengarten, 1982). Social workers also orient new staff, provide in-service education and serve on administrative committees.

Agency policy determined service eligibility, but policy is significantly influenced by funding sources; primarily Medicare and other forms of insurance. Medicare regulations specify conditions of eligibility as well as types of service (Mundinger, 1983). In 1986, Medicare paid $2.5 billion to home health care providers that benefitted 1.5 million patients. A person must be homebound, in need of skilled care and not receiving such care from another health care organization. According to Medicare, nursing, physical therapy and speech therapy are primary services while social work, occupational therapy and home health aid service are secondary. Reimbursement is made only while a primary service is involved; thus, with the exception of occupational therapy, which can continue to work with a patient after primary service ends, secondary service must be provided in conjunction with a primary service. For example, if Mrs. Smith who is recuperating from a stroke no longer requires the services of a nurse, she may continue to work with an occupational therapist in retraining for activities of daily living, but she may not continue to work with a social worker in managing her depression or the problems she is having in her marriage as a result of the stroke. Medicare's criteria for social workers in home health are a Master of Social Work degree from an accredited institution and at least one year of experience in a medical setting.

New Legislation

Much new legislation has an impact on home health care. The *Omnibus Reconciliation Act of 1980* allowed proprietary agencies to apply for Medicare certification in home health. Ten years ago, there were ten home health care agencies in the Greater Delaware Valley encompassing Philadelphia and the contiguous areas; now there are fifty-four (Gilbride, 1983). Thus, home health agencies are competing for the referrals which will determine survival.

The *Tax Equity and Fiscal Responsibility Act of 1982* (TEFRA) changed the basis for reimbursement to hospitals. Before, it was the cost to the hospital of providing daily care for the patient. Now it is the diagnostic category of the patient. The resultant system, *the Medicare Prospective Payment System*, established a patient classification system of 468 diagnosis-related groups (DRGs) which determines the amount which Medicare will reimburse the hospital for the care of a patient. Consequently, the length of hospital stay for patients has been dramatically shortened with patients being discharged in a more debilitated state (Feller, 1986).

Initially, home health referrals increased as a result of TEFRA and the DRGs, but as the census of hospitals began to decline, so did the number of referrals for home health. Thus, the competition for referrals was further escalated. Concerned about their own survival, hospitals have begun to diversity services and to form coalitions with home health agencies among others (Kuntz, 1983). Initially, they contracted with home health agencies, but many have now hired their own staff. Free standing home health agencies such as CHHSP now are trying to increase referrals by appealing directly to physicians. In addition, all of the Visiting Nurse Associations (VNAs) which are based in a charitable rather than a business tradition have formed a consortium to provide home health services in the Eastern Region of the United States.

In 1985, the Health Care Financing Administration (which under the Department of Health and Human Services is responsible for Medicare, federal participation in Medicaid, and other health programs) created a uniform system for physician orders — and a prodigious amount of paper work: It introduced several new comprehensive forms (485-88) for physician orders and treatment plans for Medicare patients which must be completed by all disciplines after the initial visit, signed by the physician within thirty days, updated by staff and recertified through new forms prior to the sixty day validity limit (Holloway, 1984).

An elaborate system through intermediary insurance companies which pay claims under contract to the federal government monitors these forms and uses them to deny payment for services. The National Association of Home Care reports that "The contractors must return at least $5.00 in denials for every $1.00 that they spend in order to retain the government contract" (*Home Health Line*, National Association of Home Care, 1987). A medical denial means that the service provided did not meet Medicare's requirements for skilled nursing services; a technical denial means that the physician did not sign the form, the form was completed incorrectly, or the patient was not homebound. Payment for part or all of the service period may be denied. All home health agencies have experienced an increase in denial of payment. From 1983 to 1986, the Health Care Financing Administration (HCFA) which governs Medicare shows a 300% increase on payment denials for home health care (Rainer, 1987). In addition, the Gramm-Rudman Act, 1986, reduced CHHSP's payment from Medicare by one percent.

Denials have caused agencies to be more stringent about service provision. Shorter and less frequent visits are being made. Specifically, social workers have less time to intervene with multiproblem, emergency situations which often require protective services, referral to nursing homes which have long waiting lists, and to underfunded, understaffed community agencies for additional in-home services.

While Medicare limits in-home social work services, Medical Assistance and many private insurance companies do not reimburse for social work services at all. Thus far, attempts to rectify this problem have not been successful. States which do not reimburse for social work services through Medical Assistance say they cannot afford the cost and want the federal government to contribute through block grants.

Many coalitions have been formed in response to the needs of home care patients and professionals. The National Association of Home Care and its state chapters, the National Association of Social Workers, and several congressmen are working to remedy the problems and increase monies available for home health care. NASW is making a concerted effort to change home care policy in regard to social work. Testimony has been sent to the House and Senate with recommendations for social work representation on Bill S1076 which proposes to increase the availability of reimbursable home health care (*NASW News*, 1987). Introduced by Senator Bradley (Democrat, New Jersey) S1076 would allow patients to receive daily home care services under Medicare for sixty days. Under exceptional circumstances, this coverage could be extended through physician prescription (Rovner, 1987).

For ten years, there has been a local home care social workers' group which provides in-service education, peer support and advocacy activities. More recently, NASW has also established a Home Health Care Group (*NASW News*, 1987). In 1986, the Social Workers in Home Care Coalition was created to interpret and influence the new regulations.

In light of these policies, CHHSP establishes the conditions of service; nursing and therapy protocols, hours of service, productivity standards (the average number of home visits expected each day from each employee, according to discipline). Social workers are expected to make 2.5 to 3.5 visits each day.

CHSSP has always taken pride in being able to offer care to the indigent and others without health insurance. To maintain this mission, CHHSP created the Indigent Care Program which in 1986 raised more than $700,000 for this purpose.

Technology

Technology has enabled CHHSP to improve its services medically and professionally. Living at home with advanced chronic illness or trauma convalescence often requires some equipment and assistive devices which reduce architectural or physical barriers. Patient's mobility and independence can be improved with equipment such as hospital beds, wheelchairs, walkers, commodes, raised toilet seats, bathtub seats, stairlifts, and ramps; assistive devices such as braces, longhandle tongs and sponges, button hookers, and large print telephone dials; removal of architectural barriers such as throw rugs and some doors; and help with activities of daily living (Arthritis Health Professions Section, 1980; *Up and Around*, n.d.; Kerson, 1985).

Prior to a patient's discharge home, appropriate equipment is ordered by the hospital social worker or discharge coordinator. When CHHSP staff finds other equipment to be necessary, they obtain a prescription from the patient's physician and order the devices. Some equipment is covered for payment by insurance plans. When coverage is not available, families pay suppliers. Those who cannot afford to pay do without the equipment.

Providing service in the home calls for creativity and collaboration (Sitt, 1985; Weinstein, 1984). For example, the rehabilitation staff can often increase a person's functional ability and independence using everyday household items, such as an old handbag filled with canned goods used as a weights for exercises to strengthen arms and legs. In addition, each profession combines new techniques with traditional ones. For example, nurses perform intravenous therapy and use (and teach family members) sophisticated techniques such as enteral and perenteral feedings, and tracheotomy care. Physical therapists teach patients how to use a TENS (transcutaneous electrical nerve stimulation) to reduce pain without drugs or penetration of the body; social workers have incorporated new theories about care of the terminally ill drawn from the hospice literature.

Organization

In 1979, CHHSP was established as a non-profit corporation to provide multidisciplinary home health care including patient education, social services, and health maintenance and rehabilitation services. This entity succeeded Community Nursing Services, an unincorporated, non-profit association formed in 1959 by agreement between the city of Philadelphia and the Visiting Nurse Society of Philadelphia (VNS).

Recently, CHHSP was also compelled to reorganize. In 1984,

Medicare had diminished the definition of a home health agency to only nursing and one other discipline, thereby dramatically increasing CHHSP's competition; also, caseloads of patients who could not afford to pay for services were increasing. The establishment of DRGs as the basis for hospital reimbursement prompted many hospitals to establish their own home care affiliates, again heightening CHHSP's competition (Ginzberg, 1984; Eaton, 1984; Benjamin, 1986; Lerman, 1987). In order to survive financially, CHHSP sought additional funding sources.

In response, a parent corporation, Philadelphia Home Care (PHC), was established. CHHSP and two new affiliates, Home Care Specialists and the Philadelphia Equipment Company are under PHC's domain. Home Care Specialists offers private pay nursing, homemakers, and companion services. The Philadelphia Equipment Company leases and sells medical supplies and equipment needed by the home care patient. The revenues from these two organizations can be used to offset the deficits created by CHHSP.

CHHSP is governed by a board of trustees comprised of governmental, community, medical and business representatives. CHHSP's performance and policy promulgation are the primary responsibility of the Board. The president and her staff implement the policies. The administrative staff is divided into three areas: financial and administrative services, patient services and human resources (personnel).

CHHSP's social service component is small; therefore, the three workers are responsible to the vice president of patient services who oversees the area offices from which the field staff operates. In each office, an associate director of patient services is responsible for the daily operations and is the person to whom the social workers report. A social work consultant provides clinical supervision.

Essentially, CHHSP remains a nursing agency (Fessler and Adams, 1985). Cooperation between nursing, social work and therapy staffs remains a difficulty in the informal organization. Blending and blurring of professional roles create problems on cases. Social work depends on other disciplines for referrals and, more importantly, for the closing of cases. Therefore, quality care depends on open communication and cooperation. The social worker is responsible for teaching the rest of the staff about the appropriate role of social work by fostering positive work relationships and informal case discussions and demonstrating her contribution through joint home visits.

Case Description

Mrs. Burden, aged fifty-nine, is a black woman who has multiple medical problems (Palley and Oktuy, 1983). Hospitalized as the result of a stroke, Mrs. Burden was referred to CHHSP on discharge, bedridden and unable to care for herself. Previously, Mrs. Burden was diagnosed as having lung cancer and received chemotherapy treatments. Presently, the cancer is in remission. Her secondary diagnoses are hypertension, seizure disorder and non-insulin dependent diabetes.

Since she was discharged from the hospital, Mrs. Burden has lived in the home of her son and his family in an inner-city neighborhood. Before her illness, she lived alone in her apartment in an unused rectory of the church to which she belonged where she taught Sunday school and enjoyed the children. A devout Catholic, Mrs. Burden finds great comfort in her religion. She is very talkative and peppers her conversation with religious themes. The mother of two grown sons, she worked as long as she was able and now receives Social Security Disability payments.

Mrs. Burden is a small, wiry woman with large shining eyes. Her decaying teeth and noticeable breath are due to years without dental care. She is friendly and exudes a willingness to cooperate. Only the constant fingering of the cross she is wearing around her neck betrays her nervousness.

During the two months that CHHSP was involved in Mrs. Burden's care, her son's family participated fully in the home care plan (Haug, 1985; Moseley, 1986). With the help of the nurse, physical therapist and home health aide, Mrs. Burden learned to transfer from bed to chair independently and to ambulate with a walker, and began to climb stairs with supervision. With some assistance and encouragement, she was able to perform most activities of daily living such as eating, bathing and dressing.

As Mrs. Burden became stronger, her son and his girlfriend allowed her to do more for herself. Mrs. Burden then became angry and complained that her family was no longer providing her care. At this point, the care plan began to break down. The nurse, physical therapist and home health aide were concerned about Mrs. Burden's complaints but were uncertain about what to do because Mrs. Burden refused to confront her family. Aware that the care plan would continue to deteriorate if no action were taken, the nurse requested a consultation with me. From the discussion, I realized that Mrs. Burden was giving double messages and taking no responsibility. Instead, the nurse was feeling responsible. I suggested that the nurse ask Mrs. Burden how she would solve the problem.

When she returned from the next home visit, the nurse said when Mrs. Burden began to complain again, they both decided the problem would only worsen unless everyone discussed it. Eventually, Mrs. Burden would be independent enough for CHHSP to terminate the service, and the problem would remain. When Mrs. Burden agreed, the nurse asked me to facilitate a family conference in the patient's room, attended by her nurse, home health aide, son, and son's girlfriend. The physical therapist was on vacation.

Definition of the Client

The agency defined the client as Mrs. Burden. Once I became involved as a consultant to the nurse, I defined the client as the family and caregiving unit. After the family meeting, Mrs. Burden became my client for brief work so that we could address her response to her illness and disability.

Goals

Mrs. Burden made becoming totally independent her long range goal. Staff and family's goals for Mrs. Burden were independent self-care and unsupervised or minimally assisted stair climbing. The goal of the family meeting was to assess Mrs. Burden's progress, to have everyone involved discuss feelings, concerns and responsibilities and to reestablish a coordinated care plan (Kaye and Sager, 1983). We all agreed that Mrs. Burden was progressing beautifully. As Mrs. Burden required less help, the family stopped waiting on her. What Mrs. Burden viewed as rejection was the family's reaction to her growing independence (Silverstone and Burack-

Weiss, 1982). Before that meeting, no one in the family had discussed their relationships. Lucille was pleased to hear that her son still cared for her and wanted to help her to reach her goal. A bonus to the meeting was some resolution of the earlier conflict between mother, son and son's girlfriend (Getzel, 1981).

Contract

The contract for this patient and family was established during the family conference. We all agreed to try the plan for one week. As part of the family meeting, a new treatment plan was written which identified specific responsibilities for Mrs. Burden and each caregiver as well as how long each discipline would provide service (Dobrof, 1984). I offered Mrs. Burden brief social work intervention to help her think about her ambivalence and anger concerning her illness (Berger and Anderson, 1984). She agreed to the new plan. The following week, everyone involved agreed that the plan was realistic and workable.

Meeting Place

CHHSP is a home visiting agency, therefore, all contacts except discharge planning meetings, interdisciplinary team meetings, and professional conferences occur in the patient's home. After agency hours, a staff member is always available by telephone. Unless it has been prearranged to meet in a particular room, the meeting place is usually determined by the patient's location when the social worker arrives. The family conference and our first four meetings took place in Mrs. Burden's bedroom because she was not able to climb stairs, and it was too difficult to carry her downstairs. Our final visit took place in the dining room; Mrs. Burden was now able to climb stairs with assistance and had walked downstairs to eat her lunch just before I arrived.

Use of Time

In order to coordinate services, one week after the family conference an interdisciplinary team meeting was held at which each discipline projected duration of service. The consensus of the group was that Mrs. Burden would reach "maintenance" level of care in five or six weeks. This information was shared with the family at the next home visit.

Generally, duration of service is determined by medical condition, Medicare regulations and the amount of care which the agency can absorb beyond the limits of insurance. Extended hours now enable CHHSP to provide dressing changes twice a day and to teach care techniques to family members with normal working hours.

Treatment Modality

Social work intervention includes counseling, advocacy, coordination of services and referrals for concrete services to other agencies. Due to Medicare and Medicaid reimbursement policies, the social worker must utilize a brief, crisis oriented approach (Everstine and Everstine, 1983). Family treatment methods are employed when appropriate (Pinkston and Linsk, 1984).

Stance of the Social Worker

My stance depends on whether I am acting in the role of clinician or collaborator, and on the phase of the relationship. With staff, I was active and direct because I had to obtain specific information. My role was to listen and recommend appropriate interventions. During the family meeting, my role was to facilitate sharing information, identification and clarification of problems, and problem resolution (Snow, 1980).

In individual work with Mrs. Burden, I moved from an active to a more passive stance. I structured the interviews and provided resource information. Mrs. Burden enjoyed talking about the past and avoided the present. As she began confronting the present, I supported her and became her advocate with staff, family and the recreational program to which she was referred.

Outside Resources

I gave Mrs. Burden information about recreational and social activities, transportation services, and housing, and she chose a recreational program for physically handicapped older adults which also provided rehabilitation. The physical therapist ordered Mrs. Burden's walker.

Reassessment

Agreement to evaluate the treatment plan was included in the contract, and I was responsible for obtaining evaluation information from each person involved. I asked Mrs. Burden, her son and his girlfriend for feedback each time I visited the home. Staff reassess cases each week during team meetings (Brill and Horowitz, 1983). This exchange is helpful in planning the termination of services.

When goals are attained and termination is contemplated, my client and I review our work together. Reassessment helped Lucille to understand her contribution to reaching goals and to plan for the future.

Transfer or Termination

Frequently, CHHSP patients are referred to a community agency for follow-up in-home and social services. Mrs. Burden's stable medical condition and referral to the recreation program meant that she was ready to terminate. She knew what she had to do to maintain her health and activity level.

Case Conclusion

With a lot of support and encouragement from staff and family, Mrs. Burden continued to progress slowly and steadily. Although she was hesitant about joining the recreation program, she was anxious to get out of the house. The recreation program represented the next step of many Mrs. Burden would have to take in order to become independent. When she realized that she could again have a life outside of her son's house, much of her anxiety was reduced, and she was able to mobilize her strength for rehabilitation. At the time the case was closed, Mrs. Burden was independent in self-care and could climb stairs with minimal assistance. In time and with more practice, she would climb stairs independently.

Differential Discussion

Throughout the case, I made several decisions about my role that affected outcome. Initially, I was asked to consult. The turning point came when I was asked to facilitate the family conference.

Had I refused, I would have had minimal involvement, Mrs. Burden would have made little progress, and she and her family would have become increasingly angry with one another. By shifting roles, I was able to address the psychosocial needs of the patient and identify an ongoing role for myself. I was uncertain about future contact with the family until everyone agreed to reestablish a coordinated plan. Because I facilitated the meeting, I was able to redefine the problem as a family problem.

Once the crisis was resolved, I began to focus on Lucille's individual feelings and needs. The son's work schedule prevented his attending regular family meetings, and individual sessions would provide Mrs. Burden with the recognition she needed to work toward her goal of independence; so, I agreed to individual work with her. During these sessions, Mrs. Burden verbalized her need to be involved in activities away from home. The program I found had a short waiting list, provided transportation and met Mrs. Burden's needs for socialization and rehabilitation. Without this follow-up referral, terminating the service would have been difficult for patient and staff because Mrs. Burden's rehabilitation would have been interrupted. According to agency policy, she would no longer be eligible for CHHSP services. She was enrolled in the recreation program within two weeks of CHHSP's closing her case. Being able to leave her son's home represented independence to Mrs. Burden and reduced some of the responsibility her son carried. Everyone was proud of the progress Mrs. Burden had made. This choice of treatment alternatives contributed to a coordinated and mutually satisfying termination.

PRACTICE IN CONTEXT

Social work in home care is greatly affected by policy, technology and organization, with policy the most significant factor. Federal and state regulation dictate specific eligibility criteria as well as types and duration of services. Home care social workers must be aware of pending legislation and call for primary status and payment from all health insurance plans. Regulations and standards for professional service are incorporated into CHHSP's policies, which in turn affect the status of the social worker within the agency and the relationship between worker and client.

Because social work is considered a secondary service, it is impossible for social workers to continue treatment with patients who no longer need skilled nursing or rehabilitation services, even though illness-treated social or emotional problems remain. In these situations, the social worker tries to transfer the client to another community agency, but there are few such services for home-bound people. When services exist, transfer must be managed delicately.

Practice decisions are affected by all aspects of context. One area in which home care differs from many other kinds of health social work is meeting place. That the social worker is a guest in the client's house has many ramifications. Initially, patient and family may feel threatened especially when the referral for service comes from outside the family. Often, patients are living in a dining room or living room, and the lack of privacy makes the establishment of a helping relationship more difficult. A positive aspect of seeing people in their homes is the opportunity to observe daily living and to meet other members of the patient's support system. Understanding how this and other practice decisions are affected by context allows the social worker to plan fine services within the demands and realities of bureaucratic life.

REFERENCES

Austin, C.D. and Seidl, F.W. "Validating professional judgement in a home care agency." *Health and Social Work*, 6(1), Feb. 1981, pp. 50-56.

Baer, N. et al. "Home health services social work treatment protocol." *Home Healthcare Nurse*, 2(4), July/Aug. 1984, pp. 43-49.

Black, R.B. et al. "Challenges in developing health promotion services for the chronically ill." *Social Work*, 31(4), July/Aug., 1986, pp. 287-293.

Benjamin, A.E. "Trends and issues in the provision of home health care: Local governments in a competitive environment." *Journal of Public Health Policy*, 7(4), Winter 1986, pp. 480-494.

Berger, R.M. and Anderson, S. "The In-home worker: Serving the frail elderly." *Social Work*, 29(5), Sept./Oct. 1984, pp. 456-461.

Brill, R.A. and Horowitz, A. The New York City home care project: A demonstration in coordination of health and social services." *Home Health Services Quarterly*, 4(3/4), 1983, pp. 91-106.

Dobrof, R. (ed.). *Gerontological social work in home health care*. N.Y.: The Haworth Press, 1984.

Eaton, B.J. "Hospital improves service through diversification." *Home Health Journal*, 5(2), March 1984, pp. 3, 9-10.

Everstine, D.S. and Everstine, L. *People in crisis: Strategic therapeutic interventions*. N.Y.: Brunner/Mazel, 1983.

Feller, B.A. *Americans needing home care*. U.S. National Center for Health Statistics, Program Division of Health Statistics. Pub. No. PHS 86-1581. March 1986.

Fessler, S.R. and Adams, C.G. "Nurse/social worker role conflict in home health care." *Journal of Gerontological Social Work*, 9(1), 1985, pp. 113-123.

Garner, J.D. "From hospital to home care: Who goes there? A descriptive study of elderly users of home health care services post hospitalization." *Journal of Gerontological Social Work*, 7(4), 1984, pp. 75-85.

Gelman, D. "Staying home, feeling better." *Newsweek*, 108, July 7, 1986, pp. 48-49.

Getzel, G.S. "Social work with family caregivers to the aged." *Social Casework*, 4(9), Sept. 1983, pp. 201-209.

Gilbride, N. "Philadelphia home health expanding market boom." *Home Health Journal*, 4(9), Sept. 1983, pp. 6, 15.

Ginzberg, E., Ostow, M. and Balonsky, W. *Home health care: Its role in the changing health services market*. Totowa, N.J.: Rowman and Allanheld Pub., 1984.

Hatch, O.G. "Home health care: Necessary option for older Americans." *Hospital Progress*, 62(4), 1981, pp. 6, 10.

Haug, M.R. "Home care for the ill elderly: Who benefits? (Editorial). *American Journal of Public Health*, 75(2), Feb. 1985, pp. 127-128.

Hoffman, J. "Medical social services offer agencies a greater flexibility in the provision of in-home services." *Home Health Journal*, 4(2), Feb. 1983, p. 13.

Holloway, V.M. "Documentation: One of the ultimate challenges in home health care." *Home Healthcare Nurse*, 2(1), Jan./Feb. 1984, pp. 19, 22.

Home Health Line. National Association of Home Care, 1987.

"Home health social work standards get NASW nod." *NASW News*, 32(7), July 1987, p. 10.

Jacobs, P.E. and Lurie, A. "A new look at home care and hospital social worker." *Journal of Gerontological Social Work*, 7(4), 1984, pp. 87-99.

Kaye, L.W. "Home care for the aged: A fragile partnership." *Social Work*, 30, July/Aug. 1985, pp. 312-317.

Kirschner, C. and Rosengarten, L. "The skilled social work role in home care." *Social Work*, 27(6), Nov. 1982, pp. 527-530.

Kuntz, E. F. "Alternative services: Hospitals move into home care by striking partnership deals." *Modern Health Care*, 13(12), Dec. 1983, pp. 116-118.

Lerman, D. "Home care payer mix: Referrals need expansion." *Hospitals*, 61(2), Jan. 20, 1987, p. 98.

————. "Room to expand home care business in 1987." *Hospitals*, 61(1), Jan. 5, 1987, p. 51.

Liu, K., Manton, K.G. and Liu, B.M. "Home care expenses for the disabled elderly." *Health Care Financing Review*, 7(2), Winter 1985, pp. 51-58.

Livengood, W.S., Smith, C. and Hallstead, S. "The impact of DRGs on home health care." *Home Healthcare Nurse*, 1(1), Sept./Oct. 1983, pp. 29-34.

Moskowitz, D.B. "Getting hospital-quality care at home." *Business Week*, March 9, 1987, p. 121.

"NASW makes point on nursing home, home health bills." *NASW News*, 32(7), July 1987, p. 11.

Palley, H. and Oktuy, J. *The chronically-limited elderly: The case for a national policy for in-home and supportive community-based services*. N.Y.: The Haworth Press, 1983.

Pinkston, E.M. and Linsk, N.L. *Care of the elderly: A family approach*. N.Y.: Pergamon Press, 1984.

Rogatez, P. "Home health care: Some social and economic considerations." *Home Healthcare Nurse*, 3(1), Jan./Feb. 1985, p. 38.

Rovner, J. "Long-term care: The true 'catastrophe'?" *Congressional Quarterly Weekly Report*, 44, May 31, 1986, pp. 1227-1231.

————. "Expansion of Medicare sought to improve home health care." *Congressional Quarterly Weekly Review*, 45(17), April 25, 1987, p. 790.

Sager, A. *Planning home care with the elderly: Patient, family, and professional views of an alternative to institutionalization*. Cambridge, MA: Ballinger, 1983.

Silverstone, B. and Burack-Weiss, A. "The social worker function in nursing homes and home care." *Journal of Gerontological Social Work*, 5(1/2), 1982, pp. 7-33.

Sitt, P.G. "Home health care innovations in health care delivery." *Hawaii Medical Journal*, 44(5), 1985, pp. 168-169.

Smith, J.B. "Home care is more than Medicare regulations." *American Journal of Nursing*, 3, March 1987, pp. 304-306.

Trager, B. *Home health care and national health policy*. N.Y.: The Haworth Press, 1980.

United States House, Select Committee on Aging. "The 'black box' of home care quality: A report." 99th Congress, 2nd Session, Pub. No. 99-573, August 1986.

————. "Out 'sooner and sicker': Myth or Medicare crisis?" Hearing, 99th Congress, 2nd Session, Pub. No. 99-591, April 10, 1986.

United States House, Select Committee on Aging, Subcommittee on Human Services. "Exploring the myths: Caregiving in America; a study." 100th Congress, 2nd Session, Pub. No. 99-611, January 1987.

————. "Home health care: Present and future options." Hearing, 99th Congress, 1st Session, Pub. No. 99-539, September 30, 1985.

United States, Medicare. *Home health manual*. Washington, D.C.: Government Printing Office, March 1983.

_____. *Use of home health services*. Washington, D.C.: Government Printing Office, 1982.

United States, Social Security Administration. *Medicare; Health insurance for the aged: Length of stay by diagnosis*. Washington, D.C.: Government Printing Office, 1983.

Weinstein, S.M. "Specialty teams in home care." *American Journal of Nursing*, 84(3), 1984, pp. 342-345.

Zimner, J.G., Groth-Juncker, A. and McCusker, J. "A randomized controlled study of a home health care team." *American Journal of Public Health*, 75(2), Feb. 1985, pp. 135-141.

Group Work with Institutionalized Elderly: The "Being Old" Group Revisited

Phyllis Braudy Harris

Group work with institutionalized elderly is now recognized as a viable treatment of choice for many institutionalized elderly. From examining the geriatric social work literature over the past ten years, the amount of reported social group work services with the institutionalized and community based elderly has increased dramatically. There seem to be two major reasons: First, the number of elderly in the population is growing rapidly. In 1975 the over 65 segment of the population comprised 23 million people, 11% of the United States population, with the oldest segment of this group, the 85 and over cohort, numbering 2 million people or .8% of the population. By the year 2050, there will be 67 million people, or 22% of the population, over 65; the 85 and over cohort will number 16 million, 24% of the total elderly population in the United States. The "Graying of America" is upon us, with the 85 + group, the frailest elderly, increasing in the greatest proportions (DHHS, HCFA, 1985; Suzman and Riley, 1985).

The second reason for this increase in social group work services with the elderly, especially with nursing home residents, is the unique contribution social group work can make. The central tenet of social group work is the concept of the group as a mutual aid system where new behaviors, roles, and relationships can be explored in an accepting environment (Schulman, 1985). The opportunity this type of experience affords the institutionalized elderly is extremely important, since as a function of reaching an advanced age with chronic health problems, many elderly have experienced a series of losses: roles, home, health, friends, family, finances, etc. Participation in a social group work experience affords the elderly nursing home resident the possibility of redeveloping a new peer social support network. As Abels and Abels (1980) have stressed, the major focus of social group work should be the strengthening and developing of social networks. "Social group work has demonstrated that carefully designed group work programs can contribute effectively to meet the therapeutic, socialization, and development needs of the institutionalized elderly" (Cohen and Hammerman, 1974, p. 124). This treatment modality can give the elderly a chance to develop or relearn social interaction skills, to make new contacts, and to develop mutual aid peer support systems. It also offers the elderly a chance for therapeutic ventilation, for personal growth and development, and to evaluate their own life situation in terms of comparable others (Lowy, 1982; Cohen and Hammerman, 1974).

Groups with institutionalized elderly can be of different types. Priscilla Ebersole (1976) lists such examples as: (a) discussion groups, (2) reality orientation groups, (3) remotivation groups, (4) bereavement groups, (5) self-help groups, (6) instruction groups, (7) psychotherapy groups, (8) self-image groups, and (9) social groups. Group work can also be a combination of different types, as will be illustrated by the case presented here, the "Being Old" group. This was a combination discussion, instructional, self-help, social, and psychotherapeutic group. It gave elderly nursing home residents with adequate social interaction skills the opportunity to openly and honestly confront the problems they were having with aging and also to redevelop some new peer social support networks. The name "Being Old" was given to the group in its first session by a participant who suggested we call the group what it really was—"We're old so the group should be called the 'Being Old' group."

DESCRIPTION OF THE SETTING

The "Being Old" Group was held at the Jewish Home for Aged, a 310-bed nursing home serving elderly Jewish residents of the state of Michigan. It is a non-profit organization that started in 1907 as a charitable burial society and fifty-six years ago evolved into a home for the aged. It is an Orthodox Jewish Home that operates according to traditional Jewish laws and rituals, but uses the most modern nursing care. It provides medical, educational, social, psychological, nutritional, recreational, religious and cultural services for its residents and day program participants, over 50% of which are Medicaid participants.

The philosophy of the Detroit Jewish Home for Aged has always been that the home operates on a social, not a medical model, because it is a permanent residence for chronically ill aged, not an acute care hospital. The social work department has always played an important role in the home.

The age of the resident population ranges from 66 to 100, with 85 the average. The length of stay for an elderly resident averages 4.5 years. Most of the population was born in Eastern Europe, coming to the United States in the pre- and post-World War I immigration waves. Though Yiddish is the native tongue, most of the residents speak English fluently. Not well-educated themselves, they see education as a very important family value, and most of their children are well-educated professional or business people.

Policy

The policies that most affect this institutional setting are those of the home; and of the federal and state government. The home's policies are set by the Board of Directors comprised of 42 lay members of the Jewish community. These policies reflect the charter of the facility: The purpose is to establish, provide, and maintain a Jewish Home in the state of Michigan for the aged and chronically ill. An acceptable applicant must be Jewish, a resident of Michigan, and at least 65 years old. The person must be in need of twenty-four-hour supervision, and requires a physician's statement that he or she is in need of closely supervised medical care. The applicant must not be severely mentally impaired at the time of admission and must be cognizant of the fact that he is moving into a home for the aged on a permanent basis. The admission policy limits the type of resident entering the Jewish Home for Aged to those who are able to some extent to avail themselves of the social, recreational, educational, and religious services the home can provide.

This admission policy's effect upon social work practice is to promote the use of social work services. The social worker meets the elderly resident and his family at a time when the resident is able to communicate to the social worker his needs and concerns and can form a worker-client relationship. As this frail elderly resident becomes more dehabilitated and in need of more supportive services, the social worker's relationship with the resident and family is already established and thus promotes a better understanding of the situation and a more effective service delivery (Getzel and Mellor, 1982).

In terms of federal policies influencing social work practice, the Detroit Jewish Home for Aged receives federal funding through Title XVIII of the Medicare Act and Title XIX of the Medicaid Act. The home follows the regulations stipulated by these Acts for skilled nursing facilities. One which promotes social work practice in the home is the stipulation that social work services must be made available to nursing home residents. The medically related social needs of the patients are to be identified during admission, and services to meet these needs are to be provided during the patient's stay in the facility and in the planning of his discharge. This gives the social work department the legal mandate to provide services within the home, but it is up to the social workers to creatively and effectively use this sanction. The Medicaid and Medicare Acts also put constraints upon the social worker in terms of the type of services and medical equipment they will fund (Kaufman, 1980; U.S., 1981).

Licensed by the state of Michigan, the Jewish Home for Aged also follows the laws and policies for the Michigan Department of Public Health. These affect every area of the operation of the home, from the administration to how often a piece of machinery is checked. The other state agency that influences the relationship of social worker and client is the Michigan Department of Social Services. This agency implements the reimbursement of federal and state monies and checks regularly on the type of care the nursing home resident is receiving in the institution. It also evaluates whether the elderly patient could manage in a non-nursing home setting.

Thus the home itself, and the state and federal governments all create constraints and supports for the social worker and her relationship with the client. The social worker must learn to recognize and identify these constraints and supports, and to take a creative approach toward working within them.

Technology

Another category of constraining factors that affect the social worker-client relationship is technology, in this instance the technology of geriatric medicine and chronic illness. The nursing home setting is quite different from the acute care hospital setting where the focus of medical care is on curing the patient. The goal of long-term care is upon rehabilitation and maintaining the level of patient functioning. Therefore, a different approach is needed with geriatric patients. Yet, geriatric medicine in the United States is still a fairly new and not very popular specialty in hospitals and medical schools. Even with the recent emergence of geriatric assessment units in medical centers (47% of the 114 units in medical centers only began in 1983 or later), only 50% of the physicians primarily servicing these units are trained in geriatric medicine (Epstein et al., 1987).

The importance of the primary physician taking extra time with the geriatric patients and reaching out to them cannot be overemphasized. The art of listening to their complaints, aches, and pains is essential to understanding exactly what the patient is saying. Especially important to consider when communicating with the elderly, is their high incidence of impaired vision and hearing, which hampers their communication skills. Also, better patient education is needed in order for the elderly resident to have a clearer understanding of his chronic illness. The limited interest and concern on the part of the medical community places a serious constraint and burden upon the geriatric social worker (Aging in the Eighties, 1980).

Organization

Factors within the organizational structure can also act as constraints or supports on social work practice, depending upon the social worker's approach. There are strong formal and informal structures within the Jewish Home for Aged that greatly affected the "Being Old" Group. Even though the nursing home is small in comparison to a hospital setting, the informal networks play an important role and it is necessary for the social worker to understand them in order to effectively help her clients. One of the major roles of the social worker in this particular institution is to be an advocate for the resident and to act as a mediator or go-between for the resident and the various departments within the home (Wells and Singer, 1985). It is essential for the social worker to establish a good rapport with the various department heads, charge nurses, and nurses aides in order to perform her job. More often than not, problems can be solved more quickly and effectively by using the informal networks than by going through the bureaucratic channels. Mastery of these informal channels was quite useful in avoiding the scheduling of the "Being Old" Group members for baths, physical therapy, beauty shop appointments, etc., at times when group meetings were held.

The formal organizational structure of the home supported the formation of the group. The executive director had a social work orientation and gave the social work department a great deal of freedom and latitude in performing and implementing innovative therapeutic ideas (Boissenau and Kirschner, 1982). This orientation was reinforced by the director of the social work department, an ACSW who also had considerable group work experience. Thus, this official philosophy of the nursing home created a positive environment that lent itself to the formation of a "Being Old" group.

DECISIONS ABOUT PRACTICE

Definition of the Client

Little group work has been done in most nursing homes that deals specifically with problems of aging. In this home, there were orientation groups, diabetes groups, reality orientation groups, a resident council, but nothing that specifically gave the elderly nursing home residents the opportunity to openly discuss and confront the problems they were having with being old (Boling, 1987). The author, after talking with different residents, decided such a group was needed. The residents who could best benefit and participate in this type of confrontation group would be the more alert ones who had adequate social interaction skills and limited sensory impairment. As Priscilla Ebersole (1976) states in her article on group work with the aged, both sensory loss (hearing and vision) and mental alertness should be assessed since a great many sensory deficits in group members will greatly affect the expectations and goals of the group. This was kept in mind as the group members were being chosen.

The author invited the registered occupational therapist to assist in leading the group, because some of the discussions would be on physical health issues in which the therapist had expertise. Together, the author and occupational therapist decided on the group's composition. Thirty-five prospective group participants were selected from the residents living in the home. These people were approached by one of the group leaders, interviewed, and invited to join the group. Only a small group of participants was expected because this type of group would not appeal to all the invited residents, and other programs and activities always occurred at the nursing home at any given time. It was also decided that the group sessions would be announced over the public address system and that anyone else who wanted to attend the group would be welcome, because only the most motivated and interested residents would be likely to respond to such an announcement. A total of twenty-eight people came to the group, but the usual attendance was nine to twelve people, consisting mostly of a constant core of the same nine persons. Attendance was completely voluntary, and approximately one-third of the people who attended at least one session continued to come regularly. The age range of the participants was sixty-nine to ninety-one. The majority were women; this reflected the higher percentage of women in the home's total population.

Goals

The goals of the group were briefly explained to each resident (Toseland, Sherman, and Blivin, 1981; Newgarten, 1984) in the individual interview sessions. At the first session, they were explained in detail and reiterated again during that session and later ones. The goals of the group were the following:

1. To encourage verbalization of fears, feelings, and problems of old age
2. To encourage group members to share feelings and experiences
3. To develop the beginnings of a peer support system
4. To encourage self-help among the participants
5. To provide educational information that would clear up misinformation and misunderstandings about physical and mental health problems of old age
6. To help the members as a group and as individuals come to some self-realization and acceptance of the aging process

These goals were reassessed at various times by the leaders in their post-group evaluation meetings and with the participants themselves. This helped the residents see that progress was being made within the group.

Contract, Meeting Place, and Time Period

The group contracted in the first session to meet for a short period every week for twenty weeks. The leaders felt that this would be sufficient to meet the areas they and the residents might wish to cover. Each session lasted forty-five minutes to an hour. The meeting place chosen by the leaders was the board room of the home. This was an area of the building the residents do not usually have access to, and the leaders felt it would help give prestige and status to the group to meet there. The room had a conference table with chairs; it was quite businesslike and relayed the message to the group participants that serious business was going to take place here. The room was also directly across the hallway from the executive director's office, so its location showed his acknowledgement and administrative sanction of these sessions.

Treatment Modality and Stance of the Social Worker

The problem of aging is a very broad topic to discuss, so the leaders chose as general topics for discussion the five main problem areas for the elderly as outlined in the OARS Multidimensional Functional Assessment Questionnaire prepared by the Older Americans Resources and Service Program (Pfeiffer, 1975). The five areas were: physical health, emotional health, social resources, financial resources, and independence versus dependence. Each topic could have been discussed for months, but the leaders chose the problems that the nursing home residents most commonly experienced in each area. The occupational therapist led the discussions in the area of physical health, which covered, among other topics, cardiovascular disease, arthritis, diabetes, and sensory loss. The book *Aging and Mental Health* by Butler and Lewis (1975) was used as a reference for the discussion on emotional health, which dealt with the attitude of giving up, loneliness and losses, ageism, mental impairment, death and dying, and coping mechanisms. The discussion of social resources included such topics as sexuality, loss of friends, family, status, and prestige in the community. Financial resources included the topics of retirement and lack of financial reserves. The last problem area discussed was independence versus dependence. This dealt with the elderly persons' increased dependencies on their adult children and the institution; it is discussed by Edna Wasser as the stage of filial maturity (Wasser, 1966).

The stance the leaders decided to take with the group had a big influence upon the progress of the group itself. From the beginning, the atmospheric tone of the group was one of warmth and acceptance. It was felt this would help the residents feel more comfortable in opening up and expressing their thoughts and feelings. The leaders also stated in the first session that they would be active members and give the group a great deal of support and direction, but it was expected that as the group evolved and coalesced, group members would become increasingly active. It was hoped that the residents' conversations would become more directed toward one another and that perhaps they would eventually initiate topics for discussion and lead them (Weiner, 1986; Yalom, 1985).

At times the leaders felt it would be appropriate and help stimulate discussion if they expressed their own feelings about aging and related life experiences. The modeling technique described by Authier and Gustafson (1976) was used, and it was quite beneficial in moving the group along when members were stuck or exhibited a great deal of resistance. A great many of the Rogerian treatment model techniques of positive, supportive, empathetic listening were also used, although at times the leaders became more directive than traditional Rogerian models would advocate in order to stimulate discussion. The technique of confronting certain feelings was also used at certain times in the group sessions, though it needed to be done with the elderly in a gentle, accepting manner. Appropriate reminiscing was also an important technique used throughout the session.

William Schwartz (Schwartz and Zalba, 1971) suggests the best way to understand the movement of a group is to examine the group process by dividing it into four separate phases. The first stage is a preparatory phase the worker goes through in organizing the group. The second phase is when the worker helps the group in its beginning process. The third phase is the work phase, containing the essential happenings of the group, and the final phase is the separation and termination phase. The "Being Old" Group followed these phases in its evolution.

The first, or preparatory, phase was described above. The second phase was embodied in the first three meetings of the "Being Old" Group. These initial meetings were the most difficult sessions for the leaders to control for a number of reasons: (1) The participants, though familiar with each other's faces since they resided together, were for all practical purposes strangers to each other; (2) They felt uncomfortable sharing feelings and ideas with strangers; (3) Many of the group members had never participated in a group such as this before and were unclear about what to expect; (4) There is a social taboo among the elderly about talking openly about such subjects as death, dementia, and sexuality; (5) There is such a negative stereotype about old age that it also presented an area of social taboo not easily discussed, and (6) There was a fear that if they did open up and discuss such topics, they would meet rejection and ridicule. As Lawrence Schulman (1979) discusses, each group member brings to the group the norms of behaviour and taboos which exist in his culture. One of the tasks of the group leader is to help members develop new norms and feel free to challenge some taboos so that the group can become more effective. The leaders used this technique, and out of this initial beginning stage came some important statements that laid the foundations for the later stages. One woman named the group, saying: "Let's say it as it is—we are old. People talk but never listen to each other; here we should be willing to listen to each other.'' Another woman confided, ''I was a very independent person once; I never understood how many problems old people had until I became old.'' Group participants displayed their various coping mechanisms, but no one denied that they had problems with growing old.

By the fourth session the group had moved into the third stage of the group process, the work phase. Group cohesion had begun to develop, and the elderly members were ready to open up and discuss their feelings more freely. They were willing to share feelings and take risks, as was demonstrated by one woman expressing her feelings on the topic of sexuality:

> Is there anything wrong with having a certain person of the opposite sex that you enjoy just talking with, just sitting together and conversing? Is there anything wrong with it? I have done nothing I would be ashamed of, but as I sit in the lobby or walk through the halls, people talk about me as if I have done a terrible thing and it hurts me.

Other participants reacted to this woman's statement, some supportive of her and others not (Hobson, 1984). But there was definite movement in the group toward direct conversation with each other and away from directing the conversation toward the group leaders. In later sessions dealing with ageism and society's attitude toward old people, the members shared their feelings and were quite supportive of each other. One participant stated:

> I never felt old and I don't feel old now at eighty-seven years old. Yes, I feel weak, unsure of my footing, but I don't feel old and I don't like being stereotyped.

She vented a great deal of her angry feelings by also saying:

> I'm younger than a lot of young people. You see a lot of young people who are old, absolutely old, because their minds are asleep.

During this stage members emerged as group leaders and took responsibility for running some of the sessions and bringing topics in for discussion. One member asked, "What as residents can we do to help people who have given up?" The underlying feeling of the group was, Yes, I am my brother's keeper. As one member stated:

It is the responsibility of everyone living here at the home to help each other. It makes a difference when we old people try to help each other in any way and as much as we are capable of.

The termination phase, according to Schwartz, deals with the member's development of self-realization and acceptance of aging, with its fears and joys (Simons and West, 1984-85). In relationship to the topic of mental impairment, the most difficult for the elderly group members to discuss, one participant stated:

I can't go visit the people on the third floor (the section of the building where the most mentally impaired residents reside) because it upsets me too much. I go up there and get sick of it, and I must come down.

Another member stated: "What is most frightening is that this may happen to any of us. A close friend of mine became senile." Unlike earlier sessions, most of the group members were willing to admit their fears of this aspect of aging and be supportive of each other. The final session dealt with acceptance of the aging process and with positive aspects of it. The member who emerged as the group leader remarked that at the age of eighty-seven there were less societal expectations placed upon her and she felt a new degree of personal freedom and expression.

Case Conclusion

A number of significant outcomes resulted from the "Being Old" Group. One was the establishment of a camaraderie and closeness among its members that carried beyond the group sessions. A new peer social support network was being established. This is a definite accomplishment in a nursing home setting where the atmosphere generally promotes self-preoccupation and an unhealthy competition for attention.

Another significant outcome was the "Positive Aspects of Being Old" bulletin board that still remains in the lobby of the Detroit Jewish Home for Aged. The member who developed into the group leader came to the author with the suggestion of placing a bulletin board in the lobby of the home, where all the residents, staff, and visitors could see it. She was specifically aiming it toward the resident population, which she labeled as having given up. This was a board that she, a resident, would take the responsibility of maintaining. She would find articles about the positive aspects of being old, put them on the bulletin board, and write captions underneath them, changing them regularly. She wanted to reach and educate as many people as possible. She asked the author to help her arrange for the bulletin board and get administrative sanction for it. She stated she did not want the effect of the "Being Old" Group just to fade away after the group ended.

The most important outcome, though, was that through the group work process, elderly people who at first showed great resistance to sharing their feelings and talking about being old progressed to the point of sharing feelings, supporting each other, and accepting responsibility for themselves and others. The participants had to examine, to share, to work through and to come to terms with their feelings about being old. The leaders felt the goals of the group were reached and that the "Being Old" Group was a successful experience for the elderly nursing home residents. Other nursing home residents have asked the leaders to run another "Being Old" Group at a different time so they, too, can have the opportunity of this experience.

Differential Discussion

The "Being Old" Group was a positive social work group experience for these institutionalized elderly. In re-thinking possible explanations for this group's success, a number of reasons emerge. There were also some problems in the running of the group that need to be examined.

There were a number of decisions made by the group's leaders which seemed to contribute to its success. First of all, the group's goals were relevant for its members and met their needs, aspirations, and capabilities. As Louis Lowy (1982) discusses, there are differential needs within the life span of an older person that social group work can address. Such needs are: coping needs, which come into play as the older person adapts to changes in himself and his social environment; expressive needs, those strivings associated with fulfilling oneself by participating in activities for one's own sake; contributory needs, wanting to give to others; and the need to exert some degree of influence over conditions in one's environment. The "Being Old" Group addressed these needs, and it gave to the members a better understanding of the problems associated with aging, as well as a chance to express their fears and realities.

A second reason for the group's success was its ability to discuss extremely pertinent topics that are considered taboo for the elderly, such as sexuality and dementia, in an accepting, non-threatening atmosphere. An unstated norm of behavior existed in the nursing home, mirroring the society at large, that prohibited an open and honest discussion of these topics (MacLean and Bonar, 1983). As Lawrence Shulman (1985) states, the mutual expressing and sharing of feelings about such topics allows group members to become in touch with their feelings and to confront them, which is necessary for continued growth and development.

Thirdly, the group composition positively affected the nature of the group's development. Gitterman (1982) suggests that in terms of composition, groups ideally require homogeneity (stability) and heterogeneity (diversity). Homogeneity refers to common background: age, sex, ethnic and religious backgrounds, comparable life experiences and also common personality capacities and capabilities. According to Gitterman, these commonalities tend to stabilize a group and help in the quick development of group identity and cohesiveness. Too much homogeneity though, can also be a problem reflected in the lack of diversity and vitality in the group. Gitterman states that groups that are overly homogeneous do not create the necessary tension for change to take place or provide the necessary models for alternate attitudes and behaviors. The "Being Old" Group with its constant core of nine people was able to fulfill both the heterogeneous and homogeneous needs for group composition, which aided the group in meeting its goals.

Another structural aspect that added beneficially to the group process was the decision by the leaders to have a time-limited group, a group formed for a specific purpose with the time length specified in advance to the members (Alissi and Casper, 1985). By choosing this type of group structure, a sense of urgency and immediacy was established within the group, which helped give it an impetus and push it forward.

The decision to have two leaders from complimentary professional disciplines also aided the group process. Since the size of the group was not predetermined, and the leaders wanted the members to have the opportunity for maximum participation, it was decided two leaders would be necessary. A given rule of thumb in group work is not to have more than seven members for one group leader. This decision worked for this group, for the few times one of the leaders was absent, the group did not run as smoothly. Having an occupational therapist and a social worker lead the group led to a more thorough and accurate discussion of the various topics, since the leaders' gerontological knowledge base was complimentary.

Perhaps the final reason this group was so successful was the type of group work approach that was used. This focused on group process and stages of group development. Issues and problems were handled by discussion and confrontation, rather than by structured tasks involving role play and learning techniques. The techniques of reflection, clarification, reminiscence and support were used. It was an effective method for working with the institutionalized elderly to develop mutual support groups and deal with some of their concerns and fears. This group work approach appears to be the most effective way of treating the elderly (Lowy, 1979; Toseland, Sherman, and Bliven, 1981).

There were two major limitations in the running of the group that need to be addressed. First of all, this type of discussion confrontation group was directed toward the highest functioning residents in the home. Thus, the leaders were directing their group membership toward a very select group of clients, whose capacity and capability to benefit from a social group work experience was enormous. The ability of this type of group experience working with other types of institutionalized elderly needs to be further explored.

The second major limitation in running the "Being Old" Group was the high drop-out rate. Only one-third of the people who attended the sessions remained as active group members. People dropped out for such reasons as ill health, prior commitments because of scheduling in the nursing home, and the inability to face the subjects being discussed. The leaders talked individually with the elderly residents who dropped out, and extended an open invitation for them to come back. However, a strong recruitment of these residents to rejoin the group was not done. Perhaps if it had been, more people would have benefited from the group experience (Carlton, 1986).

PRACTICE IN CONTEXT

Any social work practice is affected by the environment in which it practices. In terms of the "Being Old" Group, the group was strongly influenced by the agency's policies, organizational structure and philosophy, and geriatric technology. The Detroit Jewish Home for Aged was established as a non-profit nursing home to provide a full spectrum of sociomedical care to the elderly and chronically ill, which has been this facility's building block. Within this framework, all aspects of the home are guided by state and federal legislation, which place both inhibiting and promoting factors on social work practice.

The "Being Old" Group did have the agency's administrative sanction to establish this type of social group work for the residents, an important impetus for group progress. This sanction was reflected by the use of the home's board room for the group sessions. Thus, the formal organizational structure did have a crucial positive impact upon this group. And by using the informal organizational network, the leaders were able to obtain support for the group on all organizational levels and assure that group members would be available at the time of the group meetings. Thus, a clear working knowledge of the organization's formal and informal structures was imperative in order to be effective in the role of resident advocate, therapist, and mediator.

The area of technology most influencing resident care is the fairly new specialty of geriatric medicine. In addition to the specialized knowledge needed about certain medical procedures with the elderly patient and the different effects of certain drugs, a whole different doctor-patient manner and approach is needed in dealing with the geriatric patient. This understanding has to be incorporated into the nursing home's total resident care practice. Geriatric medicine is lagging behind other specialties in its knowledge base and in the number of physicians specializing in this area. This places a constraining factor on the geriatric social worker's role with the client (Green and Monahan, 1981; Solde and Manton, 1985).

Thus, there were three major contextual factors which hindered or supported the "Being Old" Group. It is within this context that the social group work experience took place. It was a successful group work experience for the nine core members who attended the group regularly. The group goals were met and a peer social support network was established among the members. If this support network will last remains to be seen. There were some limitations with the group: it only serviced and addressed the needs of a select group of nursing home residents, the highest functioning ones, and only one-third of the group remained active participants. However, the "Being Old" Group clearly demonstrates that given the opportunity, institutionalized elderly have the ability for continued learning, individual growth and development, the capacity to confront their fears constructively and to adjust to new life situations, and lastly the ability to still give and care about others.

REFERENCES

Abels, S. and Abels, P. "Social group work's contextual purposes." *Social Work with Groups*, 3(3), 1980, pp. 25-37.

Aging in the eighties. Advanced data from vital health statistics. Hyattsville, MD: National Center for Health Statistics, 1986.

Alissi, A.S. and Casper, M. "Time as a factor in group work." *Social Work with Groups*, 8(2), 1985, pp. 3-16.

Authier, J. and Gustafson, K. Group intervention techniques: A practical guide for psychiatric team members." *Journal of Psychiatric Nursing and Mental Health Services*, XIV(7), July 1976, pp. 19-22.

Boissoneau, R. and Kirshner, A.N. "The behaviorally-oriented long-term care administrator." *Journal of Long-Term Care Administrator*, 11(1), 1983, pp. 15-20.

Boling, T.E. "Growing old: Adjustments to change." *Nursing Homes*, 36(2), March/April 1987, pp. 20-23.

Burnside, I. (ed.). *Nursing and the aged*. N.Y.: McGraw-Hill, 1976.

Butler, R. and Lewis, M. *Aging and mental health*. St. Louis: Mosby, 1975.

Carlton, T.O. "Group process and group work in health social work practice." *Social Work with Groups*, 9(2), 1986, pp. 5-20.

Cohen, S.Z. and Hammerman, J. "Social work with groups." In *A social work guide for long-term care facilities*, E.M. Brody (ed.). Rockville, MD: National Institute of Mental Health, 1974.

Cormican, E.J. "Social work and aging: A review of the literature and how it is changing." *International Journal of Aging and Human Development*, 11(4), 1980, pp. 251-267.

Ebersole, P. "Group work with the aged: A survey of literature." In *Nursing and the aged*, I.M. Burnside (ed.). N.Y.: McGraw-Hill, 1976.

Epstein, A.M. et al. "The emergence of geriatric assessment units." *Annals of Internal Medicine*, 106, 1987, pp. 299-303.

Getzel, G.S. and Mellor, M.J. (eds.). "Gerontological social work practice in long-term care." *Journal of Gerontological Social Work*, 5(1/2), Fall/Winter 1982.

Gitterman, A. "The use of groups in health settings." In *Social work with groups in health settings*, A. Lurie, G. Rosenberg and S. Pinsky (eds.). N.Y.: Watson Academic Publications, Inc., 1982.

Greene, V.L. and Monahan, D.J. "Structural and operational factors affecting quality of patient care in nursing homes." *Public Policy*, 29(4), 1981, pp. 399-415.

Harris, P.B. "Being old: A confrontation group with nursing home residents." *Health and Social Work*, IV(1), Feb. 1979, pp. 153-156.

Hobson, K.G. "The effects of aging on sexuality." *Health and Social Work*, 9(1), 1984, pp. 25-35.

Horner, J. *That time of year: A chronicle of life in a nursing home*. Amherst: University of Massachusetts Press, 1982.

Huttman, E.D. *Social services for the elderly*. N.Y.: The Free Press, 1985.

Kaufman, A. "Social policy and long-term care of the aged." *Social Work*, 25(2), March 1980, pp. 133-137.

Lowy, C. *Social work with the aging: The challenge and promise of later years*. N.Y.: Harper and Row, 1979.

Lowy, L. "Social group work with vulnerable older persons: A theoretical perspective." *Social Work with Groups*, 5(2), 1982, pp. 21-32.

MacLean, M.J. and R. Bonar. "The Normalization Principle and the Institutionalized Elderly." *Canada's Mental Health*, 31(2), 1983, pp. 16-18.

Newgarten, B.L. "Psychological aspects of aging and illness." *Psychosomatics*, 25(2), 1984, pp. 123-125.

Novick, L.J. "The function of the social worker in the long-term hospital." *Long-Term Care and Health Services Administrations Quarterly*, III(3), 1979, pp. 181-193.

Nursing home law handbook. Los Angeles: National Senior Citizens Law Center, 1975.

Palmore, E. "The future status of the aged." *The Gerontologist*, 16, 1976.

Peterson, K.J. "Changing needs of patients and families in long-term care facilities: Implications for social work practice." *Social Work in Health Care*, 12(2), Winter 1986, pp. 37-49.

Pfeiffer, E. *OARS multidimensional functional assessment questionnaire*. Durham, N.C.: Duke University Center for the Study of Aging and Human Development, Older Americans Resources and Services Program, 1975.

Pincus, A. "Reminiscence in aging and its implications for social work practice." *Social Work*, XV, July 1970, pp. 47-53.

Scharlach, A.E. "Social group work with institutionalized elders: A task-centered approach." *Social Work with Groups*, 8(3), 1985, pp. 33-47.

Schulman, L. "The dynamics of mutual aid." *Social Work with Groups*, 8(4), 1985, pp. 51-59.

_____. *The skills of helping: Individuals and groups*. Itasca, Ill.: F.E. Peacock Publishers, 1979.

Schwartz, W. and Zalba, S.R. (eds.). *The practice of group work*. N.Y.: Columbia University Press, 1971.

Silverstone, B. and Hyman, H.K. *You and your aging parent: The modern family's guide to emotional, physical and financial problems*. N.Y.: Pantheon, 1976.

Simons, R.L. and West, G.E. "Life changes, coping resources, and health among the elderly." *International Journal of Aging and Human Development*, 20(3), 1984-1985, pp. 173-189.

Soldo, B.J. and Manton, K.G. "Health status and service needs of the oldest old: Current patterns and future trends." *Milbank Memorial Fund Quarterly*, 63(2), 1985, pp. 287-317.

Sperbeck, D.J. and Whitbourne, S.K. "Dependency in the institutional setting: A behavioral training program for geriatric staff." *The Gerontologist*, 21(3), 1981, pp. 268-275.

Spitz, II.I. "Contemporary trends in group psychotherapy: A literature survey." *Hospital and Community Psychiatry*, 35(2), 1984, pp. 132-142.

Suzman, R. and Riley, M.W. (eds.). "The oldest old." *Milbank Memorial Fund Quarterly*, 63(2), Spring 1985 (entire issue).

Toseland, R., Sherman, E. and Blivin, S. "The comparative effectiveness of two group work approaches for development of mutual support groups among the elderly." *Social Work with Groups*, 4, Spring/Summer, 1981, pp. 137-153.

U.S. Department of Health and Human Services, Health Care Financing Administration. *Long-term care: Background and future directions*. Washington, D.C.: U.S. Printing Office, 1981.

Wasser, E. "Family casework focus on the older person." *Social Casework*, XLVII, July 1966, pp. 423-431.

Weiner, M. "Group treatment with the aged." *Journal of Jewish Communal Service*, 62(4), 1986, pp. 307-317.

Wells, L.M. and Singer, C.A. "A model for linking networks in social work practice with the institutionalized elderly." *Social Work*, 30(4), 1985, pp. 318-322.

Wetzel, J.W. "Interventions with the depressed elderly in institutions." *Social Casework* LXI(4), 1980, pp. 234-239.

Yalom, I.D. *The theory and practice of group psychotherapy*, 3rd ed. N.Y.: Basic Books, Inc., 1985.

Alzheimer's Disease: Intervention in a Nursing Home Environment

Susan O. Mercer
Betsy Robinson

Alzheimer's disease (AD) is a progressive, relentless dementia characterized by cognitive impairment, disorientation, personality changes, and, ultimately, death (Kerson, 1985). It is rapidly becoming one of the nation's most heart-rending and expensive diseases. It afflicts an estimated 2.5 million Americans, it causes 150,000 deaths annually, and is the fourth leading cause of death (Thornton, Davies, and Tinklenberg, 1986). It usually strikes persons over age 65 and, as the proportion of older Americans rises, the absolute number of AD patients will increase. The annual U.S. bill for the disease is estimated to be greater than $20 billion (Stipp, 1987).

There are only hypotheses, including the possibility of a genetic factor, as to the cause, and there are no known cures (Forsythe, 1987; Heyman et al., 1983). Ante-mortem diagnosis is an exclusionary process. That is, a complete neurological, physical, and psychiatric evaluation should rule out other conditions associated with dementia. A detailed social and medical history will help reveal whether there has been an insidious onset and gradual progression of symptoms which suggests AD (Dahl, 1983; Wells, 1984).

There are stages and phases of AD. The disease typically begins with memory loss, mistakes in judgment, and affect changes. The person may lose car keys, leave the stove on, and generally appear absent-minded. As the dementia progresses all the senses are affected. If the person lives long enough, complete disorientation will occur, in addition to night restlessness, increased aphasia, failure to recognize family, general loss of socially acceptable behaviors, and perseveration. Eventually, the symptoms progress to a point where the person is bedridden, incontinent, unresponsive, and mute. The progression of the disease may take from 2 to 14 years or more. Eventually the person requires total nursing care within an institution (Kerson, 1985).

DESCRIPTION OF THE SETTING

The case intervention occurred with a resident placed at Riley's Oak Hill Manor South in Little Rock, Arkansas. Riley's South is a 224-bed skilled care nursing home serving (primarily) the elderly residents of the state. It is a private-pay, for-profit, modern facility. Riley's can accommodate the ambulatory resident who needs regular medication and minimum supervision as well as the resident requiring intensive care. The one-level facility is nine years old, 63,000 square feet in area, and purpose built.

In the minimum care wing, residents require little supervision, may bring their own furniture and may come and go as they please. The intermediate and skilled care wings provide a more structured environment. There are four intensive care beds for residents who must be monitored 24 hours a day or require intravenous feeding, five furnished patios for visiting and outside activities, and three large day rooms for activities, meals, and socialization. A large central dining room serves cafeteria-style meals, and is also used for activities. There is a large, well-equipped physical therapy room, and an arts and crafts center where residents can pursue ceramics, painting, and woodworking. One section of the yard is fenced to provide a safe "wandering" space for residents.

The facility is centrally and conveniently located in the state and community. It is within five minutes of the four major hospitals and medical centers, and yet is at the end of a private cul-de-sac, surrounded by piney woods.

The average age of the resident population is 80, with the ages ranging from 28 to 100. Eighty-three percent are women. About 40% of the residents experience dementia and confusion with a variety of diagnoses and etiology. The average length of stay is one year which is considerably lower than the national average. Approximately 62% of the discharged residents are discharged alive. Many residents and families take advantage of the respite care and short-stay options.

Policy

The home is regulated and licensed as a skilled care facility by the Arkansas Office on Long Term Care. Since it is private pay, there are no federal or state monies involved. The home's policies are established by the Governing Board, the President of the corporation, the Director of Operations, and the Administrator.

The social work profession has always played an important role in the policies and practices of the home. The standards of excellence go well beyond federal and state requirements. Since its inception the facility has had a full-time Masters level social worker as well as a consultant with a Doctor of Social Work degree. The MSW was recently promoted to the Administrator's position and a new MSW was hired. The home has also routinely provided a field placement and supervision for two first year MSW students. Riley's is unique in the state for the quality and quantity of professional social workers. We are not too humble to tout the "social work power," and believe the social work presence has made a positive difference in the level of care and quality of life for the residents, families, and staff.

The admissions policy does not discriminate on the basis of sex, race, religion, or ethnic background. The home may refuse admission to persons who are currently abusing alcohol or drugs, anyone under age 18, persons who are actively psychotic, have a known communicable disease, require a respirator, or require a liquid narcotic administered through an IV. The administrator and social worker reserve the right to evaluate each applicant on an individual basis.

The resident's rights are strictly adhered to, and the resident and family are provided a copy of the bill of rights upon admission. Staff are trained and involved in the implementation of the policies and procedures. Living wills are available for the resident to discuss and complete with her family and physician. Upon request from the resident, the facility will maintain a confidential file for this advance directive.

The admissions packet is detailed and outlines all the services and conditions of the facility. The home provides medical nursing, pharmacy, nutritional/dietary, housekeeping/laundry, beauty shop, recreational/activity, religious, and social work services. Dental, occupational therapy, speech pathology, and physical therapy services are available on a contract basis.

Riley's, Inc., the parent corporation, also owns a nursing home in North Little Rock which participates in third party payment. The corporation also owns a retirement center adjacent to Riley's South Nursing home. Retirement center residents are provided short-term care at the nursing home as needed.

TECHNOLOGY

Technology can be addressed in a variety of ways. There is technology related to mechanical, structural, and architectural advances. The facility is responsive to whatever the physician requests in terms of special devices or beds. For example, there are clinatron beds which aid in recovery from decubitus and, for stroke patients who no longer have "internal thermometers" operating, a machine which monitors internal body temperature and adjusts a cooling pad accordingly.

There is a computer at the facility which is linked to the computers in the corporate office. Medications, physicians orders, admission and discharge documentation, care plans, and social histories are among the records stored.

The home is open to advances in how to best manage residents with Alzheimer's Disease. This includes indoor and outside free "wandering" space, the need for increased exercise, and minimal physical restraints. The facility is exploring the feasibility of developing a specialized Alzheimer's wing (Peppard, 1985). The Activity Director has special expertise in working with the visually impaired, and these skills are particularly utilized during resident orientation. The staff have regular in-service training sessions which are led by full time supervisory staff as well as by consultants.

Technology can also be measured by the facility's responsiveness to knowledge advances in geriatrics and gerontology. Riley's gets a high rating here also. The home is affiliated with the Graduate School of Social Work, University of Arkansas at Little Rock, the Geriatrics Department and the School of Nursing of the University of Arkansas Medical Sciences Campus, and the GRECC unit of the Veterans's Administration Medical Center. The Pharmacology consultant specializes in geriatrics and is affiliated with the Department of Pharmacy at the University Medical Center. Nursing students from the various University programs also rotate through the facility for training. The facility has permitted carefully monitored research projects to be completed. For example, the senior author obtained an Arkansas Endowment for the Humanities grant to fund a twelve month poetry writing project. A recent interdisciplinary study (by the senior author and nurse colleagues) examined the results of a cognitive skills remediation training program on Alzheimer's disease residents (Beck, Heacock, Mercer, & Thatcher, 1988). The residents and staff benefit from such projects through exposure to technical expertise, model interventions, and community visibility. Riley's philosophy is "resident first care," and administration places resources and actions behind the slogan.

ORGANIZATION

The Administrator, an LCSW, has the overall responsibility for the operations of the home. The social worker, director of nursing, medical records supervisor, and dietary manager all report directly to her. The Assistant Administrator reports directly to the administrator and has housekeeping/laundry and the maintenance supervisor under her direction. There are four RNs, sixteen LPNs, and forty eight nurse's aides, all of whom are under the supervision of the Nursing Director.

The Master's level Social Worker handles all admissions and coordinates room assignments and internal reassignments or reclassification of levels of resident care and payment rates. She completes all social histories on residents and is responsible for planning social work intervention with residents and families. She also coordinates the interdisciplinary care plan committee and is responsible for keeping the policy and admission manual updated. She coordinates the work of the Activity Director and her assistant (both are full time). The activity personnel plan and supervise daily activities which include exercise classes, cultural events, shopping activities, arts and crafts, book rentals, special events/parties, and so forth. The activity director also coordinates the resident council and the monthly publication of resident events and news.

The administrative and supervisory staff has been stable and experienced little turnover since the home's inception. This continuity contributes to an informal aspect of organization which makes for comfortable and trusting relationships, minimal bureaucracy, and easy, frequently quick, decision-making.

Case Description:
Client Profile, Social History, and Assessment

Emma Brown is a well-dressed, white female who looks younger than her eighty years. She is generally alert, but is frequently confused. She sometimes exhibits agitation and suspiciousness, but is generally pleasant and cooperative. Immediate family live nearby and include her sister, Mary Jones, and her niece, Mrs. Jones' daughter, Sarah. Mrs. Brown also has a step-daughter and two step-sons who live ninety miles away. They write and send gifts but do not visit.

Mrs. Brown was admitted to Riley's in the fall of 1986, following hospitalization for a broken clavicle suffered in a motor vehicle accident. She was en route to visit her sister who was in the hospital following a CVA. Details of the accident are sketchy. She was driving alone, apparently became confused and lost, and was in a "trance-like daze" when her car struck another vehicle.

Following extensive testing, she was diagnosed with Alzheimer's Disease. Her history reflects that she had an active, healthy life. Surgeries included a hysterectomy and, most recently, cataract removal. She smoked for fifteen years but quit in 1958. Her alcohol intake was minimal. She was treated for anemia and a resulting peptic disease four years ago. There is no evidence of hypertension, cardiovascular or central nervous system impairment.

A detailed social history revealed that memory loss predated the car accident. In the late spring, 1986, she relocated to an apartment complex for the elderly because of forgetfulness and mild confusion. She felt the move would help her cope and provide additional security. However, she soon became unable to find her sister's home or other familiar places. Instead of helping, the move seemed to exacerbate her memory impairment.

Mrs. Brown was discharged from the hospital at the same time as her sister Mary was released for post-CVA recuperation. They were placed together at Riley's in the minimal care unit. Her sister recovered well and was discharged in 2 months. Emma, on the other hand, remained confused and began to wander, particularly at night. She spoke frequently of having to go home, and her wandering seemed to focus around this theme. During her night wandering, Emma supposedly began to fall. The staff would find her sitting on the floor unable to tell them what had happened. The sister and niece felt Emma's problems were a result of the difficulty of being alone in the nursing home. In November, 1986, Emma was relocated to her sister's home.

Unfortunately this change did not alter the wandering or the forgetfulness. Emma's behavior became quite disruptive and unmanageable for her sister. She rummaged through drawers and closets, searching for mysterious, lost items. Her sister's frustration was heightened when she began to hoard and scatter clothes as well. Following a brief hospitalization for a severe rash, Emma was readmitted to Riley's nursing home in December, 1986, for long term, intermediate level nursing care.

Emma Brown was the second born of two daughters. After graduation from high school, she went to work as a bank clerk. In her mid-twenties she married and moved to California with her husband, a vaudeville performer. They divorced after a stormy 3 year marriage. She returned to Arkansas to live with her parents, and went to work as a secretary in a public school. Soon after her parents' deaths in 1957 she married a widower who had three children. They had a satisfactory marriage prior to his death in 1963. She returned to work until her retirement in 1971 at age sixty-five. Church work, family, and friends remained important to her.

The initial evaluation upon re-admission to Riley's revealed symptoms consistent with the early stages of Alzheimer's Disease.

Although the family had been given the diagnosis, little information had been provided and few attempts had been made to discuss with them her poor prognosis and the inevitable progressive decline. Emma was alert and ambulatory, with some insight intact. She had the ability to hide her cognitive impairments through a social facade. In fact, there was marked confusion, time and spatial disorientation, frequent periods of anxiety and agitation, and occasional paranoia regarding the staff.

Activity staff reported inconsistent participation levels, largely due to her inability to remember when and where activities took place. She exhibited increased wandering and agitation at night, a condition commonly referred to as sundowning (Powell, 1983). She suffered occasional night-time incontinence. Her affect appeared sad and hinted of her continual frustration of feeling lost and needing to "go home." She rummaged through her closet and drawers as well as those of her roommate. She was completely unable to find her way to her room or other relevant locations in the facility. She was often found to be sitting and blankly staring off in space, and would inappropriately respond to staff initiatives (Toseland, Derico and Owen, 1984).

Emma's family visited weekly. Their primary concerns centered on her reports of items being stolen and other "tales" she would recount about strange people, peculiar activities, and unusual demands placed on her. They said that their visits with Emma were not "satisfactory." They seemed unsure and uncomfortable in relating to her and her changing mental status.

Three assessment scales were administered. The Mini-Mental State or MMS (Folstein, Folstein, and McHugh, 1975) revealed a score of 20 out of a possible 30. She scored lowest in the areas of orientation and recall, and scored average in registration, attention, and calculation. She did well on questions dealing with language. The Beck Depression Inventory (Beck, Ward, Mendelson, Mock, and Erbaugh, 1961) revealed only mild depression with a score of 10. The areas of concern noted were feelings of disappointment, punishment, self-blame, level of irritation, decision-making, appearance, and interest in sex. An evaluation of her performance on Activities of Daily Living (Katz, Ford, Moskowitz, Jackson, and Jaffee, 1963) revealed independence in all but bathing, dressing, and continence. Difficulty in these areas stemmed from the need for assistance in focusing her activities, making decisions, remembering instructions, and other relevant facts surrounding the activity.

Because of Emma's verbal accessibility and her reasonably high MMS, she was assessed as a good candidate for social work interventions (Berman, 1984). Generally, these were designed to alleviate the behavioral problems associated with the early stages of Alzheimer's Disease, and the specific problems noted in ADL activities.

Goals and Treatment Modality

The treatment approach was eclectic. It included strategies from crisis intervention (with family and staff), basic problem solving, and behavioral techniques such as modeling and the principle of successive approximation or reinforcing successive steps to the final desired behavior.

A primary goal for Emma was reducing her anxiety and the resulting wandering, rummaging, and suspiciousness. Frequent, routine contacts with the social worker were established during the day. Sessions were kept brief and focused, with little decision-making required of her. Reassurance of continued care and praise for her intact, positive attributes were a major theme in all contacts. A daily log was maintained to systematically observe and record the timing and events surrounding her anxiety. Definite patterns were observed. For example, she had increased confusion and agitation following time spent trying to converse with more severely confused and disoriented residents. Her wandering behavior increased when she had to urinate, and she had heightened confusion and fear following an episode of nighttime incontinence. Her fear increased when more than one staff member approached her at once, and her confusion increased during periods of high noise levels.

Staff were instructed regarding the effects of the situations described above and were assisted in specific ways they could work to prevent such accidents. When such episodes occurred, Emma was taken out of the area and her attention was diverted in various ways. Once she attended a music concert in the activity area. Snack breaks and escorted walks outside were also helpful. The social worker used reality orientation (Kohut, Kohut, and Fleishman, 1983) and reminiscence techniques (Cook, 1984) to lessen her agitation and stimulate cognitive functioning. Care was taken to listen closely to the content of her conversation and make verbal connections with her whenever possible.

The second major goal was increasing her ability to perform selected activities of daily living, including dressing herself, and being able to find her room. Signs were made noting where to find particular pieces of clothing. The steps necessary to appropriate dressing were outlined on a poster along with corresponding pictures. Care was taken to use language and incorporate preferences familiar to her. Clothes were inventoried and placed in groups. This was redone as Emma's rummaging necessitated. The social worker was present each morning as Emma dressed to note problems, progress, and provide continued reassurance. Her progress was rewarded with verbal reinforcement, snacks, and afternoon walks. It became evident that part of Emma's difficulty in dressing was due to the type and amount of clothing she had. Her niece assisted by removing duplicate items and clothing that was too difficult to fasten. All remaining outfits were clustered so that choosing one hanger would eliminate further decision-making.

To enable Emma to find her room, a technique called backward chaining was used (Harrell, Smith, Piroch, and Goldstein, 1980). Emma's family made a wreath for her room door that included blue ribbons, her favorite color. Emma and the social worker spent two days talking about and admiring the wreath to establish that it would serve the purpose of distinguishing her room for her. Following this, she was worked backwards from her room to other major areas in the building. As Emma was able to consistently find her room from one location, the same process was attempted from further away. Repeated focus was placed on landmarks along the route in order to help her encode and recall. The landmarks were chosen according to her particular memory capabilities, i.e., colors and objects were easier to retain and locate than numbers or letters. In one instance, a landmark was created by placing a blue arrow on one wall to indicate the direction she should take.

The third and final major goal regarded Emma's family; specifically, increasing their knowledge and awareness of Alzheimer's

Disease, suggesting ways to make their visits more rewarding, and dealing with their feelings around the diagnosis (Chenoweth and Spencer, 1986; Marples, 1986; Kerson, 1985). They were asked to come to the facility on set days each week, and to permit the social worker to be with them during their visit with Emma. In addition, the niece, Sarah, was counseled individually by the social worker. She was given copies of *The 36 Hour Day* (Mace and Rabins, 1981) and *Managing the Person with Intellectual Loss at Home* (McDowell, 1980) to read and discuss. She and her mother were made aware of specific ways in which their behaviors may exacerbate Emma's anxiety. Through modeling and counseling they were taught to defuse Emma's agitation over "tales" by responding to her feelings and the parts of her conversation that were reality based. It was important that they respond to her but not become frustrated themselves and compound the problem by asking for details of stories and events that were largely unreal and delusions. Since they were involved in some of the interventions, they felt a part of the process. One of the most difficult tasks for the family was to lower their expectation of Emma, and to allow her to be "different" than they had known her. They had to let the old Emma go in order to make contact with the new Emma. In particular, they had to accept that she could no longer handle dressing in the more sophisticated style of clothing she had previously worn. They had to modify their image of her to accommodate her needs and abilities. This meant modifying the places they took her on outings from the nursing home (Shibbal-Champagne and Lipinska-Stachow, 1986).

Contract and Time Period

The interventions took place over an eight week period. Because of the nature of the facility and the particular case goals, sessions took place where and when they were deemed appropriate. Contacts were made in Emma's room, the day area, the social worker's office, or other sites depending on the purpose of the encounter. Emma was seen at regular times throughout each day to establish a predictable routine. The intervention goals were explained to her and accepted. Emma's family, particularly her niece, was asked to commit to regular sessions during this time to facilitate goal achievement. The primary care-providing staff were consulted at weekly intervals to record observances, note progress and problems, and recruit their assistance in meeting goals.

Stance of the Social Worker

Emma and her family were open to interventions. The frustration level of each was high, and they were motivated to participate in "anything" that might prove helpful. Strategies were planned from broad to specific. It was their level of frustration that dictated, at least initially, my stance in this case. I began by presenting myself as a primary means of support, and it was necessary to come back to this supportive role frequently. Because of Emma's confusion and cognitive impairment, I was firm and direct in guiding her, careful to be specific, simple, and concrete in my requests, and always positive and complimentary. The niece and sister's lack of knowledge regarding Alzheimer's Disease required direct and straightforward education. As their reluctance to allow her a "different" image became apparent, I had to become increasingly firm and at times gently confrontative in sessions with them.

Lowering the family's anxiety while giving them more information and support was chosen as a goal because of its importance in decreasing Emma's anxiety and providing her with positive, life enhancing supports. Furthermore, a knowledgeable and supported family had fewer negative interactions with staff over misunderstood and unexpected events. Likewise, I targeted on decreasing Emma's anxiety so that she would more readily accept and succeed at other goals. It was important to use Emma's strengths to the best advantage. Since her language and appearance were reasonably intact, these became central components to the overall intervention. It was important to remain flexible. A sense of humor also helped cut through some of the more painful moments (Cole, Griffin and Ruiz, 1985).

Case Conclusion and Reassessment

It was no surprise to observe Emma becoming dependent on the support and attentions of the social worker. Each morning she would wait anxiously for my arrival to her room for our "lessons."

These lessons, as she referred to them, initially seemed to generate a fear of failure or of appearing "crazy." The consistency and trust established within the relationship as well as her own satisfaction at the increasing number of successful attempts at dressing herself with the resulting positive rewards served to allay these fears. Though Emma is still not totally independent in dressing, she does average three days a week in which she is able to manage her own dressing unassisted. Staff is conscientious in complimenting her on her actions. Her frustration about inability to do things is no longer a daily occurrence; she now refers to "having some problems from time to time." Overall, she expressed pleasure and enjoyment at the strategies.

Recently Emma's roommate began to chatter incoherently during the session. Emma turned to her and remarked, "Please be quiet, we are working on my lessons and they are important." On another occasion, Emma's sister and niece were present in the room as the groupings of clothes on a hanger were explained. The sister was confused about the activity. After her sister asked the same question for the third time, Emma remarked, "If you can't understand any better than that, maybe you should get lessons, too."

Sarah, who was the primary caregiver to her mother in addition to seeing after Emma's needs, responded well also. She not only gained much in the way of information and support, but was able to learn more effective ways of interacting with her aunt. As a result, she did not become overly concerned with Emma's confused stories and was able to defuse potentially catastrophic situations. This made her visits with Emma more enjoyable and she no longer confronted the staff about allegedly stolen items. She has also gained skills to help her with her mother who exhibits periods of marked confusion. The efficacy of the interventions is most clearly seen in her relaxed demeanor, her verbal expressions of satisfaction with Emma, herself and the facility, and the fact that the weekly number of visits to Emma have doubled (Pratt et al., 1985).

Emma is now able to find her room successfully from the hallway in all but a few instances. She still has difficulty on occasion finding the correct hallway and frequently becomes lost when venturing past the day area of her wing. She has been able to retain the knowledge that the various landmarks we have chosen along the way will help her, but is unable at times to find them.

Emma still wanders at night but significantly less often. She continues to be anxious at times but is easily diverted to more pleasant encounters. The social worker and staff continue to sort out the reality-based pieces of her conversation and this technique appears to lessen her anxiety and confusion. It was evident that careful attention to her loose verbal associations or seemingly nonsensical words would often point to an opportunity to connect to her intact parts. For example, "a crispy piece" was her way of asking for a Nestle's crunch bar. Reminiscence about her gardening efforts led her to a discussion of "erps." Through imagination, effort, and pictures it was eventually determined that she was referring to Burpee's seedless cucumbers.

Emma is not "cured," but the specific goals were achieved. Progressive deterioration is unfortunately inevitable. The social worker's support and efforts will continue and even increase as time brings further decline. New goals and strategies will be developed. It is possible that future interventions will include group contact for socialization and additional reality orientation. As her dementia progresses, her family will need even greater support and assistance.

Differential Discussion

Despite the poor prognosis associated with Alzheimer's Disease, intervention is still a viable option to practitioners (U.S. Congress 1984). As with the case described, basic education and support along with careful attention and mapping of the resident's behavior and needs produced almost immediate benefits to all involved. Too many times we seem reluctant to discuss the particulars of Alzheimer's Disease and its devastating diagnosis. That reluctance extends to physicians as well. The devastation of the disease can be offset for residents and families by active intervention to prolong and celebrate the intact functioning in addition to creating concrete strategies to reach new levels. In other words, be the eternal optimist.

Consistency is important in any intervention. To accomplish this, cooperation among the entire staff, including all shifts, is necessary. Although efforts to consult, educate, and support staff were helpful in reaching the goals, there was still evidence of inconsistencies between different staff members and different shifts. For example, the grouping of clothing needed consistent follow-through from staff in nursing, housekeeping, and laundry. This was difficult to achieve and required considerable time. In retrospect, a more thorough way to ensure this consistency would have been to schedule facility-wide inservice training to explain, model and support the strategies.

Staff approaches were sometimes counter to the interventions. On several occasions, wandering behavior was handled as a crisis in which all available staff rushed to stop and lead her back to safety. It is clear that a standardized policy regarding wandering and catastrophic reactions needs to be in place. All residents and staff would benefit from such a policy protocol, which would be reinforced through frequent training sessions.

Although the design of the nursing home follows the current architectural model for long term care facilities, the wings made Emma's attempts to find her room more difficult. There are two clusters of symmetrical wings at either end of the building. Once the correct wing is located, four identical hallways extend from the nursing station like spokes on a wheel. The halls are labeled with a letter on one wall but it can only be seen from one angle. Like Emma, many residents have lost the capacity to read or interpret the letter. The physical environment plays an important part in assisting with resident orientation. In any facility, the environment should be examined closely as to whether it supports or hinders the programs. The use of wall color or colored lines on the floor, for example, would be helpful in delineating the wings and halls.

A deliberate effort was made to include the family in goal setting and intervention strategies. This was important for their well-being as well as for the achievement of the goals. As is often the case, Emma's family felt guilty about placing her in the facility. Some of their initial efforts to be helpful and show concern only served to complicate Emma's life and behavior. I used their feelings and energy and focused them in ways that would be more beneficial. In retrospect, I could have involved them further. For example, they could have done any necessary re-grouping of clothing. Even though they did sit in on many of the reminiscence sessions, more would have been helpful; The opportunities for modeling would have thereby increased. Participation in a family group and the statewide Alzheimer's organization could have added to their support, understanding, and involvement; (Wasow, 1986; Simank and Strickland, 1985).

Inadvertently, the interventions to help Emma dress independently probably caused some additional stress. For example, in spite of her desire to please, she let it be known that the first printed signs were too complicated because they still required too many decisions. The independent dressing strategy had to be modified twice to accommodate her abilities. In order to prevent unnecessary pressure, more time should have been spent exploring what her ability level was prior to any intervention.

Emma's dementia has already had a profound effect on her and her family. Assuming she lives long enough, she will reach the unresponsive, mute stage of Alzheimer's Disease. But that is not the point of the story. Despite the poor prognosis, some well considered interventions targeting specific behaviors and concerns can ease the burden and improve the quality of life. Such interventions must be based on a thorough assessment of the problem, its context, and identifiable patterns. Emma was assisted in maintaining some of her intact parts. She has an advocate, a listener, and someone to remain in dialogue with her. She is not left alone in her confusion and anxiety.

PRACTICE IN CONTEXT

Nursing homes are a diverse grouping of institutions which share the fact that they are designed for caring for the older person and are subsequently licensed. Being diverse, they vary on a continuum from adequacy (or excellence) to inadequacy. They basically operate on a medical model, and this model defines much of the care priorities and practice. Unfortunately, there is a dearth of professional social workers in long term care facilities, even though few would deny the relevance or need.

All institutions are governed by policies, organizational structure, technology, and philosophy of care. Riley's South is no exception, yet it is not your typical nursing home for many reasons previously stated. The facility is a first class operation, but the large number of residents presents a different practice constraint. The private, for-profit status affords many additional resources but also serves to narrow the extent of social work practice at times. It exists because it generates income. That is, admissions will take precedence in a for-profit arena. And yet having a full time professional social worker direct admissions and manage casework, an administrator who is also an MSW, and a social work consultant are all indications of the facility's commitment to attending to the psychosocial needs of the residents and families.

Policy affects practice, but the inverse is also true. The analysis of the case described herein is leading to two changes within the facility: a standardized policy regarding dealing with wandering and catastrophic reactions, and a change in identification of the wings and hallways to better accommodate the confused residents. Thus a practice intervention has led to a policy change. The process is circular, dynamic, as it should be.

REFERENCES

Aronson, M. D., G. Levin and R. Lipkowitz. "A Community-Based Family/Patient Group Program for Alzheimer's Disease." *Gerontologist* 24:4 (1984): 339-342.

Beck, A. T. et al. "An Inventory for Measuring Depression." *Archives of General Psychiatry* 4 (1961): 53-63.

Beck, C. et al. "The Impact of Cognitive Skills Remediation Training with Alzheimer's Disease Patients." *Journal of Geriatric Psychiatry* (Spring 1988 publication).

Beck, J. C. et al. "Dementia in the Elderly: The Silent Epidemic" (Clinical Conference). *Annals of Internal Medicine* 97:2 (April 1982): 231-234.

Berman, S. and M. B. Rappaport. "Social Work and Alzheimer's Disease: Psychosocial Management in the Absence of Medical Cure." *Social Work in Health Care* 10:2 (Winter 1984): 53-71.

Chenoweth, B. and B. Spencer. "Dementia: The Experience of Family Caregivers." *Gerontologist* 26:3 (1986): 267-272.

Cole, L., K. Griffin and B. Ruiz. "A Comprehensive Approach to Working with Families of Alzheimer's Patients." *Journal of Gerontological Social Work* 9:2, 27-39.

Cook, J. B. "Reminiscing: How It Can Help Confused Nursing Home Residents." *Social Casework* (Feb. 1984): 90-94.

Dahl, D. "Diagnosis of Alzheimer's Disease." *Postgraduate Medicine* 73:4 (April 1983): 217-221.

Eisdorfer, C. and D. Cohen. "Management of the Patient and Family Coping with Dementing Illness." *The Journal of Family Practice* 12:5, 831-837.

Folstein, M. F., S. E. Folstein and P. R. McHugh. "Mini-Mental State: A Practical Method for Grading the Cognitive State of Patients." *Journal of Psychiatric Research* 12 (1975): 189-198.

Forsythe, J. "Alzheimer's and Down's Syndrome: A Genetic Link." *Psychology Today* 20:9 (March 1986): 9.

George, L. K. and L. P. Gwyther. "Caregiver Well-Being: A Multi-Dimensional Examination of Family Caregivers of Demented Adults." *Gerontologist* 26:3 (1986): 253-259.

Harrell, T. et al. *ADL: Level II.* Dept. of Aging and Mental Health, Florida Mental Health Institute, University of South Florida, 1980.

Heyman, A. et al. "Alzheimer's Disease: Genetic Aspects and Associated Clinical Disorders." *Annals of Neurology* 14:5 (1983): 507-515.

Katz, S. et al. "Studies of Illness in the Aged: The Index of ADL, A Standardized Measure of Biological and Psychosocial Function." *Journal of the American Medical Association* 185 (1963): 94.

Kerson, T. S. "The Dementias." In *Understanding Chronic Illness*, pp. 71-103. Edited by T. S. Kerson with L. A. Kerson. New York: The Free Press, 1985.

Kohut, S., J. J. Kohut and J. J. Fleishman. *Reality Orientation for the Elderly*, 2nd ed. Oradell, N.J.: Medical Economics Company, 1983.

Mace, N. L. and P. V. Rabins. *The 36-Hour Day.* Baltimore and London: The Johns Hopkins University Press, 1981.

McDowell, F. H. (ed.). *Managing the Person with Intellectual Impairment at Home.* White Plains, N.Y.: The Burke Rehabilitation Center, 1980.

Marples, Margot. "Helping Family Members Cope with a Senile Relative." *Social Casework* 67:8, 490-498.

Peppard, Nancy R. "Special Nursing Units for Residents with Primary Degenerative Dementia: Alzheimer's Disease." *Journal of Gerontological Social Work* 9:2 (1985): 5-13.

Powell, L. S. and K. Courtice. *Alzheimer's Disease: A Guide for Families.* Reading, MA: Addison-Wesley Publishing Company, 1983.

Pratt, C. et al. "Burden and Coping Strategies of Caregivers to Alzheimer's Patients." *Family Relations*, 34, 27-33.

Reizberg, B. (ed.). *Alzheimer's Disease: The Standard Reference.* N.Y.: The Free Press, 1984.

Schmidt, G. L. and B. Keyes. "Group Psychotherapy with Family Caregivers of Demented Patients." *Gerontologist* 25 (Aug. 1985): 347-350.

Shibbal-Champagne, S. and D. M. Lipinska-Stachon. "Alzheimer's Education/ Support Group: Considerations of Family Tasks, Pre-Planning, and Active

Professional Facilitation." *Journal of Gerontological Social Work* 9:2 (1986): 41-48.

Simank, M. H. and K. J. Strickland. "Assisting Families in Coping with Alzheimer's Disease and Other Related Dementias with the Establishment of a Mutual Support Group. *Journal of Gerontological Social Work* 9:2 (1985): 49-58.

Snyder, B. and K. Keefe. "The Unmet Needs of Family Caregivers for Frail and Disabled Adults." *Social Work in Health Care* 10:3 (Spring 1985): 1-14.

Spencer, D. L. and D. B. Miller. "Family Respite for the Elderly Alzheimer's Patient." *Journal of Gerontological Social Work* 9:2 (1986): 101-112.

Stipp, D. "New Findings about Alzheimer's May Offer Insights into Its Cause," *The Wall Street Journal*, Feb. 23, 1987.

Thornton, J. E., H. D. Davies, and J. R. Tinklenberg. "Alzheimer's Disease Syndrome." *Journal of Psychosocial Nursing* 24 (1986): 16-22.

Toseland, R. W., A. Derico and M. L. Owen. "Alzheimer's Disease and Related Disorders: Assessment and Intervention." *Health and Social Work* 9:3 (Summer 1984): 212-215.

U.S. Congress, Subcommittee on Investigations and Oversight, Committee on Science and Technology, House of Representatives. *Alzheimer's Disease*, 1985. 98th Congress, Second Session, December 1984. Washington, D.C. U.S. Printing Office.

Wasow, M. "Support Groups for Family Caregivers of Patients with Alzheimer's Disease." *Social Work* 31:2 (March/April 1986): 93-97.

Williams, L. "Alzheimer's: The Need for Caring." *Journal of Gerontological Nursing* 12 (1986): 12-29.

Zarit, S. H., N. K. Orr and J. M. Zarit. *The Hidden Victims of Alzheimer's Disease: Families under Stress*. N.Y.: University Press, 1985.

Hospital Based Case Management for the Frail Elderly

Renee Weisman Michelsen

DESCRIPTION OF THE SETTING

Morristown Memorial Hospital is a voluntary, non-profit teaching hospital in Morristown, New Jersey. It consists of two divisions, a 541 bed acute care hospital and a 78 bed facility specializing in short-term skilled nursing and rehabilitation. The acute care facility serves as a medical and surgical regional referral center. Morristown Memorial Hospital is located in middle- to upper-middle-class suburban Morris County, however the patients served represent a variety of income levels. Morris is among four New Jersey counties with the highest percentage of residents age 75 and older.

Morristown Memorial Hospital was selected by The Robert Wood Johnson Foundation as one of 23 sites nationwide, to participate in the Hospital Initiatives in Long-Term Care project. The receipt of this grant established The Center for Geriatric Care in January, 1984. The purpose of the grant to encourage hospitals to shift from their traditional stance of focusing on acute care, toward establishing a continuum of care that includes the long term care needs of the increasing elderly population. Long term care refers to the combination of health and social services that are provided in a variety of institutional and noninstitutional settings, including the home, over an extended period of time to functionally impaired, chronically ill persons (Pollack, 1979). The Hospital Initiatives in Long-Term Care Program is designed to address the hospital's role in maintaining the frail elderly in the community.

The Center for Geriatric Care extends the spectrum of services the hospital offers to the elderly. The Center provides an outpatient multidisciplinary (MD, MSN, and MSW) Comprehensive Assessment to evaluate and diagnose the elderly patient as well as counsel the family on long term care planning; an inpatient geriatric evaluation team to help improve acute care; case management to plan, coordinate and monitor community services post discharge; educational programs for professionals, elderly citizens and caregivers; and respite services to temporarily relieve families from the burdens of home care. This article will focus on the case management service.

Policy

The policy issues which impact The Center for Geriatric Care and its clients are primarily financial. In 1983 the Social Security Act was amended to shift the way that Medicare would reimburse hospitals for inpatient acute care thus creating the DRG system (Diagnosis Related Groups). In 1984 the majority of states were phased into the federal DRG system. New Jersey, however, was one of the minority states that was operating under a model DRG waiver program since 1980. The DRG system mandates that hospitals be reimbursed based on the patient's diagnosis. Each diagnosis is assigned a particular number of days, with allotments made for patients over age 70 or those with multiple medical problems on admission. If the patient stays longer than the specified number of days the hospital still only gets the fixed payment. The patient is then considered an outlyer in the DRG system and the hospital loses money. If the patient's length of stay is less than the time assigned by the DRG, the hospital receives the same amount, and this is revenue gain (Brody and Magel, 1984). The DRG system was developed as an incentive program to contain health care costs. Under the traditional system, prior to DRGs, hospitals were reimbursed solely on their expenses.

Prior to the DRG system elderly patients sometimes lingered in the hospital for social reasons while arrangements were being made. Under the DRG system acute care hospitals can no longer be used for extended care (Friedman, 1986). It must be emphasized that the DRG system is not a product of the nation's hospitals, but of the Medicare system.

The rising costs of health care, the growth in the elderly population, and the increasing utilization of hospital services by the elderly have imposed a heavy burden upon the Medicare system. In 1980, 25 million people were over age 65. Projections for the year 2030 indicate a doubling of the over 65 population and a tripling of those over age 85, the most frail group (Lechich, 1984). In 1985, 42% of acute care patient days at Morristown Memorial Hospital and 76% of days on the inpatient skilled nursing and rehabilitation units were consumed by Medicare patients. The DRG system is a national response to these phenomena.

The DRG system creates a greater need for alternate health care services, primarily home care. Many people look to Medicare to provide these services. But Medicare was set up in 1965 to provide insurance coverage for acute care; it was not designed to be a long-term care program. Medicare does reimburse for home care (nurse, home health aide, physical therapy, occupational therapy, speech therapy, dietician and social worker), but in a limited way. There are four conditions which must be met to qualify for home care benefits under Medicare: the patient must need skilled nursing care or physical therapy, the patient must be homebound, a physician must order the service, and the agency which provides the service must be a Medicare participating agency (Friedman, 1986). Each of these conditions is very firmly defined and the specific criteria have not changed, but the interpretation of each has become more stringent. There is a misconception among the elderly and their families as to what defines "skilled care," there are many chronically ill people who cannot perform the essential activities of daily living, like toileting, who do not qualify due to the chronic nature of their problem. The home care agencies have been forced to become more conservative in providing service because Medicare will deny payment retroactively. If the patient is denied by Medicare the agency incurs the cost, resulting in more restrictive eligibility for services.

Where does the client who is ineligible for Medicare home care services turn? Most of the clients of The Center for Geriatric Care represent the majority of aged Americans, the middle-income group. These people do not meet the eligibility requirements of the Medicaid home care programs, yet do not have the funds to pay for services over an extended period of time, as is often necessary with chronic illness. This group is put in the precarious position of paying for long-term home care or institutional care until they impoverish themselves and end up on Medicaid for the first time in their lives.

The frail elderly are being squeezed by a system where acute inpatient days are being decreased, Medicare regulations for home care are more restrictive, and the private cost of in-home services is increasing. These circumstances are a challenge for social work with this population in terms of policy reform as well as casework.

Technology

The elderly population in the United States is one of the largest consumers of health care services. This is the result of more people living longer with a variety of chronic illnesses. As Mundinger (1983) describes, 40% of the elderly population suffer from some chronic illness, and this percentage increases with age. Although people are living longer they often are faced with debilitation and dependency resulting from chronic disease.

Chronic illness often involves complicated "high tech" regimens, surgical and diagnostic procedures. These include CAT scans, nuclear medicine, renal dialysis, joint replacements, bypass surgery, parenteral and enteral nutrition, chemotherapy, restrictive diets, and respiratory therapy. Chronic illness can result in functional impairments in Activities of Daily Living (ADLs) and Instrumental Activities of Daily Living (IADLs).[1] Technological advances in assistive devices such as bathroom equipment, incontinence products, stair gliders, and prostheses, help the client cope with living with the disease.

The procedures, regimens and devices associated with chronic illness represent a level of technology unfamiliar to both the family and the client. Lechich (1984) points out that technology in home health care offers the client greater independence in the face of restrictive regimens, but each technology requires understanding to resolve the problems that the technology itself creates. Much case

---

1. ADLs—Bathing, dressing, toileting and continence, transferring, eating and walking.

IADLs—Shopping, meal preparation, housekeeping, laundry, medications, financial management, use of the telephone, and mobility outside of the household.

management intervention is focused on helping the client and family to cope with these aspects of life, as well as the fact that although the client undergoes many procedures and regimens there is no cure for his ailment.

Organization

The Center for Geriatric Care is a department composed of a director (MSW), medical director-geriatrician (MD), two geriatric clinical specialists (MSN), social worker-senior case manager (MSW), and two case managers (BSW). There are also a variety of social work, nursing and medical residents training at the Center.

The climate and policies of cost containment emphasized the need for a hospital based system of coordinated care through case management. Case management fits into the organization by picking up where discharge planning leaves off. The discharge planner, nurse, or physician identifies the frail patient who is likely to require multiple community services post discharge. Initial plans for services needed immediately after the patient leaves the hospital are made by the discharge planner. The case manager then picks up to facilitate the implementation of the plan after the patient goes home. This provides a continuity of care that is delivered in a collaborative manner. The case manager then continues to provide ongoing monitoring of the patient in the community.

Having a hospital based case management program is beneficial to the organization in a variety of ways. Case management helps to facilitate the discharge of elderly patients, potentially reducing the likelihood of the patient becoming an outlyer in the DRG system. When a case management client is readmitted valuable data on prior functioning, service utilization, home environment and emotional supports is readily available to facilitate discharge and provide appropriate patient care. It also relieves the patient of having to repeat information on his situation each time he is admitted, as well as saving the acute care social worker time in getting a history and developing a plan. A goal of case management is to reduce fragmentation. Through close monitoring of the frail client in the community inappropriate readmissions can be avoided.

In an effort to be valuable to all disciplines in the hospital system, referrals for case management can be made by acute care social workers, nurses, physicians, clergy and other hospital staff. Family members, friends and clients themselves can also request the service. Frail elderly individuals, not hospitalized but residing in Morris County, may also be referred for case management services.

The grant received by the Center does not permit funds to be used to purchase home care services for clients. The goal is to coordinate and maximize existing resources, as well as promote the development of new resources.

Case Description

The case of Mrs. O'Malley is representative of one type of case where the client lives alone and has minimal family support. It is an example of the type of case that requires long-term case management to maintain the client in the community.

Mrs. O'Malley is an 85-year-old Irish woman who was born in the United States. She has lived in an apartment in senior housing for 17 years. Her husband died 11 years ago and she has lived alone since that time. She has no children. Her only relative in the area was an elderly niece who was planning to move and had been minimally involved. Mrs. O'Malley does know many people in her building and had previously been socially active. In the last three years, when many of her friends died and since her health worsened, she has become more isolated.

The client was referred to The Center for Geriatric Care by the social worker on the inpatient unit who is responsible for discharge planning. Mrs. O'Malley had been in the hospital for one month and had well exceeded the amount of time allotted by DRGs. She was admitted to the hospital with failure to thrive, congestive heart failure, and open leg ulcers due to edema. She also suffers from many chronic conditions such as diabetes, effects of polio, abdominal hernia, severe hearing loss and arthritis. The client's physician was experiencing pressure to discharge her because her acute problem had been resolved. It was the chronic nature of her disabilities that made the discharge more complicated. She was weakened from her acute illness and had been marginally safe receiving home delivered meals, and a home health aide four hours every day. Case management from the Center for Geriatric Care was part of the discharge plan. As Brody and Magel (1984) state, "Case management differs from discharge planning in that it assumes responsibility for mobilizing medical, social and health services to assure continuity of care as the patient returns to the community" (p. 677).

There were obstacles to setting up the initial home care services, that the discharge planner had to confront. Agencies that the client had been known to felt they could not serve her adequately because she had been a difficult patient. Other agencies felt the situation was too risky and still others knew of the client's hesitancy to pay and the fact that she did not have a guaranteed payer, such as a relative. After great effort, the discharge planner was able to arrange services. The hospital staff (MD, RNs and social worker) were relieved and reassured by the fact that The Center for Geriatric Care would provide ongoing monitoring of this frail client. The referral to the Center for Geriatric Care facilitated the patient's discharge.

Definition of the Client

The Center for Geriatric Care serves the frail elderly and their families. All clients are over age 65, live in Morris County and are having some difficulty managing in the community. Often the Center is contacted when the elderly person and/or his or her family is at a decision making point: Can the client remain at home alone? Should the client go to a nursing home or move in with relatives? The clientele have a wide range of disabilities, as well as social and economic problems.

Goals

The client's self-determination is the foundation upon which goals and objectives are developed. In this case the client wanted to return to independent living in the community and regain control over her environment. The goals of the case manger were to promote the client's independence and assist in its maintenance, prevent unnecessary readmission to the hospital, prevent institutionalization, promote functional ability (ADLs and IADLs), and enhance the client's quality of life. Rashko (1985) cites these goals as fundamental components of case management with the frail elderly.

Many short-term objectives were identified during the course intervention. In the beginning a primary objective was enabling the client to accept help, especially from home health aides.[2] In the middle phase a significant objective was to have the client become independent in taking her medications and personal case. In the current phase, which I will term maintenance, objectives focus on helping the client to seek appropriate help prior to crisis, and maintaining independence.

Contract

Initially establishing a contract with Mrs. O'Malley was very difficult. When she went home from the hospital she was overwhelmed and frightened. This resulted in her being anxious and suspicious of service providers. Although an initial relationship had been established between the client and the case manager, the client approached the alliance with hesitancy. After numerous episodes of the client "testing" the worker, for example not opening the door and being extremely uncooperative, Mrs. O'Malley began to realize the worker was going to be consistent and a relationship in which contracting was possible evolved. Rashko (1985) discusses the need for case managers to be highly skilled in establishing positive relationships with the elderly to overcome initial resistance and fear. He states that it is this relationship that is a conduit for implementing a continuum of services. The case of Mrs. O'Malley verifies this concept.

All contracts with the client have been verbal. Many contracts have been carried out over time. The contracts have been concrete in nature; for example, the case manager will set up the home health aide and change the aide if the client wishes, but the client must let the worker know when. Another contract revolves around bill paying; if the client collects all the bills in one place the case manager will assist her with paying them monthly. This type of contracting gave the client structure, and helped her regain control over her

---

2. In Morris County, there is not a distinction between homemaker and home health aide services.

environment through participating in accomplishing these activities.

Meeting Place

All sessions with Mrs. O'Malley were held in her apartment. This is necessary with most clients due to frailty and disability. Conducting sessions in the client's home has many advantages. The worker is able to observe the client in her environment and is then better able to fine tune the service plan based on how the client interacts and manages her environment. This is a luxury the hospital discharge planner does not have. Where the client is in her home she feels more comfortable and much more in control.

Use of Time

Initially multiple home visits were made per week to assist the client through the crisis of returning home and accepting in-home services. A substantial amount of time was also spent with collateral contacts regarding the client. By the third month of contact weekly visits were sufficient, although there were stressful events which required additional interventions. At the one year marker biweekly home visits were made. In recent months Mrs. O'Malley has required only monthly visits. The average length of time for each visit is one hour.

The change that evolved was related to two main factors, the client's improved health and the well established relationship between the client and the worker. As Goldmeier (1985) describes, the work is ". . . time-limited in that it is focused on the problems of the moment, and ongoing in terms of readiness to deal with the continuing problems of aging that do not end with one episode of case activity successful though it may be" (p. 323). The case manager became the client's anchor and the mortar that held the conglomeration of services together. Through the course of time the client learned when to call the case manager, and the case manager became more familiar with the client's limitations and the specific areas in which she needed ongoing assistance.

Treatment Modality

Case management is being recommended with increasing frequency as an approach to caring for the multiple needs of the disabled (Johnson and Rubin, 1983), whether they be frail elders or the chronically mentally ill. Exactly what composes case management varies based on the setting. Many agencies do case management within their own agency, coordinating the particular services they offer. A broader model of case management involves coordinating services of multiple agencies (formal services) as well as family, friends and volunteers (informal services); this is the approach of the Center for Geriatric Care.

Case management involves assessment, care planning, arranging services, monitoring and reassessment. The first thing the case manager did when she saw the patient at home was a comprehensive assessment of Mrs. O'Malley's mental status, functional ability (ADLs and IADLs), financial status and eligibility for various entitlements, and an analysis of her social network. Mrs. O'Malley was much more alert and functional than she appeared to be in the hospital. The case manager worked with her to develop a care plan of services she would accept. The case manager then implemented the care plan by arranging the services and providing ongoing monitoring.

Many talents and skills are needed to put case management into action; it is not the mechanistic approach it is often simplified to be. An eclectic approach was taken with Mrs. O'Malley. She benefited greatly from behavioral techniques surrounding issues such as taking medication, meal preparation, and finances. Behavior techniques helped her become incrementally more independent. Ongoing supportive counseling was needed to help Mrs. O'Malley work through her losses and regain control of her environment. Crisis intervention techniques were valuable when the client experienced an exacerbation of a chronic illness. Reminiscence therapy (Hughston, 1982; Kaminsky, 1984) was highly effective in helping her adapt. It seemed to improve her life satisfaction as it strengthened her self-concept and improved her cognitive functioning.

Reminiscence therapy with the elderly is a valuable resource; it helps the worker and client join in the therapeutic relationship. Mrs.

O'Malley had wonderful historical stories to tell which fascinated the worker. The worker was able to engage the client and help her deal with "unfinished business" through use of this technique. Having someone to listen to her stories made Mrs. O'Malley feel her life had been valuable and that she had someone to pass along her wisdom to. This desire is a natural part of the stage of life Erikson called Integrity vs. Despair (Edinberg, 1985), the therapeutic relationship can help the client successfully complete this stage. When the worker got married Mrs. O'Malley gave her a souvenir plate she had gotten on her honeymoon in Niagara Falls.

Stance of the Social Worker

The case of Mrs. O'Malley is typical in that the worker assumes three roles—coordinator, advocate, and counselor (Austin, 1983). The roles are not mutually exclusive and the worker often finds herself performing them at the same time. In this case balancing the three roles was often challenging.

The service coordinator role requires one to take a very active stance. The worker is responsible for setting up and maintaining all of the needed services. When Mrs. O'Malley experienced problems such as the home health aide being late, the home delivered meals not arriving, or the walker needing replacement, the case manager did an active investigation of the circumstances and was responsible for resolving the problems.

In the role of coordinator the case manager found that she needed to provide support for the cadre of aides that were sent to the client. Frequent mediation sessions between the aide and the client were needed. Mrs. O'Malley would frequently complain that the aide did not do enough and the aide felt the client was too demanding.

The role of advocate is intertwined with that of coordinator, and is also one in which the worker needs to be direct. The case manager was constantly advocating for why Mrs. O'Malley needed a particular service, at a specific time, and how much of that resource should be allocated to her. Often there are many people competing for the same service and it is up to the worker to present the client's care convincingly. Mrs. O'Malley also needed an advocate to speak to her physician regarding physical therapy, and to inquire with the pharmacist about a payment schedule.

In the role of counselor the stance varied from directive behavioral therapy to therapeutic listening. Time and patience were essential to making counseling effective.

At different points and in different roles, the worker took a variety of stances ranging from very active to contemplative. The roles of coordinator and advocate require political savvy; the worker is continually balancing her relationships with the client and the service providers.

Outside Resources

Concrete services have been heavily utilized by Mrs. O'Malley. Services such as home health aide, visiting nurse, home delivered meals, senior transportation and chore service, have made it possible for her to remain in her apartment.

When Mrs. O'Malley was discharged from the hospital Medicare provided a Visiting Nurse and a home health aide for two weeks. The nurse monitored the client's physical status and instructed her on the new array of medications. Because Mrs. O'Malley qualified for this skilled level of care she was also entitled to a home health aide for two hours, three times a week. The client needed four hours daily of the aide service and paid privately for the additional hours.

After service under Medicare terminated, Mrs. O'Malley continued to need a home health aide to assist her with bathing, dressing, shopping, housekeeping, and meal preparation. It was difficult to convince the client to pay for these services because she feared spending all her money. As Jenkins (1984) points out, as well as completing essential tasks the aide provides socialization and eases the client's isolation. This was very important in the early stages of her readjustment to being at home. She did eventually pay for the aide. The worker got her to agree by establishing a contract with the client which included a review every two weeks to negotiate the level of care needed. This situation created a balance where the client received needed support in decision making yet remained in control.

As Mrs. O'Malley's condition improved the case manager decreased the frequency of her home health aide service. She continued to require chore services, transportation and home delivered meals. The Center for Geriatric Care was able to provide a dedicated volunteer to assist her with tasks that do not require a formal service provider, such as buying new shoes or holiday shopping. The volunteer also does the client's weekly shopping. The most valuable service is the companionship the volunteer provides.

Reassessment

Reassessment is a continual process. Frequent changes are made in the care plan based on the need to continue, revise or discontinue various services. A formal written reassessment is required, as a condition of the grant, three months after enrollment and then annually. Reviewed in the written reassessment are functional ability, mental status, and utilization of services.

The reassessment process is a vehicle for measuring the client's progress over time. At the time of the three month reassessment Mrs. O'Malley was eating, walking outside with a cane and bathing herself. She scored 100% on the mental status questionnaire administered. She had begun to socialize more. As her health improved she ventured out of her apartment more. Her neighbors and friends were no longer overwhelmed by her needs because the case manager and formal service providers were involved. This also reduced their hesitancy to check in on Mrs. O'Malley.

The one year reassessment verified ongoing progress. Mrs. O'Malley had become independent in taking her medication. She no longer needed a home health aide. Mrs. O'Malley was able to venture out to visit a friend in the neighboring building. She showed the ability to sustain the gains she had made over time.

At the two year marker, Mrs. O'Malley is reading the newspaper daily to keep up with current events. She requires less help with financial management. At times she does her grocery shopping and goes to doctor's appointments by utilizing senior transportation. She has made significant progress and continues to demonstrate that returning to her apartment was the correct decision.

Transfer or Termination

Termination is considered when the goals toward functional independence are reached. At this point the client is able to sustain herself by utilizing formal and informal networks without ongoing assistance. Termination also occurs if the client is placed in a nursing home or other facility. In the case of Mrs. O'Malley, she continues to require active assistance and support and remains an open case.

Case Conclusion

The case of Mrs. O'Malley was successful. The primary goal of restoring her independent living through improving her functional ability was achieved. Mrs. O'Malley's strong will to remain in the community motivated her to join in a partnership with the case manager. The client responded positively to the variety of approaches the worker implemented. The worker helped her establish an environment that she could master, which in turn helped her to deal effectively with her feelings about aging and illness. Mrs. O'Malley's resilience, the case manager's efforts, as well as the formal and informal supports came together to make a fragile situation work.

Differential Discussion

Mrs. O'Malley needed an intense form of case management. Without the case management service the conclusion to the case is likely to have been quite different. Mrs. O'Malley might have been placed in a nursing home. She also might have had numerous emergency room visits and potential inappropriate admissions to the hospital.

This is a classic case of an elderly person whose family is unable to provide day to day assistance. If the client had a primary caregiver the worker's approach would have varied. It has been the Center's experience that with ongoing support and guidance the caregiver can assume many of the tasks the worker took on in the case of Mrs. O'Malley. In cases where there is a primary caregiver the case management service tends to be of a shorter duration.

The community in which the client lives shaped the outcome of the case. Morris County is a service-rich community, but the fact that Mrs. O'Malley had the money to pay for the home health aide care she needed facilitated receipt of the service. There were other services such as chore service for which she waited a considerable period of time, but proved invaluable. The case manager is put in the situation of only being able to manage the services that exist in the community, and must continually advocate for those in short supply.

Throughout the case, the flexibility the Center allotted the worker allowed her to be creative and perform many untraditional tasks. It has often been said around the office that case management is doing what no one else does. Case management can not be done in the confines of the weekly 50 minute hour.

PRACTICE IN CONTEXT

The Center for Geriatric Care was a new agency in the community three years ago and has made significant strides in becoming an integral part of the service delivery system for the frail elderly. The Center was given the mission of promoting a county-wide case management system without the funds to purchase services for clients. Many community agencies were skeptical about the value of such a program. The Center accomplished its mission by becoming a resource to the key actors—clients, families, service providers and the hospital. The Center added a dimension that had not previously existed, and which facilitated continuity of care.

Currently The Center for Geriatric Care operates in the context of a grant which mandates that case management be done in the manner described throughout the chapter. It can be said that this is the ideal method of conducting the service. The realities of cost containment make it questionable whether the current method of service delivery will continue when the grant expires.

Future funding will play a major role in defining the service. If the Center is funded solely through the hospital it will be likely to be more short-term in nature. Future clients will be those patients being discharged from Morristown Memorial Hospital, and patients identified through the geriatric outpatient consultation service. No longer will the Center be able to accept referrals from community agencies. If community and hospital funding are combined the service will be more likely to retain its current characteristics and expand. The costs and the number of clients to be served will probably place restrictions on the number of long-term cases. In either scenario a sliding scale fee for service will likely be implemented.

These factors will have a major impact on practice, especially in the area of termination. One school of thought is expressed by Butler and Lewis (1982) who state that rather than focusing on termination, case management should be ongoing and varied according to needs until the client's death. Fiscal pressures may not allow for this type of practice. After the client is stabilized and the initial goals are reached the case would be closed. It could be re-opened at any point, but the case manager would have lost that essential ongoing connection and would be less likely to prevent crises.

In some form or another, case management services will continue to be an essential component of the long-term care system, especially as the elderly population increases. This opens up a vast arena of opportunity for the profession of social work. The skills of psychosocial assessment, counseling and community organization, combined with an unmatched ability to understand and negotiate the service delivery system are unique. Historically social workers have downplayed the concrete service element of practice, but it is this expertise which makes social workers unquestionably valued in the long-term care system. Social workers also have an opportunity to impact on the development of national long-term care policies.

Hospital based case management programs linking acute and non-acute care are likely to become more prolific. As Brody and Magel (1984) state, "development and utilization of a short-term long-term care system is more than a marketing idea — it is a strategy for hospital survival" (p. 678). A flexible short-term case management program that can carry a small percentage of long-term clients is the anticipated wave of the future.

REFERENCES

Abrahams, J.P., and Crooks, V.J., Eds. *Geriatric Mental Health*. Orlando, Florida: Grune and Stratton, Inc., 1984.

Austin, C.A. Case Management in Long Term Care: Options and Opportunities. *Health and Social Work*, 8:16-30, 1983.

Berenson, R.A., and Pawlson, L.G. The Medicare Prospective Payment System and the Care of the Frail Elderly. *Journal of the American Geriatrics Society*, 32:843-848, 1984.

Berger, R.M., Anderson, S. The In-Home Worker: Serving the Frail Elderly. *Social Work*, 29:456-461, 1984.

Berkman, L.F. The Assessment of Social Networks and Social Support in the Elderly. *Journal of the American Geriatrics Society*, 32:743-749, 1983.

Brody, S.J., and Magel, J.S. DRG — The Second Revolution in Health Care for the Elderly. *Journal of the American Geriatrics Society*, 32:676-679, 1984.

Brody, S.J. and Persily, N.A., Eds. *Hospitals and the Aged*. Rockville, MD: Aspen Systems Corporation, 1984.

Butler, R.N., and Lewis, M. *Aging and Mental Health: Positive Psychological and Biomedical Approaches*, 3rd ed. St. Louis: C.V. Mosby Co, 1982.

Capitman, J.A., Haskins, B., and Bernstein, J. Case Management Approaches in Coordinated Community-Oriented Long-Term Care Demonstrations. *The Gerontologist*, 26:398-404, 1986.

Carrilio, T.E., and Eisenberg, D. Informal Resources for the Elderly: Panacea or Empty Promises. *Journal of Gerontological Social Work*, 6:39-46, 1983.

Cole, E. Assessing Needs for Elders Networks. *Journal of Gerontological Nursing*, 11: 31-34, 1985.

Edinburg, M.A. *Mental Health Practice with the Elderly*. Englewood Cliffs, N.J.: Prentice-Hall, Inc., 1985.

Friedman, J. *Home Health Care*. New York: W.W. Norton & Co., 1986.

Goldmeier, J. Helping The Elderly in Times of Stress. *Social Casework*, 66:323-332, 1985.

Haber, P.A.L. Technology in Aging. *The Gerontologist*, 26:350-357, 1986.

Hughston, G.A., and Merriam, S.B. Reminiscence: A Non Formal Technique for Improving Cognitive Functioning in The Aged. *International Journal of Aging and Human Development*, 15:139-149, 1982.

Jenkins, E.H. Homemakers: The Core of Home Health Care. *Geriatric Nursing*, 5:28-30, 1984.

Johnson, P.J. and Rubin, A. Case Management in Mental Health: A Social Work Domain? *Social Work*, 28:49-55, 1983.

Kaminsky, M. The Uses of Reminiscence: A Discussion of the Formative Literature. *Journal of Gerontological Social Work*, 7:137-156, 1984.

Kermis, M. *Mental Health in Late Life*. Boston: Jones & Bartlett Publishers, 1986.

Kerson, T.S. and Kerson, L.A. *Understanding Chronic Illness*. New York: The Free Press, 1985.

Lechich, A. *High Technology and Home Health Care* (Proceedings from The Pride Institute Conference 12/8/83). Pride Institute Journal, 3:6-7, 1984.

Liu, K., Manton, K.G. and Liu, B.M. Home Care Expenses for The Disabled Elderly. *Health Care Financing Review*, 7:51-57, 1985.

Mundinger, M.O. *Home Care Controversy*. Rockville, MD: Aspen Systems Corporation, 1983.

Pollack, W. *Expanding Health Benefits for The Elderly, Volume I*. Washington, D.C.: The Urban Institute, 1979.

Northern, H. *Clinical Social Work*. New York: Columbia University Press, 1982.
Raschko, R. Systems Integration at The Program Level: Aging and Mental Health. *The Gerontologist*, 25:460-463, 1985.
Sherman, E. *Counseling the Aging*. New York: The Free Press, 1981.
Spivack, S.M. *The Aged: A Demographic Imperative*. A Major Health Care Market in Hospitals and the Aged. Eds., Brody, S.J. and Persily, N.A. Rockville, MD: Aspen Systems Corporation, 1984.
Teri, L. and Lewinsohn, P.M., Eds. *Geropsychological Assessment and Treatment*. New York: Springer Publishing Co., 1986.

Hospice:
Terminal Illness, Teamwork and the Quality of Life

Nina Millet Fish

"Hospice" is a medieval word meaning a resting place for sick and dying travelers on their journeys to and from the Holy Land. The modern concept of hospice is a formal program of palliative and supportive care for persons in the last stages of a lingering, progressive illness (Munley, 1983). St. Christopher's Hospice in London, generally considered to be the first such program, has been in existence less than 20 years. New Haven's Connecticut Hospice, Inc., modeled after St. Christopher's, is the oldest program in the United States and has been providing home care for only a little over a decade, and in-patient care in their free-standing facility for about 5 years (Lack and Buckingham, 1978). During the 1980s, hundreds of hospice planning groups have sprouted across the country. Some have succeeded, others have not. Some provide only home care, others, combine both home and in-patient care. Difficulties in financing and operating such programs led to a variety of organizational models of delivery, and until recently had prevented the development of a definitive model for hospice care in this country. For example, in-patient units may be autonomous and free-standing, or they may be hospital based either as an entirely separate unit within the existing structure or as a smaller unit within a hospital ward (Buckingham and Lupu, 1982). Home care programs may be entirely volunteer, be supported by grants, have contractual agreements with a Medicare certified home health agency or be a Medicare certified home health agency itself.

The early 1980s were years of great change and progress for the hospice movement. A specific Medicare hospice benefit was passed by Congress and subsequently implemented. State licensure laws have been passed in many states, and the Joint Commission on Accreditation of Hospitals (JCAH) has developed guidelines and standards for hospice programs. (See Policy section.) All of these regulatory bodies have served to set minimum standards of care to the extent that, for example, a hospice program in Arizona must offer the same components of care as a hospice in Maine. The result has been the beginning of more definitive models, with the majority of programs being either hospital or home health agency based. Some remain as free standing agencies or facilities, but many, including all volunteer programs, have merged with hospitals or other existing agencies for financial or organizational reasons (Torrens, 1985).

Despite the model, the basic philosophy and concept of care remain the same — palliative and supportive care for both patient and family, and bereavement care for the family after the death of the patient.

Description of the Setting

The Hospice of Madison County (HMC) is in a heavily industrial community, surrounded by a rural area, in Southern Illinois. The area's population is largely of German descent, and numbers about 250,000.

Numerous changes have occurred at HMC in recent years. In 1986, an agreement was reached whereby HMC would merge with and become a department of the local hospital, St. Elizabeth Medical Center (SEMC). HMC's Board of Directors, by-laws and incorporation status were dissolved, according to the laws of the State of Illinois. HMC is now a state licensed, JCAH accredited, Medicare certified hospice. Palliative and supportive care is still provided at home, with inpatient care available on the oncology unit of the hospital. There, admission criteria have been broadened to include diagnoses other than cancer.

All hospice programs continue to share a number of characteristics, which, when provided within the context of a formalized program, differentiate hospice from traditional health care (Hospice Standards Manual, 1986). These characteristics are as follows:

1. physician directed services
2. emphasis and expertise in control of symptoms
3. interdisciplinary team approach
4. availability of emergency care at all times
5. patient and family together as unit of care
6. emphasis on home care as long as the patient and family can cope
7. bereavement follow-up

Hospice patients have illnesses which have progressed to the stage where palliative rather than curative treatment is considered most appropriate. Patient/family care is provided by an interdisciplinary team which includes the patient and family, a physician, nurse, social worker, clergy and volunteers (Gardner, 1985). All team members work in close collaboration with each other to ensure delivery of comprehensive care. Such teamwork and collaboration are essential because of the nature of problems being dealt with. The result is a certain amount of "role blurring," with professional roles less clearly defined than in most health settings. As might be expected, this has implications for social work practice (Kulys, 1986).

Referrals for hospice care come from physicians, social workers, clergy, family members or patients themselves. Physician consent is necessary before care can be initiated, because patients remain under the care of their own physician while in the program.

Approximately 2/3 of HMC's patients are over the age of 60. The youngest to date was 19, the oldest 99. Average length of stay is 49 days (usually from admission to the Program until death). The shortest stay has been 1 day, the longest approximately 2 years. Most patients are from white, working class families employed by or retired from one of the heavy industries in the area. Many patients, about 65%, are able to die at home.

The social worker sees and evaluates patient and family's psychosocial and environmental situation from the perspective of their ability to cope with an impending death in the family as well as the need for concrete services (Lusk, 1983). In collaboration with other team members, an interdisciplinary plan of care is developed, individualized to each patient/family situation, and revised frequently as needed.

Policy

The organizational structure largely defines the policy that affects social work practice in individual programs. Beyond this, the most crucial policies affecting social work practice, as well as the existence and functioning of entire programs has been that of reimbursement from both public and private carriers, and development of regulations and standards on the state and national levels (Federal Register, 1983). Recent changes in these areas are no less than phenomenal.

As a result of earlier demonstration projects funded by both the United States Department of Health and Human Services and some private carriers, the Medicare hospice benefit was passed as part of the Tax Equity and Fiscal Responsibility Act (TEFRA) in 1982. At the same time, JCAH was developing standards for hospice care, and numerous states were passing licensure laws regulating hospice programs. Obviously, all of this has had far reaching effects on individual hospice programs and how care is delivered. One result has been the changing image of hospice, from that of a group of grass roots volunteers barely on the fringe of the health care system, to that of an accepted specialty area within the mainstream of health care (Wald, Foster and Wald, 1980). Many issues have been raised about how these regulations affect the delivery of care. A detailed analysis from this perspective is beyond the scope of this paper, but overall, hospice has now become a business faced with the same economic, legal and quality of care issues as the rest of health care.

Under the Medicare hospice benefit, which is primarily a reimbursement program, Medicare eligible patients who are terminally ill may elect (choose) hospice care from a Medicare certified hospice program. In so doing, they waive their right to reimbursement through traditional Medicare except for problems unrelated to their terminal illness. They may also choose to rescind their "hospice election" at any time while in the program, and return to care under traditional Medicare coverage. Under this system, the hospice is organizationally and fiscally responsible for all care related to the terminal illness, including home care, physician, social work, counseling, home health aides, in-patient care, volunteers, supplies and equipment and medications. For financial, legal and ethical reasons, this benefit has been a controversial one, and to date, only about 20% of the nation's hospice programs have chosen to participate. The remainder receive reimbursement under traditional Medicare for both home care and in-patient care (Brooks and Smythe-Staruch, 1983).

In April 1986, legislation was passed that made the Medicare hospice benefit a permanent part of the health care system. (It had previously been scheduled to sunset in November 1986.) Contained in the same legislation was authorization for individual states to amend their own Medicaid plans to make hospice care available to its low income terminally ill Medicaid recipients.

JCAH standards were developed over a three-year period through a grant from the Kellogg Foundation, with input from hospice programs of all types and sizes, nationwide. Again, their purpose is to insure minimum standards of care on a national level. JCAH accreditation is mandatory for all hospital based hospice programs, voluntary for others. However, standards of care for Home Health Agencies are also in the process of development, so it is conceivable that Home Health Agency based hospices will be required to meet JCAH guidelines in the future. Currently a cooperative effort between Medicare and JCAH is in process whereby programs accredited by JCAH will also receive Medicare certification.

Other developments in the health care field such as the growth of Health Maintenance Organizations, Preferred Provider Organizations and the advent of Diagnosis Related Groupings (DRGs) are also having a profound effect on hospice care. The latter has revolutionized health care reimbursement, and deserves a closer look.

The development of DRGs and their integration into the health care reimbursement system is arguably the most significant change since Medicare was introduced in the 1960s. Simply, DRGs are a listing of all illnesses and complications into separately numbered categories with a specific dollar amount allowed for reimbursement of each diagnosis. For example, an uncomplicated appendectomy is reimbursed at $4835 for patients under 70 years of age. For those over 70, it is $6377. The figure has been arrived at by determining how many days hospitalization should be required, and the cost for that amount of time. If patients are hospitalized for *less* than the allotted number of days, the hospital will make a profit. If they stay longer, the hospital loses money. The amount reimbursed is the same regardless of the length of stay in the hospital, i.e., it is based on the diagnosis rather than the number of days treated. In addition, payment may be denied altogether if an admission is not "justi-fied," i.e., the patient did not require acute level care. Hospice programs are affected by this in two distinct ways: admission to and discharge from the hospital. A terminally ill person also must meet the requirement for needing acute level care to be admitted to the hospital, and if admitted, the goal is to discharge as quickly as possible (Caputi and Heiss, 1984; Veatch, 1986). Frequently, hos-pice patients need only custodial care, and the greatest need is res-pite care for the exhausted family. Creative use of community re-sources by the hospice team, especially the social worker, is necessary to help alleviate or prevent crisis situations when families are exhausted, yet the patient's condition does not justify a hospital admission (Christ, 1983).

What does all of this mean for the social worker in hospice care? All recent regulations require the availability of psychosocial care for patients and families, and Medicare defines social work as one of the "core" services, along with nursing, clergy and volunteers. JCAH and some state licensure laws requires its availability, but allow its provision by other than a social worker, i.e., by psycholo-gist, counselor, or psychiatric nurse. Minimum standards for edu-cation and experience are specified (*Hospice Standards Manual*, p. 6-7).

How this care is provided continues to depend on organizational structure and policies of individual programs and agencies. Hospital based programs may share a social worker with a hospital's social work department. Home health agency based programs may share a social worker with the rest of the agency. Still others may utilize a psychiatric nurse, counselor or psychologist, depending on state regulations and program policy.

More than ever, leaders in the hospice movement need to be mindful of the uniqueness and vulnerability of the population they serve. For this reason, the social work role remains crucial, either as a manager or as staff involved with patients/families and other staff. More and more, hospice directors are business persons with expertise in financial management. The danger is that the original compassionate element of care may be lost in the midst of very real fiscal and regulatory issues (Gibson, 1984).

Despite the model of care, the intervening years of experience with hospice patients and families have emphasized the need for well educated, highly skilled persons to deal with the myriad and often complex psychosocial issues involved in almost every family situation.

Technology

The primary goals of hospice care are to relieve physical suffering and to provide support to patients and family members, thereby enhancing the quality of remaining life. According to Sylvia Lack (1978),

"there is far too much talk in this country about psychological and emotional problems, and far too little about making the patient comfortable. Any group concerned with care of the dying should be talking about soothing sheets, rubbing bottoms, relieving constipation, and sitting up at night. Counseling a person who is lying in a wet bed is ineffective." (p. 44)

Technology, then, is concerned with patient and family comfort. Control of symptoms (usually pain) is the priority, and all symptoms are constantly monitored. A problem oriented approach to symptom management is used, treating each symptom almost as a disease in itself. Pain can be relieved by a variety of medications, differing in strength from very mild to very strong, depending on individual needs. After determining the appropriate medication and strength, a schedule for administration (usually every three to four hours) is planned, and medication is given on this schedule around the clock. This keeps pain from recurring yet leaves the person alert and able to interact with his or her surroundings and social environment. Patients and families are reassured that stronger medication is available if needed, so they need not worry about the medication becoming ineffective.

Medically, patients have been subjected to the range of curative treatments for their particular illness and are at the stage where continuance of such treatment is no longer considered appropriate (Lynn, 1986). Radiation and chemotherapy are sometimes given, but primarily for palliative reasons.

In recent years, the treatment of chronic pain has received a great deal of attention by researchers, and much has been learned, with new medications and treatments developed. It is necessary for those in hospice care to keep abreast of the changes and new developments in the field, not only in physical care, but new treatment options and approaches on the part of the social worker (Kerson, 1985).

The major goal of hospice care remains assisting families to provide comprehensive nursing and supportive care to patients. Technologically, this means performing tasks necessary to care for the patient. It also means teaching family members how to perform them, since most of the day-to-day responsibility for care belongs to the caregiver. More specifically to the social worker, it means teaching patients and families that their feelings, concerns, fears and anxieties are a normal part of the process of letting go of a loved one. It means helping them deal with their feelings in constructive ways, facilitating communication among family members as well as helping with concrete services. Experience continues to show that families are capable of learning and performing highly technical tasks amazingly well when provided with proper teaching, reinforcement and support (Buckingham, 1983).

Organization

HMC was organized as a community based program and functioned in this manner for 7 years. In 1986, for organizational and financial purposes, the decision was made to merge with SEMC, a 475 bed acute care Catholic hospital, incorporated as a not-for-profit corporation in the state of Illinois.

Medical direction for the program is provided by a licensed, practicing physician in the state of Illinois. Paid staff consists of a full complement of professional and clerical persons to provide all components of hospice care. A public relations staff member helps

with fund raising and marketing. The social worker, an MSW, reports to the Director of Social Service for the hospital, and is assigned to the oncology unit and the hospice program. In addition to
her patient and family responsibilities, she helps with the bereavement program.

The staff is a cohesive group of persons who are responsible for
the day to day functioning of the program. Their responsibilities
include all aspects of patient care and its accompanying functions.
Office staff do the record keeping, correspondence, dissemination
of public information and education, coordinating of volunteer efforts and the bereavement program, speaking engagements, and are
involved in marketing and fund raising events and efforts. A corps
of sixty trained volunteers are available to help in areas of patient
and family care, clerical support, fund raising events, speaking engagements and bereavement care.

Case Description

In the spring of 1980, Angie was referred for hospice care by a
hospital social worker while she was hospitalized for weakness,
symptom control and evaluation of the progression of her disease.
She was in her late thirties, had been married only a few years, and
had a two to three year history of carcinoma of the breast, for which
she had undergone a radical mastectomy two years previously. She
and her husband Bill had apparently made a satisfactory adjustment
after the mastectomy. During the two years since her surgery, however, she had failed to follow through with prescribed courses of
chemotherapy because of a strong religious belief that she had been
healed of her disease. There were no children in the family, and
both sets of parents lived in distant states. During the time we cared
for her, Angie's parents visited her twice, briefly.

When initially contacted in the hospital by hospice staff, Angie
was anxious to return home, despite continuing weakness. However, there was no one at home to care for her during the day while
her husband worked. With some financial help from her parents,
arrangements were made for her to return home with a paid "sitter"
(caregiver) who stayed during the day while Bill was at work. Bill
agreed to care for her at night and on the weekends. A hospital bed

and other necessary equipment were obtained from the local American Cancer Society office. After initial nursing and social service assessments at home, a care plan was developed. Because her insurance did not reimburse for any home care, and because finances were a problem, a hospice trained volunteer nurse was assigned to see her twice a week.

This arrangement lasted only a short time, however, because Bill was unable to continue with the responsibility of both her care and his work. Angie was admitted to the hospital briefly, with complaints of weakness, lack of appetite and depression. During her hospital stay, she indicated some marital problems related to her husband's inability to accept her illness and his fear of caring for her by himself. She would not elaborate any further on the problem and remained depressed and withdrawn during most of her hospital stay. Bill said he felt he was coping well, but he did indicate anxiety about caring for Angie at home (Yasko and Green, 1986).

At the interdisciplinary team meeting, it was decided to arrange for a volunteer to contact Bill to provide additional support, since his work schedule made it difficult for the staff to remain in continual contact with him. Because it was felt that Bill might relate better to another man, and because of Bill's religious beliefs, a minister with a background in psychology was contacted and agreed to serve as a lay volunteer to be a friend and support to Bill.

Through the volunteer, we began to learn more about Bill's background. He was the youngest of several children and the only boy in the family. As a child, he had been shielded and protected from all possible stresses of life. Now, he faced a devastating situation, without having developed necessary coping skills. His reaction was to try to escape, both physically and emotionally, and as Angie's condition worsened, he became less and less able to assume responsibility for helping with even routine household tasks.

Angie wanted to return home, so arrangements were again made, this time with two caregivers who arranged their hours so that one of them was with her at all times (Reveson et al., 1983). By now, her condition was deteriorating, and care of her physical needs required increased time and effort. She was less depressed at home, however, and enjoyed listening to her stereo and having poetry read to her. She indicated an interest in painting or drawing and was supplied with pastels and paper. She was, however, unable to accomplish this task because her hands were becoming increasingly affected by the spread of the disease to her spine. A tape recorder was provided in the hope that she might tape some of her thoughts and feelings, but while expressing verbal interest in doing this, she never followed through. Her volunteer nurse was now visiting her two or three times a week, and close telephone contact was maintained between her caregivers, the volunteer nurse and the hospice office. Angie's pain was managed with "hospice mix," a special preparation of oral morphine, a special ingredient to prevent nausea, and flavored syrup. (This was prior to the development and availability of the commercial oral morphine products now on the market.) Doses were increased as her pain increased but were kept at a level that did not cause excessive drowsiness.

During this time, Bill's behavior was becoming more erratic. He began missing work, spending large amounts of money, much of it on himself, and staying away from home for long periods of time. He seemed to have built a wall around himself that could not be penetrated despite efforts by various members of the team, including the social worker and Bill's volunteer. Telephone contact was maintained with Angie's parents, and they were able to make a brief visit a few days before her death, although they were not with her when she died.

Much effort was now given to caring for her physical needs, and during the last week of her life, her volunteer nurse visited her every day. Angie remained emphatic about wanting to stay at home and was fully aware of her condition. She remained lucid and alert until her death, which occurred quietly and peacefully one weekend morning. Her caregiver was with her, as were her husband, her own minister, and two friends from her church who sang her favorite hymns as she slipped away. She said good-bye to her husband and friends and died with a beautiful smile on her face which remained with her to the grave.

DECISIONS ABOUT PRACTICE

Definition of the Client

Initially, Angie and her husband were the clients, as is customary in hospice care. This eventually expanded to include first one, then both caregivers. As Bill withdrew, physically and emotionally, the caregivers essentially became her family.

Cicely Saunders, medical director of St. Christopher's in London, describes the terminally ill person as being on a journey from this life to the next. In this context, the family is also on a journey, and they need help to accomplish the tasks involved in caring for their loved one and in being able to let go at the end of the journey.

Related to this concept, studies done at New Haven's Connecticut Hospice, Inc., have shown that the family member carrying the burden of care suffers more anxiety, depression and social malfunctioning than does the patient (Lack and Buckingham, 1978). This was certainly the case with Angie and Bill, and seven years of hospice experience since that time have only emphasized the necessity of including the family with the patient as the unit of care.

Goals

Families vary a great deal in their need for social work involvement beyond the provision of practical needs (Moore, 1984). Often, the need for further intervention becomes more apparent as time progresses and the patient's physical condition deteriorates. Through collaboration with other team members, needs are constantly reassessed and a course of action planned. In Angie and Bill's situation, there were several goals:

1. To provide physical comfort for Angie and emotional support for both Angie and Bill.
2. To allow Angie to remain at home, since this was her wish. (This meant continuing evaluation of the stamina and coping abilities of her caregivers, since their task was demanding and they worked long hours. A mutual dependence developed between the staff and caregivers—we depended on them for Angie's care, and they depended on us for advice, reassurance, support and availability in emergencies.)
3. To help Bill deal with the reality of the situation and strengthen his coping abilities.
4. To facilitate improved communication between Angie and Bill.

5. To remain in contact with Angie's parents, keep them informed of her condition, and provide as much support as possible.

Contract

The contract with this family, as with all hospice families, was two-fold. At the initial nursing assessment, a formal consent form explaining the nature of hospice care and services provided is signed by the patient or family member. Thus, the patient and family consents to the full range of hospice care, which includes social work.

An informal, verbal agreement occurs at the time of the initial social work assessment, when specific needs and problems are recognized and alternative approaches discussed with the patient or family (Rainey et al., 1984). In Angie's case, this involved both specific, concrete needs related to care at home and a broader agreement of availability if further assistance was needed either for additional concrete needs or for supportive intervention as time progressed. Both of these were needed and provided during the course of Angie's care.

Meeting Place

Meetings with Angie took place both in the hospital and at her home. The significant differences in these settings must be realized, since they have important implications for the worker-client relationship.

Upon entering a hospital, a person becomes a "patient" and is expected to conform to the "patient role": giving up individuality and control; being subservient; recognizing staff authority; being cheerful and cooperative; eating, sleeping, awakening, bathing, and visiting according to hospital routine and schedule; and, by all means, not asking too many questions. Such an artificial setting, with little or no privacy, is seldom conducive to productive meetings whether they take place in the patient's room or the worker's office.

At home, a person is in control of his or her environment again. He or she may eat favorite foods at any time, sit in a favorite rocking chair, get up and go to bed when desired, and be a person again. Familiar surroundings decrease anxiety and increase comfort. Visiting a client in the natural home setting is more conducive to verbalization of fears and concerns, and results in a more accurate appraisal of the total patient/family environmental situation.

All of this was true in Angie's case. At home, she was comfortable and content, less anxious and depressed, and she felt better. Meetings usually took place in the living room, where her hospital bed was, with the stereo on, in a cozy, relaxed atmosphere.

It should be noted, however, that in some circumstances, when meeting a client at home, the worker may be perceived as having less authority than in the hospital. When in a client's home, staff are on their "turf," and they feel (rightly so), more in control of the situation. The opposite is true when patients are hospitalized—they are on the staff's "turf." Workers who need the support of this institutional authority may find it difficult to function in home care.

Use of Time

In hospice care, the duration of the relationship is determined by several factors and is divided into two distinct phases. Customarily, the first phase begins with admission to the program and ends with the death of the patient. The second phase begins at the time of death, after which the family is invited to participate in the bereavement follow-up program.

Bereavement follow-up consists of two types of group involvement, and individual contacts by trained volunteers. One group is on-going and meets monthly. The other, more intense group, meets weekly for six weeks, providing education and support. The time limited group is held twice a year, and participants are encouraged to attend the on-going group when it ends. The purpose of both groups, which are facilitated by the social worker and bereavement coordinator, is education and encouragement of mutual self-help and support. Both are open to the community as well as to hospice families.

Volunteers with additional training in bereavement care are available to work with individuals considered to be at high risk for increased difficulties during the first year of bereavement. Referrals for additional counseling and therapy are made when indicated.

In addition, cards, notes and remembrances are sent during the first year to hospice families at holidays and other special times.

The initial social work contact with a patient and family at home to evaluate environmental and emotional needs generally lasts 1 to 1-1/2 hours, depending on individual needs and situations. Beyond this, time is spent as indicated in supportive intervention or in provision of concrete services. As indicated earlier, social service needs are frequently provided through collaboration and consultation with other team members.

Through experience, the discovery of the importance of time spent with hospice patients and families as a valuable element in hospice care cannot be diminished. After months or years of being rushed through doctor's offices, outpatient clinics, radiation departments, emergency rooms and similar places, families and patients need time to be listened to, to have questions answered and misunderstandings explained. Drinking coffee together around the kitchen table, listening while fears, hopes, memories, joys, dreams and struggles are shared is not an uncommon occurrence. This is part of building the trust necessary to provide quality hospice care. It means that hospice care can be very time consuming; yet to deny this opportunity to share is to deny the patient's humanity and dignity, which are the essence of hospice care.

Treatment Modality

In terms of social work, hospice care is generally not oriented toward "treatment" or "therapy." Approaches most frequently used include crisis intervention, task centered casework, and a nondirective, client-centered approach with much listening, supporting and teaching. The approach taken depends on individual situations, past histories, present coping mechanisms, existing support systems and similar considerations.

Stance of the Social Worker

The stance of the social worker is dependent upon many variables — the nature of the problem, the time factor (crisis, urgent, or on-going), the relationship with the patient and family, their coping abilities at the particular moment (these fluctuate considerably from day to day, from problem to problem), and their expectations of the staff (do they just need a listener, or is more direct help needed?).

Generally, in the advocacy role or in the provision of concrete services, the stance is likely to be direct and active. The caregiver is frequently so overwhelmed by the situation that an active role is indicated. In other situations, a nondirective, supportive approach is used, with much listening and reflecting. If it seems appropriate and situations are similar, personal experiences may be shared in a limited fashion (Millet, 1983).

Outside Resources

Most concrete services relate directly to necessary arrangements and equipment for care at home. Hospital beds, wheelchairs, bedside commodes, walkers, and dressings are frequently needed and are obtainable from the local American Cancer Society office. More specialized equipment is obtained from a rental company with twenty-four-hour service. When needed, help with finances is provided, and appropriate referrals made, with advocacy and assistance to follow through with referrals. Assistance is also provided in arranging for additional help at home, either in the form of a hired caregiver or volunteer help. Considerable time is also given to obtaining and explaining insurance benefits. The recent changes in types of coverage and how reimbursement is obtained have made this a major issue with patients and families as well as with programs. It is important to know what is covered and for how long, both so the program is reimbursed, and families are not left with large bills.

Reassessment

Reassessment is a continuing process because of the nature of care provided and its limited time. Formal assessment occurs at each weekly team meeting, but informally it occurs almost daily in some situations, depending on the patient's condition and the caregiver's coping abilities and support system. In Angie's case, for example, a major goal was to keep her at home as long as possible, but if her caregivers had reached their limit of endurance, hospitalization would have been necessary. During the last two weeks of her life, this was a real concern and was evaluated daily. There was a contingency plan ready to be put into effect, had it been necessary.

Transfer or Termination

Termination is difficult to define and discuss because it is more a process than an abrupt ending. Hospice care encompasses both patient and family and continues after the patient's death in the form of bereavement follow-up. Termination officially occurs at the end of the first year of bereavement, but a form of termination occurs at the time cf the patient's death. Obviously, the formalized aspect of patient care ends at this time, and families make a transition to the less intense bereavement program. Families remain in this phase of the program for varying lengths of time, but whether or not they choose to participate in the groups, contacts are made by the hospice program during the year following the patient's death, providing special remembrances of important dates and holidays.

Case Conclusion

It has now been over seven years since Angie's death. Occasional correspondence was received from Angie's parents, and they seemed to be coping fairly well. Bill apparently functioned well at work after Angie's death. His volunteer maintained contact with him, inviting him to participate in one of the groups, but Bill declined. His immaturity remained evident during this time. Shortly after the one year anniversary of Angie's death, a post card was received from Bill thanking us for the contacts, and telling us that he had remarried recently, and gave his new address in the area. No further word was heard from him, although he did indicate a desire to remain on the mailing list for the following year.

Differential Discussion

A more direct approach with Bill might have helped him to deal more effectively with his situation and the responsibilities involved. However, Bill had grown to adulthood shielded from having to deal with life's stresses and therefore had essentially no coping skills to work with. Angie was in our program for a little over three months, scarcely time to effect change in the learned responses of a lifetime, especially given the tragic nature of the situation.

Physically, Angie's needs were met and she received excellent care. Emotionally she was a private person and was reluctant to discuss her feelings and emotions in depth. She was frequently depressed about Bill's behavior but realized that she, too, had often shielded him from stress and responsibility during their short marriage. Toward the end, she seemed more able to accept his behavior.

Hospice patients come to us primarily for help with physical care and support. Some are reluctant to discuss emotional concerns and conflicts, others very open from the beginning.

This case was chosen for discussion primarily because it exemplifies the teamwork aspects of hospice care and the necessity for close collaboration to achieve desired goals. As Angie's family became less and less available, the hospice team essentially became her family. The efforts of each team member were crucial in providing quality care and allowing her to spend her last days at home in comfort and safety.

PRACTICE IN CONTEXT

The role of the social worker as a component of the hospice interdisciplinary team has been discussed within the limits of policy, organization, and technology. Within this model, organization and policy have the greatest effect on social work practice because the level of technology is relatively low, as compared to that in an intensive care unit, for example.

Since organizational structures are currently developed to maximize available reimbursement, organization and policy are very much interrelated. Both are also directly related to the fact that the hospice movement is still new and changing rapidly.

Direct service is the primary social work role discussed in this paper. It should be realized, however, that this is only one of several possible roles for social workers. Hospice programs continue to offer unique, innovative opportunities to be involved in management and administration, policy making, program development, education, research, lobbying and legislation as well as in direct service to patients and families.

In the seven years of hospice experience since Angie's death, much has been learned. One of the most important lessons has been to realize the need to work within the limits of human and organizational realities to insure the best care possible for the patient. Early in the hospice movement, there was a tendency to be overly idealistic, striving to be "all things to all people." With time and experience has come the reality that this is seldom possible. Priorities must be set, and the first priority is to help insure the best possible care for the patient in the safest environment. Ideally (and frequently) this is in the home setting with the family giving care. In reality, because of any number of human and organizational reasons, this is not always possible. In Angie's case, she was able to stay at home and receive excellent care, but her family was not able to provide that care. In other cases, the patient may have to be hospitalized or go to a nursing home for care. While less than ideal, these are the realities of our society and the health care system that are encountered daily.

Through all the changes of the recent years, the basic hospice philosophy and concept is unchanged. How it is implemented has changed, and will continue to change as it becomes more integrated with and accepted as a part of the overall health care system (Corr and Corr, 1983).

The ability to be flexible is a necessary characteristic of social workers and other staff in hospice care. Perhaps this is the trait that has enabled the hospice movement to change and grow so successfully in such a short time. Through all of its challenges and struggles, hospice continues to offer a wealth of knowledge and experience to its patients and families as well as to the rest of the health care system in areas of management of chronic pain and other symptoms, and in issues surrounding coping with all types of losses and end of life issues (Millet, 1979).

REFERENCES

Blumberg, B., Flaherty, M. and Lewis, J. (Eds.). *Coping with cancer.* Bethesda, MD: National Cancer Institute, NIH Publication #80-20801, 1980.

Brooks, C.H. and Smythe-Staruch, K. *Cost savings of hospice home care to third-party insurers.* Cleveland, Ohio: Case Western Reserve University School of Medicine, Dept. of Epidemiology and Community Health, 1983.

Buckingham, R.W. *The complete hospice guide.* N.Y.: Harper & Row, 1983.

Buckingham, R.W. and Lupu, D. "A comparative study of hospice services in the U.S." *American Journal of Public Health*, 72, 1982, pp. 455-463.

Caputi, M.A. and Heiss, W.A. "The DRG revolution." *Health and Social Work*, 9(1), Winter 1984, pp. 5-12.

Christ, G.H. "A psychosocial assessment framework for cancer patients and their families." *Health and Social Work*, 1983, pp. 57-64.

Corr, C.A. and Corr, D.M. (Eds.). *Hospice care: Principles and practice*. N.Y.: Springer Publishing Co., 1983.

Federal Register. Vol. 48, No. 243, December 16, 1983, pp. 56008-56036.

Garder, K. (Ed.). *Quality of care for the terminally ill: an examination of the issues*. Chicago: Joint Commission on Accreditation of Hosps., 1985.

Gibson, D.E. "Hospice: Morality and economics." *Gerontologist*, 24, Feb. 1984, p. 48.

Hospice Standards Manual. Joint commission on accreditation of hospitals, 1986, Chicago, IL, pp. 6-7.

Kerson, T.S. with Kerson, L.A. "Cancer." In *Understanding chronic illness*, T.S. Kerson with L.A. Kerson (Eds.). N.Y.: The Free Press, 1985, pp. 35-70.

Koff, T. *Hospice: A caring community*. Cambridge, MA: Winthrop Publishing Co., 1980.

Lack, S.A. "Characteristics of a hospice program of care." *Death Education*, 2(1-2), 1978, pp. 41-52.

Lack, S.A. and Buckingham, R. *First American hospice*. New Haven: Hospice, Inc., 1978.

Lusk, M.W. "The psychosocial evaluation of the hospice patient." *Health and Social Work*, 8(3), 1983, pp. 210-218.

Mack, R.M. "Lessons from living with cancer." *New England Journal of Medicine*, 311, 1984, pp. 1640-1644.

Meyerowitz, B.E., Heinrich, R.L. and Schag, C.C. "A competency-based approach to coping with cancer." In *Coping with chronic disease*, T.C. Burish and L.A. Bradley (Eds.). N.Y.: Academic Press, Inc., 1983, pp. 137-158.

Millett, N. "Hospice: A new horizon for social work." In *Hospice care: Principles and practice*. C.A. and D.M. Corr, (Eds.). New York: Springer Publishing Co., 1983, pp. 137-158.

_____. "Hospice: Challenging society's approach to death." *Health and Social Work*, 4(1), Feb. 1979, pp. 130-150.

_____. "Families have needs, too." In *Social work and terminal care*. L.H. Suszycki et al. (Eds.). New York: Praeger Publishers, 1984.

Moore, K. "Training social workers to work with the terminally ill." *Health and Social Work*, 9(4), Fall 1984, pp. 268-273.

Mor, V. and Lahberte, L. "Burnout among hospice staff." *Health and Social Work*, 9(4), Fall 1984, pp. 274-283.

Munley, A. *The hospice alternative: A new context for death and dying*. N.Y.: Basic Books, 1983.

Proffitt, L.J. "Hospice." In *Encyclopedia of social work*, 18th ed., Silver Spring, MD: NASW, 1987, pp. 812-816.

Simos, B.G. *A time to grieve: Loss as a universal human experience*. N.Y.: Family Service Association of America, 1979.

Torrens, P.R. *Hospice programs and public policy*. Chicago: American Hospital Publ., 1985.

Veatch, R.M. "DRGs and the ethical reallocation of resources." *Hastings Center Report*, 16(3), June 1986, pp. 32-40.

Wald, F.S., Foster, Z. and Wald, H.J. "The hospice movement as a health care reform." *Nursing Outlook*, 2(3), March 1980, pp. 173-178.

Wasow, M. "Get out of my potato patch: A biased view of death and dying." *Health and Social Work*, 9(4), Fall 1984, pp. 261-267.

Yasko, J.M. and Greene, P. "Coping with problems related to cancer and cancer treatment." In *The American Cancer Society Career Book*. Edited by A.I. Holleb. Garden City, New York: Doubleday and Company, Inc., 1986.

Zimmerman, J.M. *Hospice: Complete Care for the Terminally Ill*. Baltimore, MD: Urban and Schwarzenberg, 1981.

Part 6

Personal and Professional Roles

Introduction

No matter what the social worker's level of experience and expertise or degree of empathy, she can never stand in the shoes of the ill person or family member. Following are two chapters written by social workers who have personal experience with managing illness. The first chronicles a generation of experience with renal dialysis and the second, a like period with chronic schizophrenia. Obviously, very few of us are fortunate enough to have avoided the experience of illness, and we all apply knowledge derived from personal experience to our work. However, these contributions are unusual because both practitioners have worked in the specialties which they have experienced personally and are remarkably articulate and expressive about their experiences. I add these chapters because no matter how able the social worker, nothing is quite the same as being there. Consequently, an opportunity to learn from personally managed experience enhances one's skill.

Beyond "Survival by Machine": Reflections of a Spouse

Elisabeth Doolan
with Toba Schwaber Kerson

THE BEGINNING

In 1964, my husband, Tom, newly married, was told he had very little renal function left and would probably have only a few years to live. He was instructed to follow a very stringent diet in order to postpone total kidney failure until a program of chronic hemodialysis was established at the hospital where his physician was practicing.

Tom was the director of the export section of a small family business. Before his illness, he travelled extensively, but as he weakened he had to confine himself to desk work. During the following two years, Tom lost an enormous amount of weight and muscle tone, felt nauseated most of the time and gradually gave up all interest in life. He spent 1967 in and out of the hospital undergoing surgery and various means of dialysis, some quite crude and experimental. At the end of that year, Tom was unable to stand, walk or concentrate enough to sustain a conversation.

During this time, I had begun to learn about treatment approaches to kidney disease. One program at the University of Washington Hospital in Seattle had begun to train patients for home dialysis using a machine which required more hours of treatment but was less taxing to the patient. The Seattle group was said to be unusually supportive of patients and families and strongly committed to emotional as well as physical rehabilitation. When Tom failed to improve after several months of thrice weekly hemodialysis, I asked his nephrologist whether he would let us go to Seattle to try the Kiil

475

artificial kidney and be enrolled in the home training program. He agreed, and two weeks later, we were on our way to Seattle.

One week of treatment in Seattle improved Tom's mood and thinking. He was less irritable, more cooperative, could follow and participate in conversations for a longer time, and seemed to regain some of his zest for life. His blood studies were much better than they had been in months, and it looked as if we were going to make it. After one month in the hospital receiving daily dialysis and physical therapy to regain use of legs and feet affected by severe neuropathy, we moved to a motel apartment from which we went to the training center five days a week for treatment and education. Our choosing this institution for training meant that we accepted the policies and technological solutions of a particular group of nephrologists who were located two thousand miles away. Repercussions of that decision would be felt in our having to be more self-reliant and later retaining technological solutions which many considered outdated.

The training did not always go smoothly. The Seattle staff taught the patient first so that he would have the responsibility for his own life. He, in turn, under a nurse's supervision, was to teach his mate or helper. Then, patient and helper were to function as a team, with the patient as captain or leader. For us, however, the plan did not work very well.

Lack of adequate dialysis in the early stage of his illness had caused extremely high blood pressure, and he had experienced numerous seizures. His mind still seemed quite foggy at times, and he was slow in comprehending new ideas. The nerve damage to his feet and hands prevented his standing up or manipulating medical instruments or supplies with dexterity. Because of his physical and mental handicaps, it was difficult for Tom to learn new skills. Since he could not realistically be expected to be the leader of our team, the medical staff agreed to let me assume that role, with the condition that we would share responsibilities more equitably as Tom improved and returned to work.

I welcomed this decision. Home dialysis was our only chance of having a near normal life, and I found the procedure of dialysis an enormous challenge. It was an opportunity to learn, a test of my competence, a way of proving my love for Tom, and a means of regaining some control of our lives. After two months of training, Tom felt much better and everyone agreed we were ready to go home. I flew back to Philadelphia to set up the kidney machine and organize the medical supplies, and Tom joined me a few days later. In retrospect I am surprised that I was not apprehensive or anxious. On the contrary, I remember experiencing a sense of elation. I was actually eager to go ahead with our first dialysis.

Despite various crises, Tom made a remarkable recovery, gradually regaining strength and the ability to walk. In addition to providing stimulation, work helped him structure his days and enhanced his self-worth. Our expenses for that first year of home dialysis (1968) including treatments in hospitals, home training, and purchases of machine and supplies came to approximately eighteen thousand dollars. If Tom had not been a partner in a family business, if he had not collected a salary when he was not working, he would not have lived. I was grateful that Tom's financial situation allowed him to live, but I felt guilty about all of the other people who were deprived of live or who survived through public appeals, or by agreeing to participate in experimental treatments.

After a fairly smooth first year, dialysis was part of our lives. We decided we wanted a child and were elated when I became pregnant and gave birth to a healthy boy we named Gregory. When our son entered first grade, I entered graduate school in social work. For many years, despite the crises that most dialysis patients face, Tom felt fairly well, worked every day, thrived on the challenges of his business, enjoyed family life and did not mind his thrice-weekly dialysis schedule. After some years, I regarded dialysis as a necessary drudgery which was fit into our lives and was quite manageable most of the time. Our life had become almost "normal."

Our Dialysis Procedure

Initially, because we lived in a small apartment, the kidney machine was in our bedroom. We took off the carpeting, installed a linoleum floor and ran a few hoses to the bathroom for water supply and drainage. It was not the most romantic setting, but we managed this way for four years. Eventually, we built a house with a "kidney room" which adjoined our bedroom and was closed off when not in use. We dialyzed three nights a week for an average of eight hours. Because we did not use a blood pump, the blood flow through the dialyzer was slow.

We were often asked why we continued dialyzing for so many hours when the trend was to shorten each treatment. Tom found daytime dialyzing difficult, no matter how short the time period, and claimed that if he had to dialyze during the day, he would soon develop serious psychological problems. With our method, he could relax watching television in the first few hours of the treatment and eventually go to sleep. We both slept during dialysis, although not quite so well as on other nights.

Operating our first dialyzer was time consuming and frustrating. Sometimes hours were spent building and rebuilding the Kiil kidney before it finally tested properly. One particular hot summer Sunday, Tom was out of town attending a funeral and was to return home in time to be dialyzed. After Gregory, then an infant, was settled I proceeded to take the Kiil kidney apart to clean and rebuild it. Eight hours later, I realized I had spent the entire day taking the kidney apart and putting it together without success. The technicians at the training center were unavailable and the staff at our hospital were not familiar with the Kiil. To make matters worse, Greg had cried off and on all day. Exhausted and disgusted, I was angry with Tom for leaving me with a crying baby and a recalcitrant kidney.

On the whole, however, things were not that bad. I became adept at rapidly rebuilding the kidney and enjoyed the challenge of increasing my speed and solving problems. Preparing the machine became part of my household chores.

In the early 1970s, dialysis centers began to use artificial kidneys which were more expensive but smaller, presterilized, partly disposable, and easier to handle. Despite this advance, we persisted with our old method for eleven years because we rationalized that we were far from our training center and successful with the old procedure. In retrospect, I see that change was always difficult for me. Familiarity with the old method gave me a sense of control and security. Finally, I was forced into learning a new machine and disposable dialyzer because supplies for the Kiil were increasingly hard to find.

Transplantation

Invariably people ask why Tom never had a kidney transplant. Before the advent of immunosuppressant drugs, people in need of renal transplantation were dependent on a good tissue match of a close relative. Since Tom's only close relative, his brother, did not seem willing to be considered as a donor, transplantation was not a possibility in the earlier stages of Tom's disease. The advent of immunosuppressant therapy has made the transplantation of living relative and cadaveric kidneys highly successful, and our reasons were probably more emotional than logical. Tom remembered how close to death he had been before dialysis and was afraid to be in a similar condition again. He had seen friends reject a graft and subsequently become very ill. The transplantation statistics were not good enough for him until he became too debilitated and ill to have a transplant. Although Tom's life might not have appeared so good to others, he enjoyed every day of it. He believed that it would be foolish to "upset the apple cart" after almost two decades. While I felt sad and sometimes depressed, I recognized that his was a very personal decision.

Initially, I shared this thinking. As years went by, however, I could see the likelihood of a successful transplantation. I knew that if I had been the person with kidney disease, I would have chosen transplantation because I would have found the dependency on a machine and other people's good will for my care and survival too difficult to tolerate. Despite the risks, I would have wanted a chance to feel totally healthy and normal again.

Observations and Recommendations

People ask how we lived with End Stage Renal Disease for more than twenty years. Perhaps the best way to analyze our experience is to review the dimensions of our lives that were most supportive and those that were most difficult. At the beginning of Tom's illness we were newly married, in love, very devoted to each other. His care was at the center of our lives, and we had no other obligations. Our financial resources eased the adjustment to Tom's illness, paying for the best of medical care, as well as a nice house, a household helper and baby sitter, short pleasant trips, and graduate school tuition. All this compensated for some of the deprivations associated with renal dialysis.

Many of our personality characteristics were also helpful. There is no doubt that Tom's strong desire to live enabled him to ignore or forget that he had many limitations. He appeared surprised that anyone thought his illness influenced our lifestyle. He did, however, see himself as different from most other kidney patients, and he took pride in the fact that he had no psychological problems. His denial protected him from painful feelings and helped him to live with very real restrictions.

I would place myself in that obsessive-compulsive, somewhat parental and nurturing spouse pattern that is described in the literature as a good partner. In the dialysis situation I was often the "mother protector" and Tom was the "dependent child." This combination of roles may have contributed to our adaptation to home dialysis, but the resentment and unhealthy interactions it engendered meant we had to constantly watch and negotiate these roles.

The personality factors which served us well in dialysis also can create problems with intimacy. The patient who denies, takes pride in his independence, and acts aloof may detach himself and withdraw in order to avoid true intimacy or conflict with the nurturing, parental, perfectionistic spouse. This same spouse who appears to give excessive attention to detail, who worries and is over-sensitive and often controlling, is really in need of nurturing too. Physical and sexual limitations are also the lot of the spouse and the frustration and deprivation can stir up resentment, anger and rage followed by intense guilt. The equal give and take of a healthy marriage is much more difficult to achieve in a dialysis marriage.

We also had great confidence in the physicians and staff who treated us with respect and involved us in decision making. They knew how to rejoice in progress and support us when Tom was experiencing setbacks. While Tom was in intensive care, the renal social worker and liaison psychiatrist were willing to sit with me and let me talk about my pain, my doubts and my conflicts. Still, dependency on the medical staff and the institution for survival was threatening, and our independent and overly cautious attitude could have been viewed as offensive by the medical staff. Whenever I sensed tension and lack of support, I became defensive. I was angry at first, then sad, and finally afraid we would be abandoned.

Over the years, several groups and organizations have been important to us, and at different times, I have been an active participant and board member defining policy and instituting programs, a professional renal social worker using their services, and a recipient of service. Tom and I helped to found PAK (People on Artificial Kidneys) which acted as a support, education and advocacy group. PAK eventually became a chapter of NAPHT (National Association of Patients on Hemodialysis and Transplantation) which provides support, education and advocacy on local and national levels and publishes a quarterly news magazine for its members called *Renal Life*. NAPHT has been instrumental in the passage of PL 92-603 which allows for reimbursement for dialysis and transplant under Medicare. The American Kidney Foundation was formed in 1971 to provide direct financial assistance for individuals with chronic renal disease. Finally, the National Kidney Foundation has as its goal the irradication of diseases of the kidney and urinary tract and sponsors research and many services such as education, monitoring of programs and organ donor programs.

While organizations such as PAK, NAPHT, AKF, NKF sometimes appear to duplicate efforts or compete, they each serve a particular purpose and are beginning to see possibilities for united strength. They have each affected our experience with renal disease, and they continue to influence the experiences of thousands of patients and families by providing them with information, support and hope for improvement in the quality of their lives.

Just as returning to work was important for Tom, renewing outside interests and resuming a professional career proved to me that life did not revolve completely around a dialysis machine. Perhaps the greatest step in the direction of normalcy was having a child. Gregory was fourteen years old when his father died. He provided us (and still provides me) with many joys and continuously taught us to take our minds off ourselves. He showed us that we could have moments of fun and enjoyment despite Tom's illness and the regimen. Of course, Gregory had to live with dialysis as well. I remember once when he was a tiny boy, he told me that when he grew up and had a home of his own, it would have a dialysis room just like ours. We talk freely, Greg and I, and I think that he is a fine, healthy young man, perhaps stronger for his early experiences.

Although long term dialysis is certainly manageable, it would be wrong to give the impression that my husband and I found dialysis unstressful. Despite our inclination to be strong and capable, we often felt frustrated and anxious. The stress was real. There is never any reprieve in dialysis. If there is insufficient support from medical staff and friends, the stress builds and becomes increasingly difficult to tolerate.

Over the years, we had our share of crises which revived all the initial pain, fear and anxiety interfering with our functioning for weeks. Major surgery, episodes of internal bleeding, frightening but probably safe postponements of dialysis sessions due to mechanical problems and accidents such as serious blood loss and bad reactions while Tom was on the machine represented real setbacks.

During these crises we assumed complementary roles. Sometimes, Tom remained very calm and supported me when the situation required fast decisions and prompt action on my part, sometimes, I could calm him when he was overly anxious, and other times we lost patience with each other and fought. Although we coped, crises never became routine. Every one was frightening because it could be the last. They were a painful reminder of this precarious life.

Because dialysis is so consuming and people's reactions are often uncomfortable, patients and families can become isolated. My husband found that people did not know what to say to us or what to expect of him. To compensate for intense feelings of anxiety and deprivation, the literature says people develop "primitive urges towards psychological closeness." Spouses often use the pronoun "we" instead of referring to the dialyzed person by name. I know that while Tom was on dialysis I frequently said, "When we were on the machine last night" or "what are the results of our blood tests?" My husband sometimes asked, "Have you found out what is wrong with your machine?" This kind of closeness can perpetuate isolation and deprive one of individuality. The balance of caring and maintaining autonomy requires painful choices.

The Last Years

In the summer of 1983, two months after Tom had decided to retire, he fractured his right hip. The next year and a half was to be the most difficult of our lives. Tom underwent hip surgery three times and multiple additional hospitalizations. No sooner would he begin to recover when he would face a new fracture, more internal bleeding. After each hospitalization, he would try very hard to make a comeback, working with a physical therapist several times a week, forcing himself to go out with his walker or wheelchair, but there were constant setbacks. We were both getting tired of the struggle. Although we did not talk about it we must have felt that nothing would ever be good again.

During one of Tom's admissions to the hospital where I worked, he had bled from esophageal varices, dilated veins in which valves become incompetent so blood flow can become reversed. With great courage and sensitivity, the nephrologist on whose service I was a social worker explained that Tom might some day die from internal bleeding if these varices bled extensively. Tom did not know this. He knew how to protect himself when he sensed that not much could be done about a problem, and he only asked questions about his medical condition when there was some specific solution. For many months, we just hobbled along with Tom hoping he would never again have to be hospitalized because he was so frightened of hospitals, and me hoping that I would have enough time to get help when the varices bled.

In December, 1984, three days before Christmas, Tom woke after dialysis feeling very weak, anxious and irritable. His blood pressure was so low, I knew he must have been bleeding and convinced him to let me take him to the emergency room. He was admitted to the intensive care unit for his last and most difficult hospitalization.

The End Stage

The phone rang 8 o'clock Saturday morning, flooding me with anxiety, causing my heart to pound. The phone always made me jump when Tom was in the hospital, and this time, I was particularly weary because Tom and I had spent six weeks on a physical and emotional rollercoaster.

After eighteen years of dialysis, three hip fractures in the previous twelve months, episodes of bleeding and various surgical procedures, Tom had been admitted to the hospital for surgery to arrest internal bleeding caused by esophageal varices. The surgery had left him disoriented, confused, anxious, agitated and subject to hallucinations. Despite his confusion, he could at times appear logical. On those occasions, accusing me of never being available to him, he could forcefully demand that I be there all the time or that I convince his doctors to let him go home with me because he was better off at home. When he did that, I became confused myself and did not know what to believe or do.

It has taken me years to understand that he often behaved in this manner when he was in the hospital, and that the irritability and demands were, in fact, a protective cover for his fears and confusion. His physicians explained that the disorientation was caused by severe encephalopathy which could only be controlled with medication which caused constant diarrhea. The diarrhea left him so sore that he cried whenever he was being cleaned. He had wasted away to skin and bones, and his body ached all over. Tom's nephrologist began to vaguely discuss the possibility of discontinuing dialysis, but I had no sense of who would be responsible for making that decision if Tom was too confused to decide for himself. As a nephrology social worker, I have participated in team and family conferences where such decisions were made, and I knew I did not want to be responsible for making that decision about Tom.

As I answered the phone that Saturday morning, I was surprised to hear Tom's voice. I couldn't believe that he was alert and clear. He sounded calm, pleasant but concerned about why he was still in the hospital, why he had so much diarrhea, whether the diarrhea would persist and how assaulted he felt. I cannot remember exactly how the conversation proceeded, but I do remember that we began to talk about the possibility of discontinuing dialysis. I hurriedly dressed and rushed over the hospital, and Tom said "I think the time has come to stop everything. I want to go home. I want to be home in my nice sunny room."

As we talked, I wanted to be sure he understood that giving up dialysis meant dying. I remembered how scared he had always been about dying. Memories of his jokes about death came back to me, and I asked directly, "Do you know what this means?" I could tell by his answer that he clearly understood, and suddenly I felt an overwhelming sense of urgency. Because it was Saturday, his physician was not there, and I couldn't ask him whether we could go home right away, but I sensed that Tom might lose some clarity of thought. I wanted him to enjoy himself at home before he died, to be with us in the house he liked so much away from the cold hospital environment where he felt attacked and isolated. On the one hand, I thought we should wait until the following Monday when Tom would be dialyzed and we could discuss this with his nephrologist. On the other hand, I felt that we didn't have time to plan, time to waste. It was time to make a decision. Some weeks earlier, the nephrology social worker said, " When the times comes, you will know deep down in your heart, and you will be able to make the right decision." I asked Tom whether he wanted to go home immediately. Saying yes, he told me to call his brother so that he could say he had decided to go home and that he would not undergo dialysis treatment any longer.

After Tom spoke to his brother, I asked the floor nurse to locate the physician on call whom I informed of our decision. Because he knew us, as well as Tom's condition and prognosis, he said he would go along with whatever plan we had. In an hour, we were on our way home in an ambulance accompanied by the private duty nurse who had taken care of Tom in the hospital.

When we got home, Tom was elated to be back in his nice, sunny room and to find Gregory, our son, whom I had called earlier. It was like a happy reunion. All three of us acted as if we had escaped something terrible and this was going to last for a long time. We hugged and kissed and talked euphorically about the things we would do together during the following week. Later, when Tom rested, I realized I had to make some practical arrangements. Since I wanted to be available to him completely, I asked my social work colleague to manage my responsibilities and inform everyone that I would not be in until after Tom's death. I also decided that Gregory should continue to go to school everyday.

After Tom's first night at home, I realized I would never be able to care for him by myself. I had been up all night, holding his hand, turning him, changing his pajamas, washing him. On Sunday morning, I called my friend who directs a hospice program for a recommendation of good nurses with experience in terminal illness. An hour later, she called back to ask tactfully how I planned to manage alone. She reminded me that what I needed to be was Tom's wife, not also his nurse and social worker, and suggested hospice care.

Hospice was a crucial element during that last week. Regular attendance by a physician and nurses meant Tom did not suffer and everything could be very peaceful for him. Hospice allowed me to devote myself totally to him, be available emotionally, hold his hand when he needed me, talk, listen, and let him rest. The hospice team was there for all of us.

Tom wanted his brother, nephew and niece to come and say goodbye to him, and they visited very briefly on Sunday. In retrospect, I see that day as almost surreal. I was in such a state of euphoria that I did not quite realize what was happening. The following day, two of Tom's favorite physicians came to say goodbye: the internist who had diagnosed his renal disease twenty years earlier and the surgeon who had performed all of his procedures over that long period. Both men had become good friends of ours, and their approval was very important to Tom who needed to know that by discontinuing dialysis, he was not disappointing two friends who had fought along with him for his life for so many years. By reviewing his struggles, accomplishments and happy times, they were able to reassure him that it was right to recognize when the time had come to let go.

It was an unreal week, sad and beautiful at the same time. Even though it was February, we had some sunny days. Tom's room faced east, and when the morning sun poured in, he talked about the warmth of the sun on his face. I sat next to him. We held hands and then he would rest again. Greg would come home from school and talk about his day. That week, Greg, who had never been an athlete, played basketball and was proud to report that he had made several baskets. He received an acceptance from the high school which Tom wanted him to attend, and Tom was delighted.

I do not think that I realized that after that week he would never be with us again. Now as I talk and write about it, I'm overwhelmed with emotion. At the time, I must have totally isolated my feelings to be available to him and probably to protect my suffering.

Tom began to sleep more and more and his periods of alertness were growing shorter, but while he was alert we had wonderful conversations and I felt very close to him. He would tell me what I should do when he was no longer there. Up to the end, Tom wanted to be in control. All his life he had been a man who hade his own decisions, and now, in the last week of his life, he still behaved in the same manner. He reminded me to order baseball tickets so we would continue to attend the Phillies games and think of him. He also told me to make sure I would always have some champagne in the house since I loved champagne and it would be good to have a glass whenever I was too sad. One day, he began to cry about Gregory's being able to grow up without his parents. I reminded him that I would be there for Gregory, and with a smile, he turned to me and said, "Oh, that's right. I had forgotten you were going to stay here, that you were not coming with me."

Sometimes, Tom would start to fantasize about a wonderful miracle which would make him well. One day, he asked me if perhaps we could give our money to a charity in the hope of producing a miracle. At those times, I would hold his hand and remind him that the miracle had already happened. He was home with us, and not suffering. We loved him, and I would make sure that he would not be hurt any longer and would go in peace. After these conversations, he would rest again. I would look at him and be surprised that I still loved him so much despite all the changes in that body. I wanted to crawl into his bed and have him hold me and tell me that I had been a good wife, but I also knew that he did not want to be touched and needed to detach himself. Once he asked me why I was not letting him go home. Thinking he was confused, I told him he was home, and he replied, "You know what I mean."

Tom was intent on doing everything for himself, being in control, sitting up, eating, drinking, being washed or not washed on his terms. When the nurses at times insisted on adhering to their schedule, I had to remind them that he had the right to decide what was good for him as he always had. The night before his death, I left the house for the first time that week to get suppositories at the hospital in case Tom could no longer swallow medication. Gregory walked over with me, and we talked about Tom's imminent death. Gregory reminded me that five years earlier I had come to school to tell him that Tom had had a heart attack and might not survive. He thought then that he would lose his father, and he felt fortunate now to have had his father for fourteen years of his life.

I went to sleep late that night, and at three o'clock in the morning, I felt the nurse tapping my shoulder. She said, "It won't be long now." I quickly went to Tom's room. His breathing was very shallow. I took his hand and waited. Ten minutes later, his breathing stopped. Everything was quiet and peaceful, sad and beautiful. I felt a great sense of relief. Tom would never again have to suffer, and I would never again have to worry about him.

It has been two years since Tom's death. Although it is still painful for me to speak of the events, interactions and feelings we experienced during eighteen years of dialysis, time, some emotional distance and professional experience have contributed to my understanding how we managed to survive those years. In retrospect, I feel we functioned fairly well, and considering our lack of sophistication about the medical system at the beginning of our "career in dialysis," we made good use of internal and external resources; the new technology which was developed in time to save my husband's life and governmental policies which insured payment for treatment. Although we did not have the support of a close extended family (my family is in Europe where I was raised, and Tom has only one brother), access to organizations offering information and support allowed us to develop a network of friends and supportive professionals. Gradually, we learned to deal with the medical system. When we sensed a lack of coordination, we requested meetings to discuss Tom's medical condition and participate in decisions. We assumed responsibility for our lives.

From an emotional perspective, the road was always more difficult for me, because Tom was more adaptable than I, and I tended to assume more responsibility than he did for his treatment. It is clear to me that denial helped us to survive these years. To some extent, we believed that I would always be able to take care of him and maintain his life. I miss him.

REFERENCES

Brown, C.J. and Ryersbach, V. "Vocational rehabilitation for dialysis and transplant patients." *Health and Social Work*, 5(2), Spring 1980, pp. 22-26.

Campbell, A. and Campbell J. "Marital approach to dialysis and transplantation." *NAPITT News*, Feb. 1977, pp. 8-11.

Carosella, J. "Picking up the pieces: The unsuccessful kidney transplant." *Health and Social Work*, 9(2), Spring 1984, pp. 142-152.

Council of Nephrology Social Workers: Guidelines for clinical practice, 1986.

Evans, R.W. et al. "The quality of life of patients with end-stage renal disease." *The New England Journal of Medicine*, 312, 1985, pp. 553-559.

Faris, M.H. *When your kidneys fail*. Los Angeles, Calif.: National Kidney Foundation of Southern California, 1981.

Fortner-Frazier, C.L. *Social work and dialysis: The medical and psychosocial aspects of kidney disease*. Berkeley: University of California Press, 1981.

Green, G.J., Pedley, J. and Littlewood, J. "Coping with chronic renal failure." *British Journal of Social Work*, 16(2), 1986, pp. 203-222.

Holden, M.O. "Dialysis or death: The ethical alternatives." *Health and Social Work*, 5(2), Spring 1980, pp. 18-21.

Krakauer, H. "The recent U.S. experience in the treatment of end-stage renal disease by dialysis and transplantation." *The New England Journal of Medicine*, June 30, 1983, p. 308.

Kress, H.W. "What comes after the psychosocial assessment? Casework interventions with chronic dialysis patients." *Perspectives*, 4(1), Winter 1982, pp. 11-16.

Lancaster, L.E. (Ed.). *The patient with end-stage renal disease*, 2nd. ed. N.Y.: John Wiley & Sons, 1984.

Macklin, R. "Ethical issues in treatment of patients with end-stage renal disease." *Social Work in Health Care*, 9(4), Fall 1984, pp. 11-20.

Maher, B.A., et al. "Psychosocial aspects of chronic hemodialysis: The National Cooperative Dialysis Study." *Kidney International*, 23 (Supplement), 1983, pp. 550-557.

Mailick, M.D. and Ullman, A. "A social work perspective on ethical practice in end-stage renal disease." *Social Work in Health Care*, 9(4), Winter 1984, pp. 21-31.

Medicare coverage of kidney dialysis and kidney transplant services (booklet). U.S. Department of Health and Human Services, Health Care Financing Administration, Pub. No. HCFA 10128, 1987.

Moskop, J.C. "The moral limits to federal funding for kidney disease." *Hastings Center Report*, 17(2), 1987.

NAPHT. *The voice of all kidney patients* (pamphlet).

National Kidney Foundation, Inc. (pamphlet), 1986.

Nichols, K.A. and Springford, V. "The Psycho-social stressors associated with survival by dialysis." *Behaviour Research and Therapy*, 22(5), 1984, pp. 563-574.

O'Brien, M.E. "Effective social environment and hemodialysis adaptation: A panel analysis." *Journal of Health and Social Behaviour*, 21(4), 1980, pp. 360-370.

Palmer, S.E., Canzona, L. and Wai, L. "Helping families respond effectively to chronic illness: Home dialysis as a case example." *Social Work in Health Care*, 8(1), Fall, 1982, pp. 1-14.

———. "Finances and adaptation to illness: A study of home dialysis patients." *Social Worker-Travailler Social*, 53(2), 1985, pp. 57-60.

Peterson, K.J. "Integration of medical and psychosocial needs of the home hemo-dialysis patient: Implications for the nephrology social worker." *Social Work in Health Care*, 9(4), 1984, pp. 33-44.

———. "Psychosocial adjustment of the family caregiver: Home hemodialysis as an example." *Social Work in Health Care*, 10(3), 1985, pp. 15-32.

Piening, S. "Family stress in diabetic renal failure." *Health and Social Work*, 9(2), 1984, pp. 134-141.

Polts, A., Tokuda, K. and Fisher, D. "Renal dialysis: Two views." *Practice Digest*, 3(4), 1981, pp. 20-23.

Procci, W.R. and Martin, D.J. "Effect of maintenance hemodialysis on male sexual performance." *Journal of Nervous and Mental Disease*, 176(6), 1985, pp. 366-377.

Ruchlin, H.S. "The public cost of kidney disease." *Social Work in Health Care*, 9(4), 1984, pp. 1-9.

Sherwood, R.J. "Compliance behaviour of hemodialysis patients and the role of the family." *Family Systems Medicine*, 1(2), Summer 1983, pp. 60-72.

Smirnow, V. (ed.). *Nephrology resource directory*, 1986-1987-1988. Bethesda, MD: Virgil Smirnow Associates.

Smith, M.D., Hong, B.A. and Feldman, R.D. "An assessment of the social networks of patients receiving maintenance therapy for end-stage renal disease." *Perspectives*, 7, 1985-1986, pp. 49-56.

Steinglass, P. et al. "Discussion groups for chronic hemodialysis patients and their families." *General Hospital Psychiatry*, 4(1), 1982, pp. 7-14.

Willix, I.G. "The choice for kidney patients should be up to them." Letter to the Editor, *New York Times*, March 2, 1981.

He's Schizophrenic and the System Is Against Us: Reflections of a Troubled Parent and Professional

Mona Wasow

> What's so terrible about schizophrenia is that there is no help anywhere. And if you do get to see someone, they only ask you what you did wrong.
>
> *Parent of a schizophrenic child*

Chronic schizophrenia is a dread disease with no known cure. It strikes 1 to 2 percent of the population the world over, and there is now ample evidence that its etiology is largely genetic and biochemical. With many other serious diseases, parents usually get prompt and sympathetic help when they ask for it. Sometimes there is little that can be done, but the medical model is used to intervene as soon as possible to prevent further deterioration. Only in mental illness is this now reversed in a strange and terrible way. Mental illness seems to have fallen into the hands of the legal profession, under the name of civil rights. In our zeal to protect human freedoms, we have created a legal climate in which mentally ill patients are free to "die with their rights on." The new mental health laws prevent involuntary medications and involuntary hospitalizations. They were designed out of a scientific and humane concern "to protect the rights of mental patients and to insure that unwanted, difficult people are not dumped into mental hospitals to be forgotten" (Wasow, 1978, p. 128). This, in principal, is a good idea and no doubt has spared unnecessary loss of freedoms for many people. But the law has gone to an extreme which now prevents help to those in desperate need.

PERSONAL INVOLVEMENT

My son David was born in 1957, a beautiful, big, healthy, brown-eyed boy. It was surely one of the most joyous days of my life. My first personal encounter with the mental health system came in 1972, the year David was 15. Something was wrong: despite his desire to do well, our lovely, bright son was failing in school. He was behaving very erratically, and his moods swung from extreme happiness to acute depression. I took him to see Dr. A., a well-known psychiatrist in town. Dr. A spent one hour with the boy and referred him to a child psychiatrist. The specialist spent two hours, charged us $100, and declared David to be "a fine, intact youngster." What a relief—the specialist must be right!

By the next year, however, things were much worse. David was now a truant, and his mood swings were even greater. He was also actively hallucinating and thought that "people" were planning to destroy him. He told us with great agitation that he was going to take a gun and go north where he would find food to save all the starving people of the world.

David began to wander away from the house for days at a time — usually barefoot and without money or food. He offered no explanation of where he had been except to say that he was headed for Alaska. He looked exhausted.

We were all badly frightened and felt we had lost control over the situation. I took David back to Dr. A, who told me, "Your son has an inability to screen out sensory perceptions . . ." A year later, however, he admitted to us that he had seen that David was schizophrenic at that time. Was he afraid of labelling our son? He never shared that diagnosis with us, he only spoke of "sensory perceptions."

This fear of labeling occurs again and again in the mental health field. Labeling people is harmful, we are told. Certainly labeling has been abused, and it can be harmful. But it can also be useful. Refusal to give the disease a name will not help the schizophrenic.

In my own case, ignorance helped neither David nor myself. A paragraph from my personal journal reads:

My God, what is happening to our little David? Those were hallucinations last night! Is this what R.D. Laing calls "a different way of looking at life"? Or is David mentally ill? Is it bad genes, or bad parenting? I know these are futile, irrelevant questions. But we must get *help*! I'm so scared. (Wasow, 1978, pp. 135-136)

My case, unfortunately, is all too typical. In 1973, when David was sixteen and "schizophrenia" was finally diagnosed, we were told that medications were an absolute necessity to prevent further deterioration. At that time David was still able to function reasonably well. He said, rather typically for a schizophrenic: "I will not take meds. I am not sick."

Following is an excerpt from a letter I wrote to "that month's" psychiatrist during a period when we were able to get David admitted to the hospital "through the back door."

Dear Dr. B:

A note of explanation as to why I've temporarily stopped coming to family therapy sessions on Tuesdays. I've lost hope — it seems so futile. I'd like to suggest we try something new.

You say that David has a lifelong pattern of holding other people responsible for his life. Therefore, you will attempt to get him to take responsibility by not taking it for him. As a theory, that makes sense. But suppose he really is *not* capable of this? Then it's like insisting that a cripple walk. I've thought about this a great deal, trying to understand the pattern of David and our family over the past 16 years, and I think you have cause and effect mixed up. Perhaps other people have always directed David's life because he's been unable to cope himself. There is another case of schizophrenia in the family, and there may be a genetic component here. It seems to me, and to others I've talked to who have known David since birth, that he never "would have made it," even to age 12, without the extra protection he was given.

The reason I dwell on this is because of the rapid deterioration that has set in since we withdrew our support and direction. To me, David's deterioration indicates that we're on the wrong track. In January 1973 . . . my husband and I gave up control, and David was essentially on his own. We were friendly, but there was very little contact with David. We did stay out of his life at this time, just as you are doing at the hospital. It was between January and June that he went from "intact" to really sick.

When we put him in the hospital, he still was largely intact. It seems to us the last three months have seen steady deterioration. I was shocked when he came home last weekend — he eats like an animal, he takes no care of himself physically (unbathed, hair matted and filthy), he doesn't talk at all, and he seems profoundly depressed. Also, he has active hallucinations.

Please understand, I think you are a fine human being and a professional. God knows I missed the boat on David for years. And I know that there are no correct answers for this kind of mental problem. I am panicked. I love my kid, and I want us to try another direction before it's too late. There's nothing to lose.

. . . I truly believe (and, I guess, this is a professional difference of opinion between us) that it would be helpful to David to be told: "I am the doctor. You are the patient. You are sick. Doctors make sick people well. I am going to make you well. Do as I say." The kid is panicked and feels hopeless and helpless. I think that at this point he needs someone to take control temporarily, because he doesn't seem to have the hope, faith, or ability to do it on his own.

Please let me hear from you soon. I am writing instead of talking because I'm so terribly upset. (Wasow, 1978, pp. 139-141)

For the following four years we lived an indescribable nightmare as we watched our beloved son turn into a suffering, terrified psychotic. Every doctor said he must have medicine. Everywhere we turned the law said, "No, we must protect his civil rights." Can you imagine the law determining whether or not you could give antibiotics or a blood transfusion to a child in need of surgery? After four years our son was a psychotic vegetable, unable to feed or clothe himself, wandering about on highways in front of traffic. There really are no words to describe the pain, suffering, panic, and destruction of those days, for all of us. Madness reigned supreme, both in our son and in the mental health care system. *The dominant concern of the mental health system was to follow the law, not to help David.* Finally David stepped in front of a car on the highway and was officially judged "incompetent" under the Wisconsin mental health law that provides for involuntary commitment for treatment — four years too late.

He was committed to a hospital and responded beautifully to medications; within a few days he was without psychotic symptoms, feeling deep relief, and able to take care of his basic needs. He was certainly not normal, but he was greatly improved and remained so for the next six months.

Under the new mental health laws, a case must be reviewed in the courts every six months. Even after having gone through it twice in the last four years, I cannot quite believe what followed: David was declared "competent." He went off his medications and slowly but surely became desperately ill again. In the next three years the cycle was repeated; only it was even worse. Pleading with doctors and lawyers about what had happened in the past and what was obviously happening again was in vain.

Let me skip the horror of those seven years and get to the details of May 1980. David was wandering about in a psychotic state, eating out of garbage cans, hallucinating, living in a terror I do not suppose I understand. One night, perhaps as a desperate plea for help, he attempted to jump out of a tenth story window.

Good news! Now he could be declared "dangerous to self or others," and the crisis intervention team was called. They were called at 8 P.M. and arrived at midnight. But now there was a new problem: by midnight David was catatonic. As such, he was not considered "dangerous," and the crisis team left. The following day was a repeat, and this time the crisis team said "hospitalize him." He was then handcuffed and put in a police car, where he spent the next six hours being rejected by every major hospital in Madison, Wisconsin. Finally, he was accepted into a hospital twenty miles outside of the city.

The following week, two court hearings were held to determine whether or not he was mentally ill and in need of care. The local mental health board had lawyers there to look after his civil rights. There was no physician there to look after his health.

Therein lies the crux of this issue: the battle is civil rights versus health care. In every other illness, medical intervention is used at the earliest possible moment. Only in mental illness does the law dictate that such intervention can only be used voluntarily or at the end stage of the illness.

Now it is 1987: My 28-year-old son is a success statistic in a model community treatment program for the chronically mentally ill (CMI). He is a success because he has been rehospitalized only once in the 12 years of his mental illness. He is very quiet and unobtrusive and does not bother anyone.

He had been living on his own in a one-room apartment, but I brought him into my home a few days ago to get him ready for a National Institute of Mental Health (NIMH) research project, where I know he will get adequate food and shelter and humane care. He is filthy and very skinny; he has boils on his body and is essentially mute. There was no toilet paper in his room, no food, no sheets on the mattress; the chaos in the room was congruent with the chaos in his poor sick mind.

He has lived in 15 different places in 12 years: three times with relatives, four times in a room by himself, twice at the YMCA in two different group homes, once in jail for 6 weeks while waiting for a court hearing to determine placement (that was his only crime: truancy—no place to live), once in a room with a roommate, once in an unlocked institution for 130 retarded and mentally ill people, and now off to the NIMH project. There were also two hospitalizations, one for 4 months and one for 1 month, but I do not count those. His case is quite typical for a CMI person. Moves are stressful even for people in good health. Imagine what all that moving does to a frightened, fragile, mentally ill person.

None of our model community treatment programs would consider my son or others like him a "success." They understand that rehospitalization should not be the only outcome criterion—that quality of life, patient satisfaction, and social functioning all need to be considered. But the *reality* of the situation is that despite massive deterioration, the mental health system as a whole does not provide him asylum.

So unless he commits an outwardly violent act, my son gets listed as a "success" in the deinstitutionalization movement. That is not how he looks to me. I think he looks like a giant, broken plastic throwaway toy. And he breaks my heart. (Wasow, 1986, pp. 162-167)

There is nothing more I can say or do for my poor, desperately ill son or the thousands upon thousands of others who suffer like him.

CURRENT KNOWLEDGE ABOUT SCHIZOPHRENIA

It is not the domain of this paper to describe what the syndrome of schizophrenia is, but very briefly, according to Mendel (1976), there are three major disabilities which are present at the same time over an extended period. These are: (1) inability to manage anxiety, (2) disastrous interpersonal relationships, and (3) failure of "historicity" (the ability to learn from experience).

Biochemical and genetic research of the past thirty years or so points strongly in the direction of schizophrenia's being a physical disease. Causes are still unknown and may very well be multiple – a combination of physical and psychological. But surely, at the present time, there is little doubt that process schizophrenia is largely a genetically determined disorder. One difficulty that has plagued genetic research in schizophrenia is the lack of clearly identifiable biochemical markers. There are other difficulties having to do with problems in diagnosis that puzzle both genetic and biochemical researchers. But this research holds more water than the psychodynamic theories of the 1940s and 1950s.

Unfortunately for schizophrenics and unfortunately for the direction of research in this area, professional thinking has leaned heavily on psychodynamic theories of both causation and cure. Not only did this lead down many blind alleys, but it also has led to the unfounded assumption that bad parenting causes schizophrenia. Parents are hearing this assumption from the professionals, and it is hurting them deeply. As recently as 1969, well-known authorities (Bateson, Jackson, Haley, and Weakland) were expounding the "double bind" theory, in which schizophrenics were seen as victims being driven crazy by the double messages of their parents:

> We do not assume that the double bind is inflicted by the mother alone, but that it may be done either by the mother alone or by some combination of mother, father, and/or siblings. (Bateson et al., 1969)

All of their data came from schizophrenia patients and their families who had come in for treatment, already accepting themselves as guilty, so to speak.

When looking at psychodynamic theories, we must remember that clinical practice often lags many years behind new theoretical developments. Many of today's professionals were trained with yesterday's theories, have not kept up with the more recent research, and are consequently still blaming parents for their offspring's schizophrenia. This attitude, more than any other, is turning parents away from professionals and making them very angry.

WHY SUCH ANGER?

Why do parents of schizophrenics experience so much anger? The first thought that comes to mind is that the tendency to be angry and frustrated is just there for parents of *all* defective children — the "Why me, oh God?" syndrome. While part of this may be true, it is not enough to explain the extent of rage toward professionals found among parents of schizophrenics. In fact, in a study done on parental versus professional views of the adjustment of parents of mentally retarded (MR) children (Wikler, Wasow, and Hatfield, forthcoming), just the opposite was found to be true! That is, the professionals, in this case social workers, were feeling frustrated that they could not be more helpful to the parents. The parents, however, perceived the professionals as being quite helpful. The parents were not only not angry, they were grateful for the help.

What, then, are the differences? I would suggest several. In the first place, mental retardation is rightfully seen as a largely fixed condition. You can maximize what potential there is, but you cannot change the condition. With schizophrenia, professionals are still thinking in terms of rehabilitation and "cure." But there is, at this point, no cure for schizophrenia (Mendel, 1976), and to lead parents to believe in one is an unending cruelty. Parents are constantly being led into false hopes. "If only I did this . . . or that. If only . . . if only . . ."

There is another marked difference. Parents of MR children are not blamed for the retardation. It is accepted and known that it could happen to anyone. But parents of schizophrenics are blamed, sometimes overtly, more often subtly. However it is done, that guilt-producing blame is clearly the greatest heartache of them all, next to losing the child to mental illness.

Another major complaint from parents is the lack of knowledge about the disease on the part of many professionals. Information about schizophrenia is one of the things parents need most. Thankfully, there are organizations that provide it and more.

ORGANIZATIONS THAT HAVE PROVED HELPFUL

The National Alliance for the Mentally Ill

On September 7-9, 1979, 275 representatives of parent support and advocacy groups for the chronically mentally ill (CMI) from 28 states and Canada met in Madison, Wisconsin. In a remarkable display of unity and concern, they established the first National Alliance for the Mentally Ill. This alliance and the hundreds of local chapters from which it grew developed in large part out of dissatisfaction both with professionals and with the mental health delivery system. Its objectives are two-fold: (1) to fight for better care for the mentally ill through better legislation, better housing, adequate money, increased research, etc.; and (2) to provide emotional support for families of the mentally ill. Many local chapters of the alliance are quite new, but they are a very important resource to know about.

Nonprofessionals May Be Better Than Professionals

There are many examples of helpful and impressive work coming out of nonprofessional groups: Alcoholics Anonymous, Al-Anon, groups of parents of the mentally retarded, and so on — too many to enumerate in this paper. What makes them helpful? There is one obvious explanation. Most of these groups are made up of people who share in the experience – they have "been there." Thus, there is no credibility gap. But there may be other reasons which relate to our training of professionals.

Fisher (1975) feels that graduate schools of social work have the potential of training *out* of their students interpersonal skills that have been shown to lead to effective practice. Hence, some nonprofessionals, unaffected by such training, may communicate higher levels of interpersonal skills, especially in their understanding of and empathy with the client.

The current attack on professionalism derives in part from the consumer-advocacy movements of the 1960s and 1970s. None of the professions has escaped attack.

> But the most hopeless of all professionals in the present climate have been those belonging to the so-called 'helping professions,' the social workers, psychologists, guidance counselors, and others who run the so-called service agencies dealing with people in distress of one kind or another. The scientific basis of these professions, assuming there is one, is rather shaky, resting as it does on the social sciences, which offer only sandy footing; and developmental psychology and psychiatry, which are not much firmer. (Glazer, 1978, pp. 39-40)

Eighty-nine parents of schizophrenics, all members of a self-help group in the Washington, D.C. area, were asked to describe how they got help (Hatfield, 1978a). To meet the problems of coping with schizophrenia in the family, these parents sought out an array of professional and nonprofessional supports. They reported friends, relatives, self-help group members, and books as being most helpful and various forms of therapy as least helpful. In fact, nearly half of this sample found no value at all in therapy.

> These findings are better understood when needs of families are expressed. Of highest priority are understanding of the illness, practical guidance, inpatient management, and community resources such as housing. These are not typical functions

of therapy. Self-help groups may serve these needs better. (Hatfield, 1978a)

One reason that mental health professionals have been so limited in their capacities to meet the needs of these families is because these needs are not known. As Hatfield says:

Little is known about the crises of mental illness, how families cope with this devastation, to whom they turn for help, and how adequate is the help received. Little effort has been made to go to these families and find out. (Hatfield, 1978a)

One of the particularly salient findings of Hatfield's study is that parents found books so helpful. Clearly this was their best source of information about the disease. Why was this information not coming from the professionals? Are they perhaps ignorant? Is it still easier and perhaps more popular to learn about the psychodynamic theories of schizophrenia? If this is the case, then parents would indeed do better to turn to the books, for it is there that the more recent biochemical and genetic explanations of schizophrenia are to be found. It should be mentioned here that most self-help groups are primarily committed to the biochemical explanation of schizophrenia, and they keep their members informed of new research developments.

Parents of schizophrenic children say they learned about self-help organizations primarily through friends, by word of mouth, and from the telephone book. Only rarely were mental health professionals a referring source. Again, one has to ask why, since professionals often refer alcoholics to AA, parents of the mentally retarded to self-help groups, and so on. Perhaps self-help groups for the parents of schizophrenics are too new a development to be well known. They should be better utilized in the future.

This has been a negative tirade against professionals. When parent and professional are suspicious of each other, the patient is the loser. Unfortunately, professionals have not been trained to develop a working alliance with patient's relatives. (Hatfield, 1978b)

The ideal would be professionals and parents working together as allies and as mutually respected collaborators — the professionals as experts in the disease, as advocates linking patients to needed resources, and as developers of new resources; and the parents as experts on their child and as critical resources for the child's well-being.

Quite apart from the ideal, one must also acknowledge the fact that many schizophrenics do *not* have any family or friends who can look after them. There may be no one around who loves them. The state and its professionals then are better than no one at all.

SOME SUGGESTIONS FOR NEW DIRECTIONS

> Most of our children had experienced all sorts of treatment from total isolation and being stripped of their clothes, to massive dosages of tranquilizers rendering them vegetables. We decided to fight for better care and better treatment.
>
> *Brochure*, Parents of Adult Schizophrenics
> of San Mateo County

Families of schizophrenics contend with formidable and heart-rending burdens. They have fewer social supports and services than exist for almost any other illness. In addition, there is still a great deal of ignorance about the illness, and much prejudice is directed against both the mentally ill and their parents. Following are several suggestions which could alleviate the burdens both experience.

Self-Help Groups

Self-help groups appear to offer more in the way of social supports and crisis intervention than anything else in our society, at the moment. Self-help groups give more credence to the biochemical explanation of schizophrenia; this fact alone makes them invaluable to parents, as it takes some of the onus off their backs. In addition, by participating in self-help groups, families can support each other emotionally, exchange practical management hints, and serve as advocates for needed resources.

Professional Training

We need to update the training of professionals, especially where it comes to educating them about what is known and not known about schizophrenia. If this were accomplished, more realistic and helpful treatment goals could be set up.

In our training and teaching of professionals perhaps we can find ways of better sensitizing them to the pain and stress that parents of schizophrenics go through, so that they can develop the same understanding and compassion usually shown to families coping with other major disabilities. Toward this end I would suggest making use of some parents of schizophrenics to do part of the training. Wikler (1979) found this method useful when she used parents of the mentally retarded to help sensitize and teach social work students about what the parents were experiencing. We could do the same in the area of schizophrenia.

Hospitalization

Some people really do need hospitalization. Under our present "progressive" mental health laws, it has become virtually impossible to hospitalize involuntarily many in desperate need of such protection. There are those who really cannot care for themselves, no matter how good the community resources, and who may have no family to pick up the pieces. We need long-term, humane facilities for them. It is presently unrealistic to think in terms of "cure," and it is outrageous to have them dumped out in the streets with inadequate resources. Admittedly, in the past, too many people were indiscriminately locked up. But now we have swung to the other extreme, and many schizophrenics are living in appalling isolation and neglect.

In addition to those who need long-term or life care, there are many who need short-term crisis hospitalization. This, too, has become a complex legal issue, often to the detriment of the mentally ill, their families, and the community. The present mode of leaving the decision about commitment up to the mentally ill themselves usually makes no sense.

My suggestion, then, is for revision of the new mental health laws, making it possible to hospitalize those in desperate need.

Proving that a person is "harmful to self or others" is too arbitrarily defined. In its present form, deinstitutionalization has become an indiscriminate method by which the government washes its hands of the responsibility for its most dependent citizens. We need to develop a better way.

Community Resources

Community resources should be better developed. Community medicine in its present form throughout the United States is not working well. Lack of money, resources, community preparation, and trained people seem to be the main reason.

The basic concept of community medicine, that patients will deteriorate less outside of institutions, is a good one. We still have a problem, however, with an erroneous assumption based on the notion of "cure." Whatever our present knowledge about schizophrenia, the recent research concerning social-psychological rehabilitation of chronic scihzophrenics (Test and Stein, 1978) indicates that we should change our thrust from "preparing" to "sustaining" in the community. A good model for this has been developed in Madison, Wisconsin. Called PACT (Program of Assertive Community Treatment), its basic thrusts are the following:

1. Assertiveness with the chronically mentally ill (CMI) and involvement of them in programming. They regress when they are on their own.
2. Individualized programming.
3. Enough supports to keep the CMI going, but no so much as to smother them.
4. Relationships with the CMI as responsible citizens, for example, giving them fair money for work done and punishing them if they break the law.
5. Assertive approach to working with community resources. Agency people often need on-the-spot help in dealing with the CMI.
6. Community education concerning the CMI.
7. Retention of responsibility for patient care and follow-up when referrals are made.

As one writer so aptly put it:

We know that with some intervention people can be kept off the bottle — off the needle — off the hallucination — off the whatever — even though they cannot be made over . . . [and] cannot be cured. They can be sustained. (Loeb, 1967, p. 10)

Social Supports

Social supports are needed. The following kinds of social supports need to be developed.

1. *Crises services*. Just as we recognize that crises develop among heart patients, diabetics, and cancer patients, for example, we should recognize that crises often occur for schizophrenics and their families. With recognition would come the building of services to help cope with crises.
2. *Respite care for families*. We have this service for parents of the mentally retarded. We should be doing no less for parents of the chronically mentally ill.
3. *Professional advocates for services for schizophrenics*. The law has become so complex and help so hard to get that many parents need assistance in getting protection and care for their children.
4. *Further development of parent advocacy and support groups and more referrals made to them by professionals*.

SUMMARY

There probably has been no group of parents so badly hurt and misunderstood by professionals as parents of schizophrenics. In addition, the present mental health system works against the best needs of many mentally ill people.

Perhaps the most telling chapter in the saga of my son is that in his discharge planning (July 1986) from The National Institute of Mental Health, St. Elizabeth's Hospital, it was to the parent's group, The National Alliance for the Mentally Ill (NAMI), where we turned and finally got help. He is now well situated in a protected environment, a working farm for 8 young men with schizophrenia, run by parents of one of them. So — it is to our own that we must presently turn, not the mental health system.

But NAMI and its many state and local chapters do not have the funds or resources necessary to serve the multitude in need. Few are as lucky as my son is now.

Schizophrenia is a terrible, debilitating, and chronic disease. Little is known about its cause, prevention, or treatment. All this leaves professionals feeling terribly frustrated, discouraged, and insecure. It leaves parents feeling overwhelmed, angry, and heartbroken. Needless to say, such a combination of feelings tends to bring out the worst in everybody. Even so, could not parents and professionals pull together better than they have been? This might best be accomplished by an updating of our knowledge, or lack of it, about the disease itself; training professionals to be more sensitive toward the agonies of parents; better utilizing parent advocacy groups for the mentally ill; getting the care of the mentally ill, at least partially, out of the courts and back into the medical profession; developing better community resources; and getting better social supports for the mentally ill and their families.

REFERENCES

Bateson, Gregory et al. "Towards a Theory of Schizophrenia." In *Theories Of Schizophrenia*, Eds., Arnold H. Buss and Edith H. Buss. New York: Atherton, 1969.

Ennis, Bruce, and Loren Siegel. *The Rights of Mental Patients: The Basic ACLU Guide to a Mental Patient's Rights*. New York: Avon, 1973.

Fisher, Joel. "Training for Effective Therapeutic Practice." *Psychotherapy: Theory, Research and Practice*, XII (1975), 118-23.

Glazer, Nathan. "The Attack on the Professions." *Commentary*, November, 1978, 39-40.

Hatfield, Agnes. *The Alliance for the Mentally Ill Newsletter*. II, No. 6 (June 1, 1979), published in Madison, Wis.

_____. "Help-Seeking Behavior in Families of Schizophrenics. Paper presented at the 55th annual meeting of the American Orthopsychiatric Association, San Francisco, 27-38 March 1978a.

_____. "Providing Social Supports for the Families of the Mentally Ill." Paper presented for the *President's Commission of Mental Health*, III, 1978.

Knee, R.I. "Health Care: Patients' Rights." In *Encyclopedia of Social Work*, Ed. John B. Turner. Washington, D.C.: National Association of Social Workers, 1977, 541-44.

Loeb, M.B. "Social Worker's Responsibility in Community Mental Health Centers." Paper presented at the Community Mental Health Conference in Saratoga Springs, N.Y., 5-7 April 1967.

Mendel, W.M., Ed. *Schizophrenia: The Experience and Its Treatment*. San Francisco: Jossey-Bass, 1976.

Test, M.A. and L.I. Stein. "Community Treatment of the Chronic Patient: Research Overview." *Schizophrenia Bulletin*, IV, No. 3 (1978), 350-64.

Wasow, M. "For My Beloved Son David Jonathan: A Professional Plea." *Health and Social Work*, III, No. 1 (February 1978), 127-45.

_____. "Professionals Have Hurt Us: Parents of Schizophrenics Speak Out." Unpublished manuscript, University of Wisconsin School of Social Work, Madison, Wis.

_____. "The Need for Asylum for the Chronically Mentally Ill." *Schizophrenia Bulletin*, XII, No. 2 (1986), NIMH, 162-167.

Westman, J.C. *Child Advocacy: New Professional Roles for Helping Families*. New York: Free Press, 1979.

Whitmer, G.E. "From Hospitals to Jail: The Fate of California's Deinstitutionalized Mentally Ill." *American Journal of Orthopsychiatry*, L, No. 1 (January 1980), 65-75.

Wikler, L. "Consumer Involvement in the Training of Social Work Students." *Social Casework*, LX, No. 3 (March 1979), 145-49.

_____, M. Wasow and A. Hatfield. "Chronic Sorrow Revisited: Parent vs. Professional Depiction of the Adjustment of Parents of Mentally Retarded Children." *American Journal of Orthopsychiatry*, forthcoming.

Williams, D.H., Bellis, E.C. and Wellington, S.W. "Deinstitutionalization and Social Policy: Historical Perspectives and Present Dilemmas." *American Journal of Orthopsychiatry*, L, No. 1 (January 1980), 54-64.

Index